# Aldosterone-Mineralocorticoid Receptor - Cell Biology to Translational Medicine

*Edited by Brian Harvey and Frederic Jaisser*

Published in London, United Kingdom

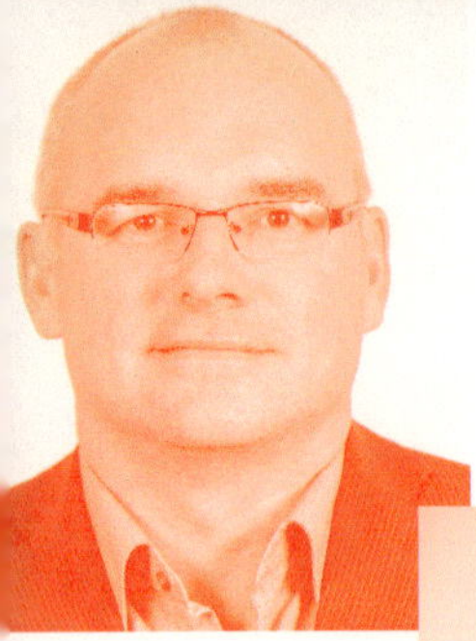
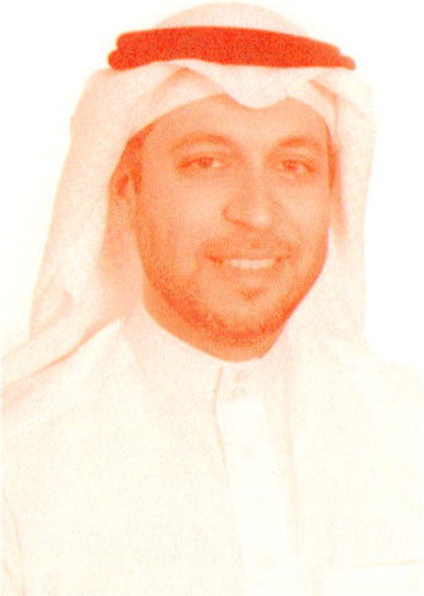
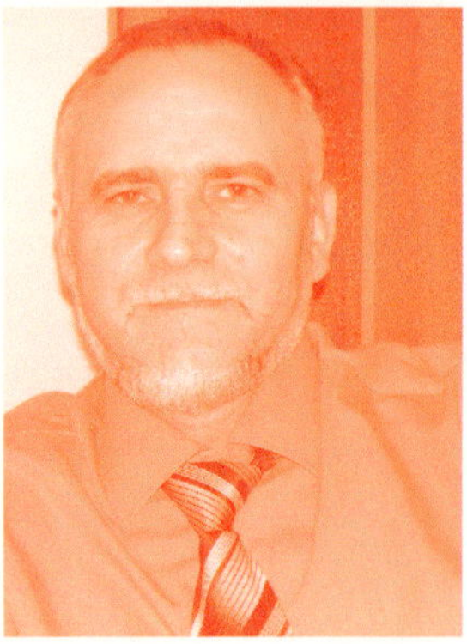
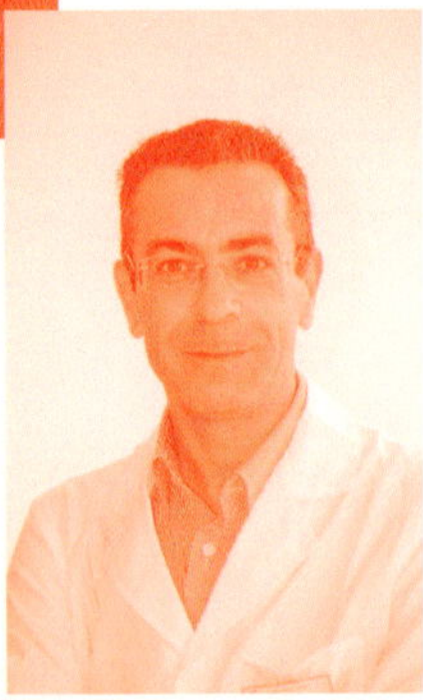
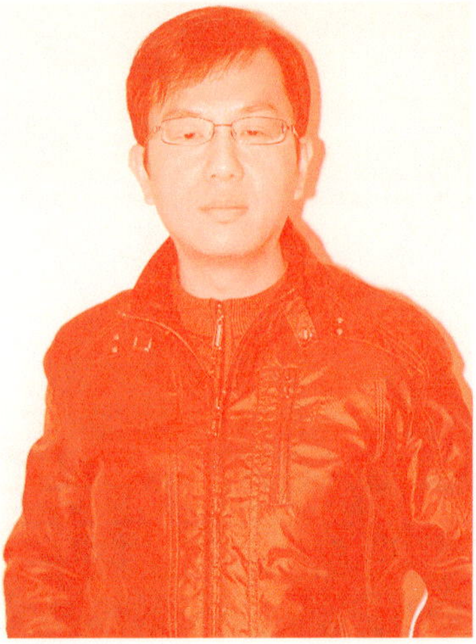
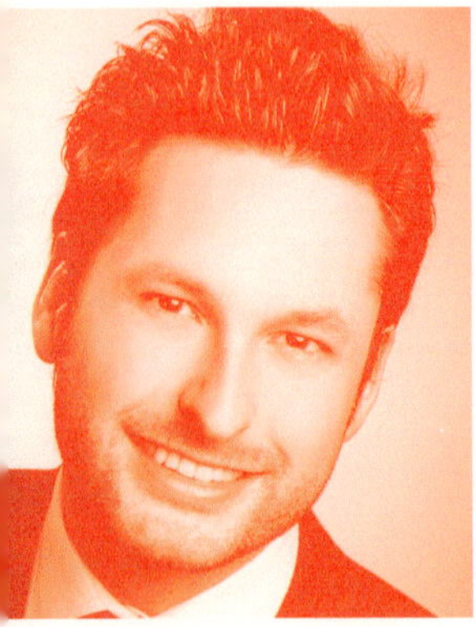
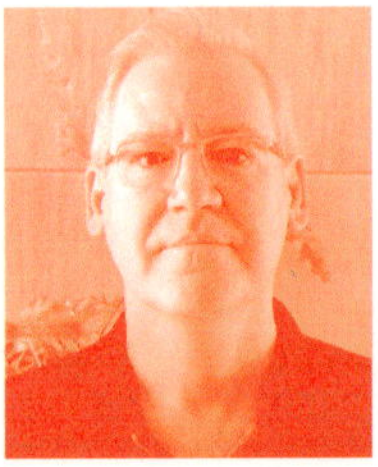

IntechOpen

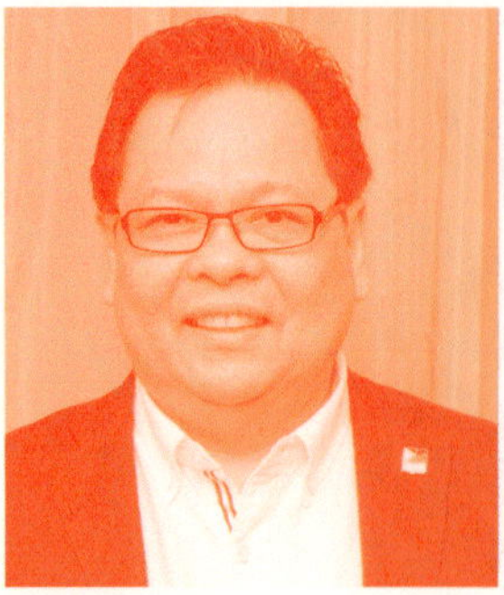
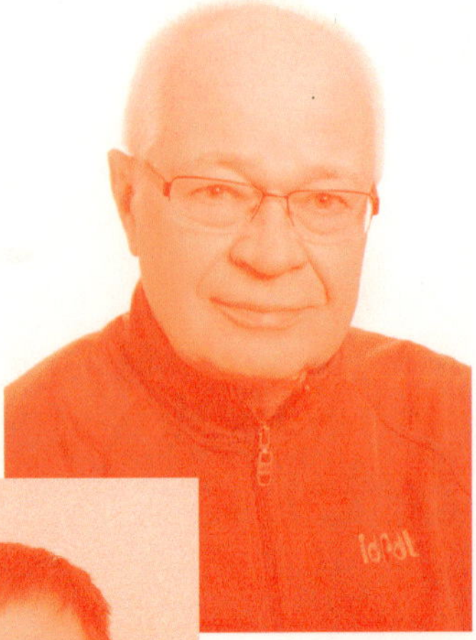
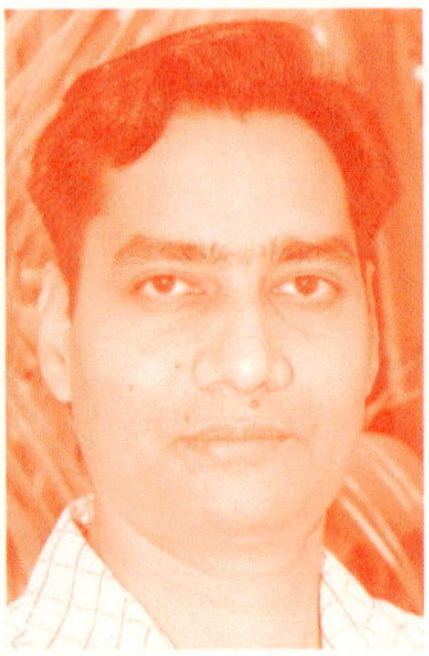
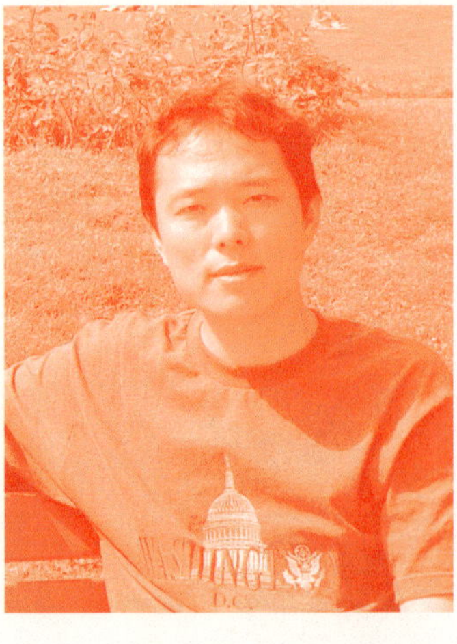
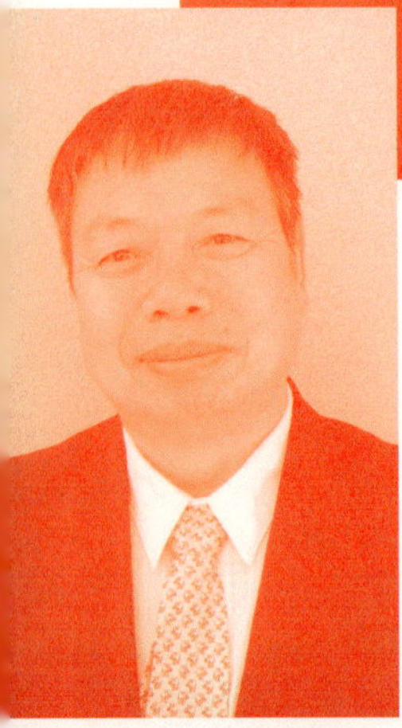
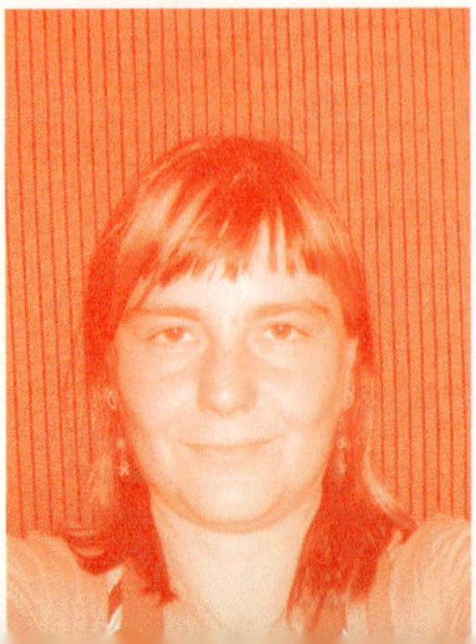

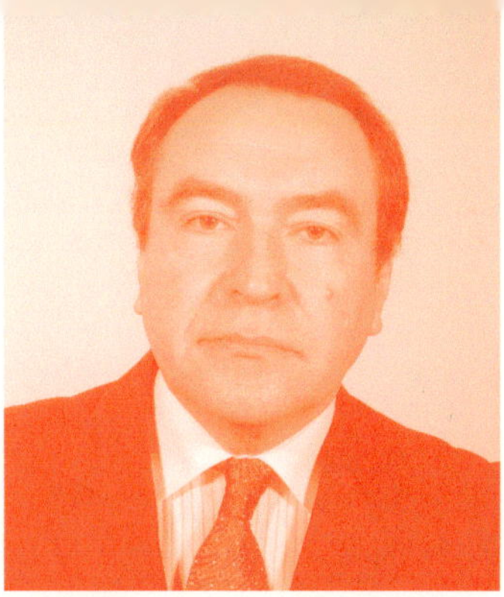
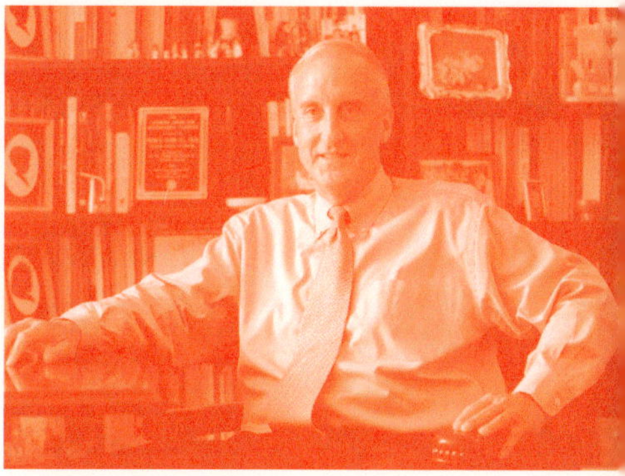
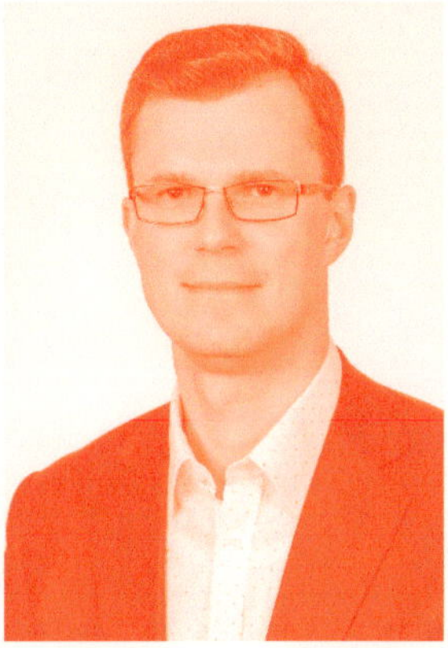
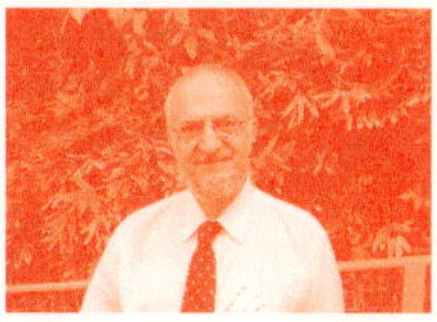
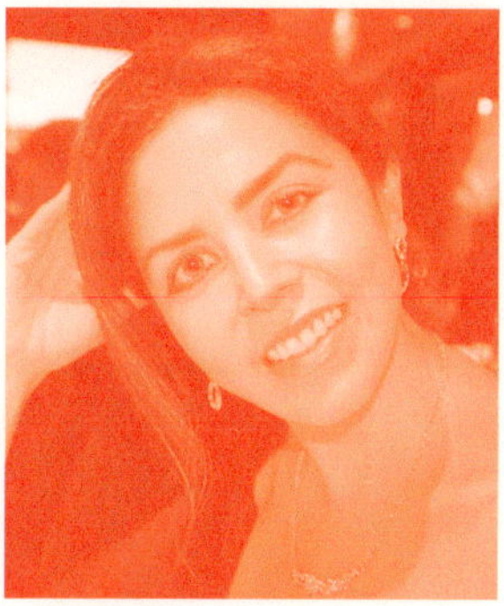

*Supporting open minds since 2005*

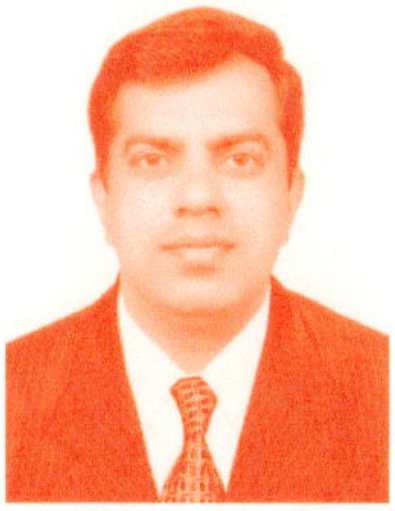
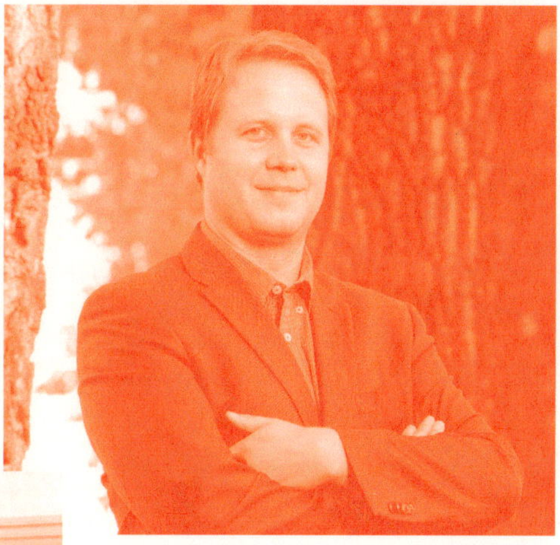
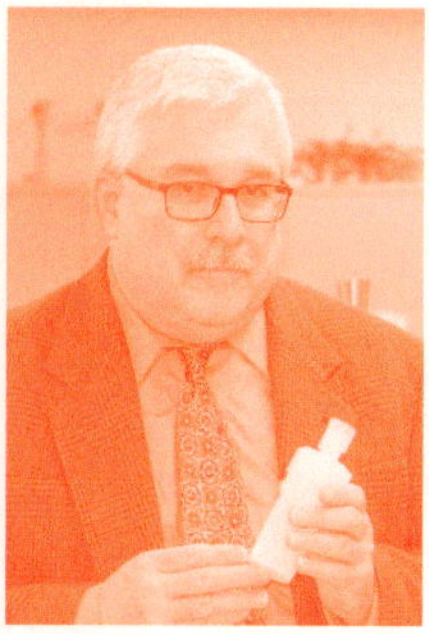
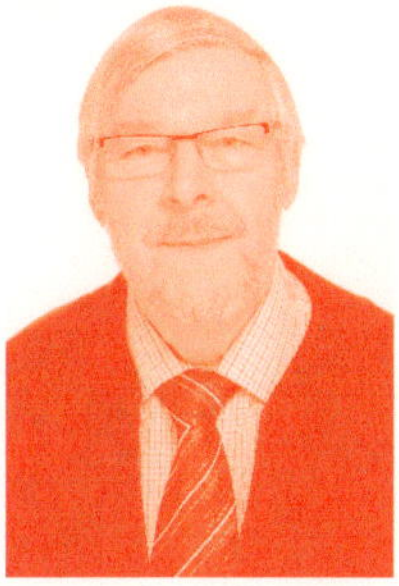
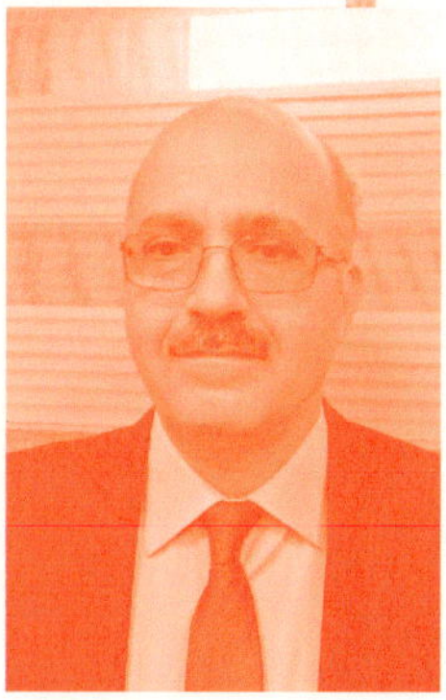
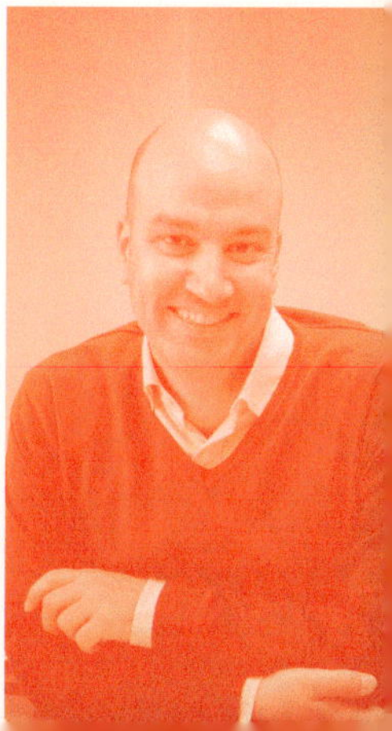
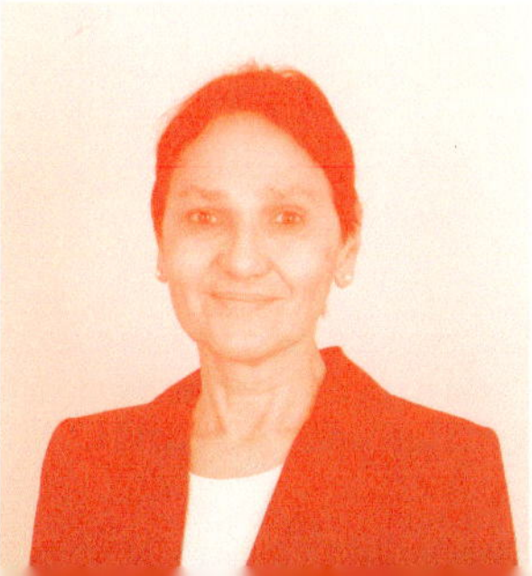

Aldosterone-Mineralocorticoid Receptor - Cell Biology to Translational Medicine
http://dx.doi.org/10.5772/intechopen.69065
Edited by Brian Harvey and Frederic Jaisser

Contributors
Brian Harvey, Johann Bauersachs, Ana M. Briones, Rhian M. Touyz, Eleanor Davies, D. Alvarez De La Rosa, Gian Paolo Rossi, Frederic Jaisser, Achim Lother, Massimiliano Caprio, Natalia López-Andrés, Ozlen Konu, E.R. De Kloet, Bernard C. Rossier, Victoria Cachofeiro, Daniela Jezova, Stefan Chlopicki, Mercedes Martín-Martínez



First published in London, United Kingdom, 2019 by IntechOpen
IntechOpen is the global imprint of INTECHOPEN LIMITED, registered in England and Wales, registration number: 11086078, The Shard, 25th floor, 32 London Bridge Street
London, SE19SG - United Kingdom
Printed in Croatia

British Library Cataloguing-in-Publication Data
A catalogue record for this book is available from the British Library

Additional hard and PDF copies can be obtained from orders@intechopen.com

Aldosterone-Mineralocorticoid Receptor - Cell Biology to Translational Medicine
Edited by Brian Harvey and Frederic Jaisser
p. cm.
Print ISBN 978-1-83962-198-7
Online ISBN 978-1-83962-199-4
eBook (PDF) ISBN 978-1-83962-200-7

For EU product safety concerns:
IN TECH d.o.o., Prolaz Marije Krucifikse Kozulić 3, 51000 Rijeka, Croatia, info@intechopen.com or visit our website at intechopen.com.

This publication is based upon work from the EU COST Action ADMIRE www.admirecosteu.com. ADMIRE is an international network bringing together more than 300 scientists, research students and clinicians from 19 EU COST member states (Austria, Denmark, France, Germany, Greece, Hungary, Ireland, Israel, Italy, Netherlands, Norway, Poland, Portugal, Romania, Slovakia, Spain, Switzerland, United Kingdom and Turkey) and 2 associated International Partner Countries (Mexico and Chile). The specific objective of ADMIRE is improving human health by "Sharing Knowledge of Aldosterone/MR Physiology and Pathophysiology".

Supported by COST (European Cooperation in Science and Technology). ADMIRE was funded for 4 years (April 2014 – May 2018) from COST funded by the Horizon 2020 Framework Programme.

# Meet the editors

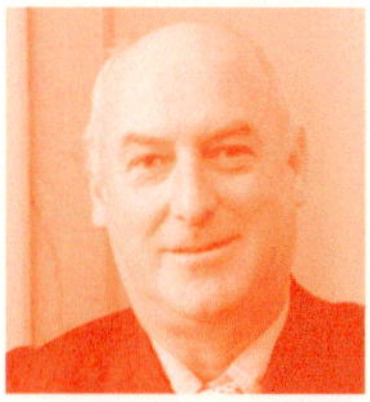

Brian Harvey is Emeritus Professor of Molecular Medicine at the Royal College of Surgeons in Ireland, Investigador Adjunto at the Centro di Estudios Cientificos, Chile, and Visiting Research Professor at the INSERM Cordeliers Research Centre, Paris. He holds a PhD in Physiology from the National University of Ireland and a DSc *honoris causa* from Michigan State University. His main research area is in cell and molecular endocrinology of rapid responses to steroid hormones on which he has published over 170 papers. He is a recipient of the International Laureat Prix Servier and Chevalier of the French Order of Merit and Member of the Ordre des Palmes Academiques, and an elected member of Academia Europaea and the Royal Irish Academy.

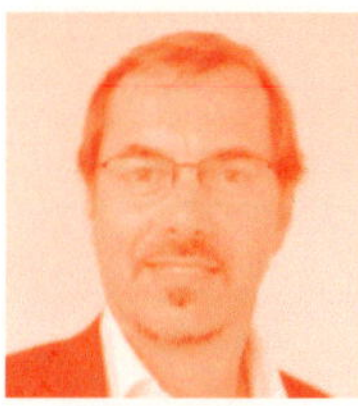

Frederic Jaisser, MD, PhD, is a director of research at the French National Institute of Health and Medical Research (INSERM). Dr. Jaisser received his medical training and degrees from Reims Medical School and qualified as a nephrologist in 1990. In 2003, he joined the Collège de France in Paris and currently manages a team of the INSERM Unit U1138 at the Cordeliers Research Centre, Paris, where he is Deputy Director and Head of the "Pathophysiology, Metabolism" Department. He was the Scientific Delegate of the Pathophysiology Committee of the French National Research Agency and is the French Coordinator for Life Sciences in the ECOS French-South America exchange programme. His research is focused on the understanding of pathophysiological roles and signaling pathways whereby the hormone aldosterone promotes pathologies in various organs, including the kidney and cardiovascular system. He was Chair of the European Network on Aldosterone (EU COST Action ADMIRE).

# Contents

# Preface

The pathophysiology of the aldosterone (Aldo) and mineralocorticoid receptor (MR) endocrine system (Aldo/MR) underpins a wide number of common diseases of high mortality and health cost. These include hypertension, heart failure, chronic kidney diseases, diabetes, and obesity disorders. The MR hormone ligand aldosterone was discovered in Europe in 1953 and since then European researchers have led the way in basic and clinical research in this area. An EU Aldo/MR network was established under the EU COST Action ADMIRE (http://www.admirecosteu.com).

The partners involved in ADMIRE have made major scientific and clinical breakthroughs in the Aldo/MR field from basic science (regulation and genetics of aldosterone production, identifying novel modes of action, novel target organs), translational research (novel disease settings related to dysregulation of the system), clinical impact (repurposing and novel indications of marketed drugs inhibiting the system), and development of new drugs targeting the Aldo/MR system.

**Aldo/MR and disease:** Aldosterone is a steroid hormone produced in the adrenal gland from cholesterol and acts via its receptor MR as a transcription factor in various organs and tissues. The main impact of Aldo/MR cell signaling is the regulation of renal sodium balance as well as biological effects, which have been reported in the last two decades in organs such as kidney, heart, blood vessels, adipose tissue, brain, eye, and skin (**Figure 1**). Increased levels of aldosterone are associated with diseases such as hypertension, heart failure, stroke, obesity, and diabetes, which are highly prevalent in the European and North American population. These conditions are known to be complex multifactorial disorders combining polygenic variations and numerous lifestyle and environmental factors. The MR is a ligand-activated transcription factor involved in renal ion homeostasis (salt reabsorption, acid/base balance), and blood pressure control. The MR is also expressed in multiple non-renal targets such as heart, vessels, adipose tissue, and immune cells where its role remains to be defined. Aldosterone is the physiological ligand activating MR; however, the glucocorticoid cortisol can activate MR under certain pathological conditions such as chronic stress.

Overstimulation of the Aldo/MR pathway is well established as a major contributor to high blood pressure. Moreover, dysregulation of aldosterone synthesis is more common than anticipated in the general population. More research is needed to better understand the underlying mechanisms (such as genetic or epigenetic) for increased aldosterone synthesis as well as the pathophysiological consequences of increased circulating levels of the hormone. The overactivation of MR is now recognized as a major targetable pathway in heart failure leading to the impressive success of the repurposing of MR antagonists in heart failure. In addition, basic research in the field by European teams in the ADMIRE consortium have very recently uncovered a novel role of Aldo/MR in various disease settings such as metabolic syndrome and chronic kidney disease. The underlying mechanisms of Aldo/MR signaling in these diseases as well as the identification of appropriate patient populations that would benefit from Aldo/MR therapeutic approaches

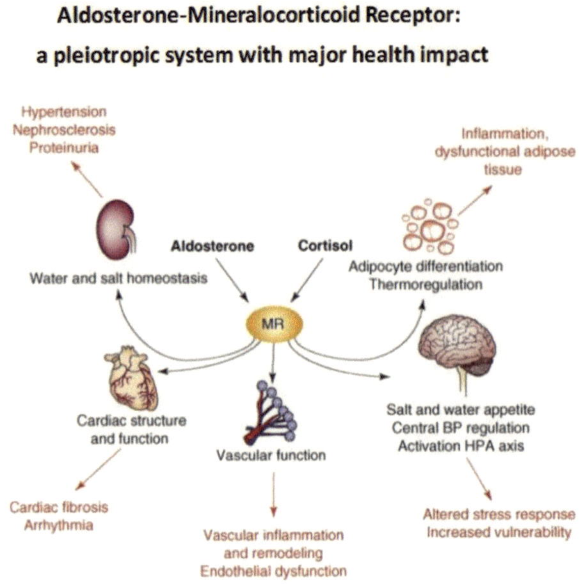


**Figure 1.**
***Aldosterone/mineralocorticoid receptor—a pleiotropic system with major health impacts.*** *Aldosterone (Aldo) and mineralocorticoid receptor (MR) (Aldo/MR) signaling regulates major body functions such as salt absorption in the kidney together with cardiovascular physiology that together regulate blood pressure. Dysregulation of Aldo/MR signaling (overactivation) is a major cause of hypertension and associated comorbidities. Novel actions of Aldo/MR have recently been found in pathologies associated with fibrosis, inflammation, and metabolic disorders.*

remain to be defined. This Open Access Intech ADMIRE book presents the latest research reviews from partners in the ADMIRE network that highlight the remarkable diversity of Aldo/MR physiology and pathophysiology.

**Brian Harvey**
Royal College of Surgeons in Ireland

**Frédéric Jaisser**
Cordeliers Research Centre INSERM,
Paris

Chapter 1

# Mineralocorticoid Receptor Antagonists in the Treatment of Coronary Artery Disease, Myocardial Infarction and Heart Failure

*Carolin Zwadlo and Johann Bauersachs*

## Abstract

Affecting sodium reabsorption and potassium excretion in the kidney, mineralocorticoid receptor antagonists (MRA) were originally developed as antihypertensive drugs. After several large clinical trials, the concept of MR blockade has nowadays become a main treatment paradigm in heart failure with reduced ejection fraction (HFrEF) and for patients after myocardial infarction (MI) with left ventricular (LV) dysfunction. Recent analyses also point to a beneficial effect of early MRA treatment in patients with acute MI without LV dysfunction, however, there is no clear evidence yet. Although promising data from preclinical settings suggest that MRAs mediate favorable anti-atherogenic effects, clinical studies in patients with stable coronary artery disease (CAD) have not been able to detect differences of hard clinical outcomes. The concept might still be pursued using the most recent MRA, like the non-steroidal MR antagonist finerenone, and larger clinical trials need to be performed. Here, we review the current impact of MRA in patients with CAD and focus on the conflicting evidence of preclinical and clinical data in patients with stable CAD and preserved ejection fraction and summarize the current indications for MRA in these patients according to the guidelines.

**Keywords:** mineralocorticoid receptor antagonists (MRA), aldosterone, heart failure, myocardial infarction, spironolactone, eplerenone, finerenone

## 1. Introduction

Because of their effect on sodium reabsorption and potassium excretion in the kidney, mineralocorticoid receptor antagonists (MRA) were originally developed as antihypertensive drugs. Over the years, it became clear that their influence on the cardiovascular system is much broader than initially thought. Spironolactone was the first MRA to be developed. Later, eplerenone followed. Nowadays, mineralocorticoid receptor (MR) antagonism consists of the steroidal first- and second-generation MRAs spironolactone and eplerenone and the non-steroidal third-generation MRAs, such as finerenone, the latter one not being in clinical use outside studies yet.

After several large clinical trials, the concept of MR blockade has become a main treatment paradigm with chronic heart failure with reduced ejection fraction (HFrEF) and for patients after myocardial infarction (MI) with left ventricular (LV) dysfunction. On the contrary, no general recommendation for immediate MR antagonism in patients without LV dysfunction is currently justified. Moreover, there are controversial data on the role of MRA in stable coronary artery disease (CAD), although high plasma aldosterone levels have been associated with increased mortality and ischemic events in patients with stable CAD with or without heart failure. Preclinical studies underline the anti-atherogenic and favorable vascular effects of spironolactone, eplerenone and finerenone via various mechanisms. These positive results, however, are largely limited to animal models and clinical studies could not confirm an improvement of markers of vascular health so far.

In the past, we have summarized the existing preclinical and clinical data on spironolactone and eplerenone in the treatment of CAD and its related complications [1]. Here, we review the impact of MRAs in these patients and supplement updated information on published clinical studies and especially the newly developed third-generation MRA, finerenone. We aim to shed light on the current conflicting evidence of preclinical and clinical data and summarize the indications for MR antagonism in patients with CAD and its complications.

## 2. Main part

### 2.1 Effects of aldosterone

The renin-angiotensin-aldosterone system (RAAS) regulates blood pressure and fluid and electrolyte balance under physiological and pathological conditions. Aldosterone is the final product of the RAAS. It is a steroid hormone produced by zona glomerulosa cells in the adrenal cortex. Traditionally, its action was thought to be restricted to sodium reabsorption and potassium excretion via activation of the cytosolic MR in epithelial cells of the distal colon, the renal nephron as well as salivary and sweat glands. However, over time it became clear that aldosterone's action is much broader than initially thought and MRs were identified in vascular endothelial and smooth muscle cells as well as in cardiomyocytes, endothelial cells, fibroblasts and macrophages in the heart [2].

Key evidence for the role of MR in the pathophysiology of cardiac diseases was derived from cell-specific overexpression and deletion studies. In mouse models of chronic pressure overload and myocardial infarction, deletion or inactivation of the MR gene attenuated left ventricular dilatation, cardiac hypertrophy and development of heart failure, whereas overexpression of the MR in cardiomyocytes induced ventricular remodeling, development of heart failure and pro-arrhythmogenic effects [3–7].

Aldosterone and glucocorticoids bind with similar affinity to MR. In the normal state, plasma glucocorticoid levels are more than 100 times higher that aldosterone levels and the majority of MRs in the heart is occupied by glucocorticoids. In patients with acute MI and chronic heart failure, not only circulating aldosterone levels but also aldosterone biosynthesis is enhanced. Moreover, the aldosterone-MR complex is more stable than the glucocorticoid-MR complex [8, 9]. Based on these findings, it is nowadays well accepted that aldosterone contributes to endothelial dysfunction, fibrinolytic disorders, inflammation, oxidative stress, fibrosis and hypertrophy leading to or at least aggravating cardiovascular diseases (CVD) such as CAD and heart failure [10–13].

Presumably, the exact molecular mechanism of aldosterone's action is still not fully understood and appears to be more complex than initially thought. For example, aldosterone has been shown to promote the formation of venous thrombosis in normotensive rats via mechanisms involving primary hemostasis, fibrinolysis, nitric oxide and oxidative stress-dependent pathways but MR blockade was insufficient to reverse the effect. Notably, other receptors, such as the glucocorticoid receptor (GR) and angiotensin II receptor type 1 are involved [14, 15]. The effects of aldosterone are mediated via classic nuclear receptors (genomic actions of aldosterone) and cell-membrane receptors (non-genomic actions of aldosterone) with alternative pathways, including activation of protein kinases or secondary messenger signaling cascades [16, 17]. Indeed, in high, non-physiological plasma conditions, aldosterone can also act via GR [18] or the G protein-coupled estrogen receptor (GPR30). The latter one plays an important role in aldosterone-mediated regulation of endothelial cell growth and in aldosterone's endothelial-mediated regulation of vasoreactivity [19].

### 2.2 Development of MRAs

The development of MRAs begun during the 1950s. At that time, the main role of aldosterone was considered to be renal sodium and potassium excretion. Spironolactone, the first steroidal MRA, was primarily developed and used for the medical control of edema and ascites and control blood pressure, respectively. With the RALES trial, the perception of spironolactone changed; spironolactone, in addition to standard therapy, substantially reduced the risk of both morbidity and death among patients with severe heart failure [20]. With eplerenone, a second-generation steroidal MRA was developed. The advantage of eplerenone compared to spironolactone is mainly the higher selectivity for mineralocorticoid receptors, therefore avoiding hormonal side effects such as gynecomastia. Despite considerable efforts to ensure a broad application of this essential medication in this defined patient collective, many clinicians were reluctant to employ MRAs in their clinical practice due to potential side effects. These side effects included worsening of renal function, hyperkalemia and gynecomastia.

Interestingly, Vukadinović et al. performed a meta-analysis. The authors emphasize that non-MRA-related rises in potassium levels might be underestimated and should be rigorously explored before cessation of the evidence-based therapy with MRAs [21].

Nevertheless, the issue of hyperkalemia and worsening renal function triggered several pharmaceutical companies to develop novel MR-antagonizing compounds. These so-called third-generation MRAs, such as finerenone or canrenone, are non-steroidal compounds with both high selectivity and high potency to inhibit MR. The first compound of these novel MRAs undergoing clinical evaluation was finerenone, formerly known as BAY 94-8862. Finerenone is even more selective than eplerenone to the MR with very low affinity to androgen, glucocorticoid and progesterone receptor. In clear contrast to spironolactone and eplerenone, which have a higher tendency to concentrate in the kidney, finerenone displays a balanced distribution pattern into cardiac and kidney tissue of healthy rats [22, 23]. This suggests a more favorable balance between cardioprotection and renal side effects, especially in populations prone to hyperkalemia such as patients with chronic kidney disease or diabetes (**Figure 1**) [24, 25].

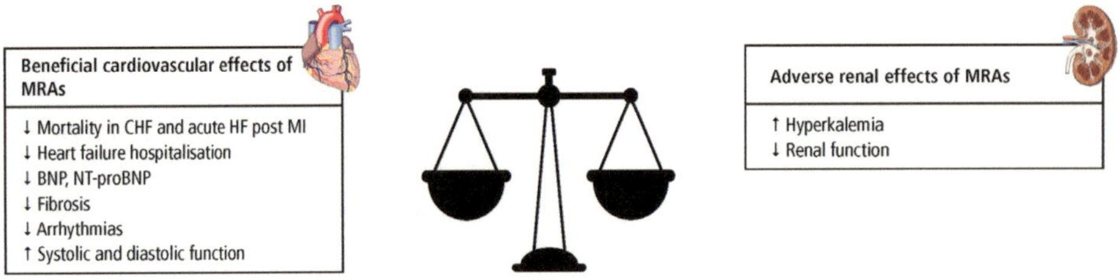
Beneficial cardiovascular effects of MRAs
↓ Mortality in CHF and acute HF post MI
↓ Heart failure hospitalisation
↓ BNP, NT-proBNP
↓ Fibrosis
↓ Arrhythmias
↑ Systolic and diastolic function
Adverse renal effects of MRAs
↑ Hyperkalemia
↓ Renal function

| Generation | Class | Example | Affinity to MR | Selectivity | Adverse hormonal effects | Tissue distribution | Assumed risk for WRF/Hyperkalemia |
|---|---|---|---|---|---|---|---|
| I. | Steroidal | Spironolactone | High | Low | + | 6-fold higher in kidney | High |
| II. | Steroidal | Eplerenone | Medium | Medium-High | - | 3-fold higher in kidney | Medium |
| III. | Non-steroidal | Finerenone | High | High | - | Equal | Low |

**Figure 1.**
*Characteristics of three generations of mineralocorticoid receptor antagonists (MRAs).*

To date, finerenone is under investigation in two large clinical trials (FIGARO-DKD: A Randomized, Double-Blind-Placebo-controlled, Multicenter, Event-driven Phase 3 Study to Investigate Efficacy and Safety of Finerenone on the Reduction of Cardiovascular Morbidity and Mortality in Subjects With Type 2 Diabetes Mellitus and the Clinical Diagnosis of Diabetic Kidney Disease in Addition to Standard of Care (NCT02545049) and FIDELIO-DKD: A Randomized, Double-Blind, Placebo-controlled, Parallel-group, Multicenter, Event-driven Phase 3 Study to Investigate the Efficacy and Safety of Finerenone, in Addition to Standard of Care, on the Progression of Kidney Disease in Subjects With Type 2 Diabetes Mellitus and the Clinical Diagnosis of Diabetic Kidney Disease (NCT02540993)). The effect of canrenone compared to other therapies on cardiovascular mortality in patients with chronic heart failure and preserved systolic function is currently undertaken in the "COFFEE-IT" study: "CanrenOne eFFects on cardiovascular mortality in patiEnts with congEstIve hearT failure" (https://clinicaltrials.gov/ct2/show/NCT03263962).

## 2.3 MRAs in chronic systolic LV dysfunction (after ischemia)

For a long time, the strongest evidence for the clinical usefulness of MRAs existed for patients with chronic heart failure NYHA III and reduced ejection fraction. In 2012, the guidelines for diagnosis and treatment of acute and chronic heart failure by the European Society of Cardiology amended the recommendation of MRAs for all patients with symptoms of heart failure class II and worse according to the New York Heart Association (NYHA)-classification and an ejection fraction ≤35% [26]. Since then, the concept of MR blockade has become a main treatment paradigm in HFrEF.

Two large clinical trials have firmly established the role of MRAs in chronic heart failure: the Randomized Aldactone Evaluation Study (RALES) and the Eplerenone in Mild Patients Hospitalization And SurvIval Study in Heart Failure (EMPHASIS-HF). Death from all causes and specifically cardiac death as well as hospitalization due to heart failure were decreased proving the efficacy of MRAs in patients with severely reduced LV function [20, 27]. Although the underlying pathophysiology is complex, the clinical effects of MRAs in these patients are thought to be mainly related to the improvement of LV remodeling with a reduction in collagen synthesis and myocardial fibrosis, seen as a decrease in LV size and hypertrophy and improved LV function [28].

With the development of the third-generation MRAs, such as finerenone, there came the necessity for further clinical trials. In rats with deoxycorticosterone acetate-(DOCA)/salt-induced heart and kidney injury as well as in a chronic myocardial infarction rat model, finerenone had proved to reduce cardiac hypertrophy, NT-proBNP and proteinuria more efficiently than eplerenone when directly comparing equinatriuretic doses [29]. Similarly, in a mouse model of pressure overload-induced heart failure treatment with finerenone compared to head-to-head with eplerenone resulted in a more pronounced prevention of myocardial hypertrophy [30].

ARTS (MinerAlocortocoid Receptor antagonist Tolerability Study) was the first randomized, controlled, phase II trial to test the safety and tolerability (Part A) of oral finerenone, at that time still under the name BAY 94-8862, in comparison with placebo and spironolactone (Part B). Finerenone was associated with significantly less increases in serum potassium concentration and fewer incidences of hyperkalemia (5.3 and 12.7%, respectively). Moreover, it decreased the levels of BNP, NT-proBNP and albuminuria at least as much as spironolactone. Adverse events related to the substance were infrequent and mostly mild. The authors concluded that in patients with HFrEF and moderate CKD, finerenone in various concentrations was at least as effective as spironolactone in decreasing biomarkers of hemodynamic stress and was associated with lower incidences of hyperkalemia [31, 32]. After these promising results, ARTS-HF (MinerAlocortocoid Receptor antagonist Tolerability Study-Heart Failure), a randomized, double-blind, phase IIb multicenter study was initiated to evaluate oral doses of finerenone given in patients with worsening heart failure and reduced ejection fraction and chronic kidney disease and/or diabetes mellitus. The trial showed a comparable efficacy between all dosage groups of finerenone and eplerenone in the primary endpoint, the decrease of >30% in plasma NT-proBNP from baseline to day 90 [33]. Similar results were obtained in the relatively small ARTS-HF Japan trial, conducted in Japan with the same regime as described for ARTS-HF [34]. Overall, finerenone showed a promising safety and efficacy profile in the so far conducted trials. However, patient numbers are too small to draw any fundamental conclusions. With FINESSE-HF, a multicenter, randomized, double-blind, double-dummy, parallel-group, active-controlled study to evaluate the efficacy and safety of finerenone compared to eplerenone on morbidity and mortality in patients with chronic heart failure and reduced ejection fraction after recent heart failure. Decompensation and additional risk factors was supposed to launch. However, the trial prematurely ended in May 2016 (https://www.clinicaltrialsregister.eu/ctr-search/trial/2015-002168-17/HU#D). To date, finerenone holds its promise of a novel MRA with greater selectivity, greater potency and fewer side effects. However, further clinical trials with enough power are needed in patients.

Currently, two clinical trials are evaluating the efficacy and safety of finerenone in patients with type 2 diabetes mellitus and diabetic kidney disease: the FIGARO-DKD and FIDELIO-DKD trial. Both trials evaluate whether oral finerenone compared to placebo is effective and safe in addition to standard of care. The primary outcome measures are, however, different. FIGARO-DKD evaluates the time of the first occurrence of the composite endpoint of cardiovascular death and non-fatal cardiovascular events (myocardial infarction, stroke or hospitalization for heart failure) in a follow-up of up to 53 months. The study is still recruiting and a total enrollment of 6400 participants with primary completion in January 2020 is estimated (https://clinicaltrials.gov/ct2/show/NCT02545049). FIDELIO-DKD aims to investigate the time of the first occurrence of the composite endpoint of onset of kidney failure, a sustained decrease of estimated glomerular filtration rate (eGFR) ≥40% from baseline over at least 4 weeks and renal death in a follow-up of up to

48 months. A total of 4800 participants and a study completion date of October 2019 is estimated (https://clinicaltrials.gov/ct2/show/NCT02540993).

### 2.4 MRAs early post infarction

Several preclinical animal studies with coronary artery disease and/or with heart failure have provided substantial evidence that activation of MR plays a pivotal role in cardiac healing and remodeling after myocardial ischemia. These studies suggested that cardiomyocyte-specific deletion of the MR gene attenuates LV dilatation, hypertrophy, fibrosis and heart failure, whereas cardiomyocyte-specific MR overexpression induced adverse remodeling and pro-arrhythmogenic effects [3, 7]. Moreover, administration of MRAs early after MI reduced the expansion of the healing infarct, attenuated early left ventricular dilatation and dysfunction and had more beneficial effects on survival, early cardiac dilatation and functional decline [3, 7, 35–38]. Indeed, after an acute MI, not only circulating aldosterone levels are increased but also the myocardium distant from the infarct zone shows enhanced activation of aldosterone synthesis [36].

In the clinical setting, Hayashi et al. demonstrated in 2003 that in patients with their first anterior STEMI and no evidence of early heart failure, intravenous canrenone followed by oral spironolactone for 6 months beginning day one post-MI was safe and associated with a significant reduction in ventricular remodeling, myocardial fibrosis and inflammatory cytokine activation [39]. In the same year, the well-planned and executed Eplerenone Post-acute myocardial infarction Heart failure Efficacy and Survival Study (EPHESUS) demonstrated MR blockade to substantially improve morbidity and mortality among patients with moderate to severe heart failure and LV dysfunction after MI [40]. More than 3000 patients with an ejection fraction <40% received either 50 mg eplerenone or placebo on a daily basis, starting 3–14 days after MI. In comparison to the placebo-group, all-cause mortality, cardiovascular mortality and sudden cardiac death were decreased by 15, 17 and 21%, respectively, in the eplerenone group.

Although EPHESUS had clearly established the clinical efficacy of MRAs in patients with heart failure after an acute MI, the value of MRAs after MI without concomitant heart failure needed to be determined. Moreover, EPHESUS suggested that an early initiation of eplerenone treatment had significant beneficial effects compared to later initiation [41]. The REMINDER trial (Role of Eplerenone in acute Myocardial Infarction-Double-blind, Early treatment initiation, Randomized, placebo-controlled, multi-center study) evaluated the potential benefit of early administered eplerenone on cardiovascular morbidity and mortality after STEMI. In this randomized, placebo-controlled, double-blind trial, 1012 patients with acute STEMI and without a history of heart failure were randomized to receive either eplerenone (25–50 mg once daily) or placebo in addition to standard therapy. Treatment was initiated within 24 hours after onset of symptoms. The primary endpoint was the composite of CV mortality, re-hospitalization or extended initial hospital stay, due to diagnosis of heart failure, sustained ventricular tachycardia or fibrillation, ejection fraction ≤40% or elevated BNP/NT-proBNP at 1 month or more after randomization. The trial showed that the addition of eplerenone during the acute phase of STEMI was safe and well tolerated. It reduced the primary endpoint over a mean 13 months follow-up mostly because of significantly lower natriuretic peptide levels [42].

Similarly, the ALBATROSS trial (Aldosterone Lethal effects Blocked in Acute myocardial infarction Treated with or without Reperfusion to improve Outcome and Survival at 6 months follow-up) randomized patients admitted for STEMI and non-STEMI to test whether administration of MRAs within 72 hours after onset of symptoms improves cardiovascular outcome regardless of heart failure and treatment strategy. In total, 1603 patients were included an received an MRA regime with a single 200 mg intravenous bolus of potassium canrenoate followed by 25 mg oral spironolactone once daily for 6 months in addition to standard therapy or standard therapy alone. The primary outcome of the study was the composite of death, resuscitated cardiac arrest, significant ventricular arrhythmia, indication for implantable defibrillator, or new or worsening heart failure at 6-month follow-up. Key secondary/safety outcomes included death and other individual components of the primary outcome and rates of hyperkalemia at 6 months [43]. However, the study failed to show the benefit of early MRA use in addition to standard therapy in patients admitted for MI, and was intensively discussed among experts. In the overall opinion, both ALBATROSS and REMINDER are undersized to detect a difference in rates of hard clinical outcomes [43, 44]. Beygui et al. therefore conducted a pre-specific meta-analysis and pooled individual patient-level data of the STEMI subgroup of the ALBATROSS and the total population of the REMINDER trial. Their analysis showed reduced rates of death in the MRA-treated group compared to standard therapy. Although the authors underline that this specific subgroup analysis should be considered "exploratory," it suggests a consistent effect of the early MRA-treatment in patients with STEMI [45]. However, under these circumstances, additional studies are needed to clarify the role of early use of MRAs in patients with MI without heart failure.

### 2.5 MRAs in stable coronary artery disease

A large number of preclinical studies indicate that aldosterone is an important stimulus for vascular disease, with inflammation and fibrosis being the key players, [3–6] and MRAs are able to inhibit atherosclerosis progression in different animal models [46–49]. Treatment with aldosterone results in increased inflammation and upregulated expression of proinflammatory cytokines, such as tumor necrosis factor-α, interleukin-1β and transforming growth factor-β1 in rat myocardium. Additionally, it leads to an increase in myocardial collagen synthesis and content, fibrosis and profibrotic factors, including connective tissue growth factor, TGF-β, plasminogen activator inhibitor-1, matrix metalloproteinase-2 and tumor necrosis factor-α [7]. Oxidative stress is well-recognized to trigger inflammation and to contribute to the development of fibrosis [7]. Furthermore, MR activation stimulates apoptosis and causes vasoconstriction and reduced blood flow in the animal heart and MRA treatment reverses these effects [7]. Especially finerenone can significantly reduce apoptosis of endothelial cells and simultaneously attenuate smooth muscle cells proliferation, resulting in accelerated endothelial healing and reduced neointima formation of the injured vessels [50]. Over the years, several clinical studies in patients with coronary artery disease pinpointed the association of high aldosterone levels with an increased risk of cardiovascular death and all-cause-mortality [51], the occurrence of an ischemic event [52] or the progression of carotid artery plaques [53]. Although clear evidence exists that there is a strong relationship between aldosterone and the progression of chronic CAD, up to now no large clinical trial has specifically evaluated the effect of MRAs on the amelioration of plaque formation. Vukusich et al. executed a randomized, double-blind, placebo-controlled trial to assess the effectiveness of spironolactone in preventing progression of carotid intima-media thickness (CIMT) in non-diabetic hemodialysis patients. Over a period of 24 months, 53 patients received either 50 mg spironolactone or placebo thrice weekly after dialysis. CIMT measurements revealed a progression in the placebo-group whereas in the spironolactone-treated patients, CIMT significantly decreased [54]. Another clinical trial is currently recruiting patients to study the effect of spironolactone on vascular atherosclerotic burden. The "Mineralocorticoid Receptor Antagonism Clinical Evaluation in atherosclerosis Trial" (NCT02169089) is a phase IV trial that aims to evaluate the efficacy of spironolactone in decelerating the worsening of atherosclerotic disease in the aorta in patients with type 2 diabetes and a previous history of CAD. The patients are randomized to spironolactone (12.5–25 mg daily) versus placebo. The primary endpoint is the atheroma volume evaluated via magnetic resonance imaging (MRI) pictures of the aortic wall before and after therapy (https://www.clinicaltrialsregister.eu/ctr-search/trial/2015-002168-17/HU#D). In another clinical approach, Garg et al. measured the effect of spironolactone on cardiovascular function in patients with diabetes and used the coronary flow reserve as a marker for coronary microvascular function. A total of 64 participants with well-controlled diabetes who were on chronic ACE-therapy were randomized to 25 mg spironolactone, 12.5 mg hydrochlorothiazide or placebo for 6 months. The spironolactone-treated patients showed a significant improvement in coronary microvascular function [55].

Endothelial dysfunction plays an important role in the pathogenesis of CAD and is a well-established marker for cardiovascular risk and prognosis [56]. Accordingly, MR blockade has been shown to improve endothelial dysfunction in patients with HFrEF [57]. Bavry et al. designed a double-blind, parallel-group, repeated measures study in women with symptoms and signs of ischemia and coronary endothelial dysfunction but no significant CAD already receiving ACE-inhibitor or angiotensin receptor blockers. Patients received either eplerenone (25 mg daily for 4 weeks, then uptitrated to 50 mg daily for 12 weeks) or placebo. The primary outcome was percent change in coronary diameter to acetylcholine and secondary in flow reserve to adenosine at 16 weeks. A total of 41 women completed the treatment period, but there was no significant difference between treatment groups [58]. Similarly, Sudano et al. randomized CAD patients with preserved ejection fraction to receive daily eplerenone (25 mg) or placebo and assessed endothelial cell function after 4 weeks of treatment. Based on brachial artery dilatation, the investigators did not find any differences in the endothelial cell function between the groups [59].

In contrast to the firmly established benefit of MR blockade in HFrEF and patients with LV-dysfunction after MI, the role of MRAs with stable CAD with preserved ejection fraction remains a matter of debate. The variety of small studies with different approaches and endpoints is not sufficient to give a general recommendation. Larger, prospective, randomized trials are needed further evaluating the role of MR blockade in stable CAD.

## 3. Conclusion

It has long been clear that the effects of aldosterone are more diverse than originally thought. High aldosterone plasma levels early after STEMI or NSTEMI or in patients with heart failure are associated with increased cardiovascular morbidity and mortality. Clinical trials have firmly established that MR blocking therapy provides considerable improvements in cardiovascular mortality and morbidity in patients with severe heart failure (RALES and ARTS-HF), LV dysfunction after acute MI (EPHESUS), as well as in patients with less symptomatic chronic heart failure (EMPHASIS-HF) (**Table 1**). With REMINDER and ALBATROSS, there is conflicting data on the role of MRAs in patients after MI without LV-dysfunction. However, one has to keep in mind that ALBATROSS and REMINDER were both underpowered and group analysis showed that patients with STEMI might benefit from treatment. As with stable CAD and preserved ejection fraction, the role of MR

| **Study** | **RALES** | **EPHESUS** | **EMPHASIS-HF** | **REMINDER** | **ALBATROSS** | **ARTS** | **ARTS-HF** | **ARTS-HF Japan** | **FIGARO-DKD** | **FIDELIO-DKD** |
|---|---|---|---|---|---|---|---|---|---|---|
| Year | 1999 | 2003 | 2011 | 2014 | 2016 | 2013 | 2015 | 2016 | Recruiting | Active, not recruiting |
| Primary end-point | Mortality | All-cause or CV mortality, hosp. for CHF | CV death, hosp. for CHF | Mortality, hosp. for CHF | Death, worsened CHF, arrhythmias | Part A: safety and tolerability; Part B: change in serum potassium | decrease in NT-proBNP >30% | decrease in NT-proBNP >30% | CV death and no-fatal CV events | Onset of kidney failure, decrease of eGFR |
| No. of patients | 1663 | 6642 | 2737 | 506 | 1603 | 65 (Part A) +393 (Part B) | 1066 | 72 | 6400 (estimated) | 4800 (estimated) |
| Inclusion criteria | Severe CHF | Post-MI (within 3–14 days), CHF or diabetes | Mild CHF, <55 years | STEMI | STEMI or high risk non-STEMI, ≥18 years | HFrEF and mild (Part A)/ moderate (Part B) chronic kidney disease | Worsening CHF, treatment with diuretics; eGFR ≥30 ml/min/m$^2$ | Worsening CHF, treatment with diuretics; eGFR ≥30 ml/ min/m$^2$ | Type 2 Diabetes mellitus, Diabetic Kidney Disease, pretreatment with ACE-I | Type 2 Diabetes mellitus, Diabetic Kidney Disease, pretreatment with ACE-I |
| | NYHA III-IV | NYHA I-IV | NYHA II | n.a. | n.a. | NYHA II-III | n.a. | n.a. | n.a. | n.a. |
| | EF <35% | EF <40% | EF <35% | EF >40% | n.a. | EF ≤40% | EF ≤40% | EF ≤40% | n.a. | n.a. |
| Major exclusion criteria | P-creatinine >220 μm, P-K >5.0 | P-creatinine >220 μm, P-K >5.0 | eGFR < 30 ml/min/ m$^2$, P-K >5.0 | eGFR < 30 ml/min/ m$^2$, P-creatinine ≥220 μm | P-creatinine >220 μm and/ or Creatinine clearance < 30 ml/m | worsening HF requiring hospitalization/ treatment with diuretucs | *de novo* HF, acute inflammation, ACS/ stroke 3 months prior | *de novo* HF, acute inflammation, ACS/stroke 3 months prior | HFrEF, NYHA II-IV, Dialysis | HFrEF, NYHA II-IV, Dialysis |
| Mean age (years ± SD) | 65 ± 12 | 64 ± 12 | 68.7 ± 7.7 | 58.5 ± 10.8 | 58 | | 69.2 – 72.5 ± 9.7 – 10.6 (different treatment groups) | 65.9 – 78.2 (different treatment groups) | | |

| Study | RALES | EPHESUS | EMPHASIS-HF | REMINDER | ALBATROSS | ARTS | ARTS-HF | ARTS-HF Japan | FIGARO-DKD | FIDELIO-DKD |
|---|---|---|---|---|---|---|---|---|---|---|
| Medical therapy | ACE-I, diuretic | ACE-I/ ARB, ß-blocker, diuretic | ACE-I/ARB, ß-blocker, diuretic | ACE-I/ARB, ß-blocker | ACE-I/ARB, ß-blocker | ACE-I/ARB, ß-blocker, diuretic | ACE-I/ARB, ß-blocker, diuretic | ACE-I/ARB, ß-blocker, diuretic | ACE-I | ACE-I |
| MRA | Spironolactone | Eplerenone | Eplerenone | Eplerenone | Bolus of K+ canreonate, then spironolactone | Finerenone versus Spironolactone versus Placebo | Finerenone versus Eplerenone | Finerenone versus Eplerenone | Finerenone | Finerenone |
| Dose (mg/day) | 25–50 | 25–50 | 25–50 | Up to 50 | 25 | 2.5–10 (Finerenone); up to 50 mg (Spironolactone) | 2.5–20 (Finerenone); up to 50 mg (Eplerenone) | 2.5–20 (Finerenone); up to 50 (Eplerenone) | 10 and 20 mg | 10 and 20 mg |
| Mean daily dose (mg/day) | 26 | 43 | 39 | 88.6% received high dose | 25 | % | % | % | | |
| Follow-up | 24 months | 16 months | 21 months | 18 months | 6 months | 1 month | 90 days | 90 days | 53 months | 48 months |
| End-point | −30% all-cause mortality | −15% all-cause mortality | −34% all-cause mortality | composite clinical endpoint: eplerenone 1.8%, placebo 3.2% | primary outcome: spironolactone 11.8%, placebo 12.2% | Part A: safety and tolerabilty confirmed; Part B: lower incidences of hyperkalaemia | 37.2% eplerenone; 30.9–38.8% finerenone | 23.1% eplerenone; 15.4–45.5% finerenone | | |
| | −31% cardiovasc. mortality | −17% cardiovasc. mortality | −37% cardiovasc. mortality | | | | | | | |
| | −33% hosp. for HF | −23% hosp. for HF | −42% hosp. for HF | | | | | | | |

**Table 1.**
*Trials of mineralocorticoid receptor antagonists in the context of myocardial infarction and heart failure: demographics and outcome.*

blockade in this highly inhomogeneous patient collective is still unclear and remains a matter of debate. The variety of small studies with different approaches and endpoints is not sufficient to give a general recommendation. Larger, prospective, randomized trials are urgently needed.

Regarding drug safety and side effects: when contraindications such as co-medication with potassium-sparing diuretics are respected and renal function and potassium levels are closely monitored, application of spironolactone and eplerenone is relatively safe and patients with mild to moderate renal insufficiency gain similar reductions in mortality and hospitalization as heart failure patients with normal renal function. Nevertheless, there are always cases in which deterioration of the kidney function or hyperkalemia requires the discontinuation of the medication. Especially with the development of the non-steroidal third-generation MRAs, such as finerenone, with both high selectivity and high potency to inhibit MR, we might be able to fulfill the hope of achieving cardiovascular benefit without or at least with fewer renal side effects than spironolactone and eplerenone (**Figure 1**).

Without any question, MRAs are nowadays one of the mainstays of current pharmacotherapy for cardiovascular diseases and are clearly indicated in patients with chronic heart failure (NYHA class II–IV and and/or an ejection fraction ≤35%) as well as in patients with evidence of heart failure/LV dysfunction early after an acute MI. On the contrary, no general recommendation for immediate MR antagonism is currently justified in patients without LV dysfunction after MI. An adequately powered prospective randomized trial evaluating the safety and efficacy of MRA administration early post-MI in patients without heart failure/LV dysfunction is still needed to finally answer that question.

## Acknowledgements

This publication is based upon work from the EU COST Action ADMIRE BM1301 in Aldosterone and Mineralocorticoid Receptor Physiology and Pathophysiology www.admirecosteu.com.

## Author details

Carolin Zwadlo and Johann Bauersachs*
Department of Cardiology and Angiology, Hannover Medical School, Hannover, Germany

*Address all correspondence to: bauersachs.johann@mh-hannover.de

## References

[1] Zwadlo C, Bauersachs J. Mineralocorticoid receptor antagonists for therapy of coronary artery disease and related complications. Current Opinion in Pharmacology. 2013;**13**(2):280-286

[2] Messaoudi S et al. Aldosterone, mineralocorticoid receptor, and heart failure. Molecular and Cellular Endocrinology. 2012;**350**(2):266-272

[3] Fraccarollo D et al. Deletion of cardiomyocyte mineralocorticoid receptor ameliorates adverse remodeling after myocardial infarction. Circulation. 2011;**123**(4):400-408

[4] Lother A et al. Ablation of mineralocorticoid receptors in myocytes but not in fibroblasts preserves cardiac function. Hypertension. 2011;**57**(4): 746-754

[5] de Resende MM, Kauser K, Mill JG. Regulation of cardiac and renal mineralocorticoid receptor expression by captopril following myocardial infarction in rats. Life Sciences. 2006; **78**(26):3066-3073

[6] Ouvrard-Pascaud A et al. Conditional mineralocorticoid receptor expression in the heart leads to life-threatening arrhythmias. Circulation. 2005;**111**(23): 3025-3033

[7] Bauersachs J, Jaisser F, Toto R. Mineralocorticoid receptor activation and mineralocorticoid receptor antagonist treatment in cardiac and renal diseases. Hypertension. 2015; **65**(2):257-263

[8] Farman N, Rafestin-Oblin ME. Multiple aspects of mineralocorticoid selectivity. American Journal of Physiology. Renal Physiology. 2001; **280**(2):F181-F192

[9] Guder G et al. Complementary and incremental mortality risk prediction by cortisol and aldosterone in chronic heart failure. Circulation. 2007;**115**(13): 1754-1761

[10] Farquharson CA, Struthers AD. Aldosterone induces acute endothelial dysfunction in vivo in humans: Evidence for an aldosterone-induced vasculopathy. Clinical Science (London, England). 2002;**103**(4):425-431

[11] Brown NJ et al. Aldosterone modulates plasminogen activator inhibitor-1 and glomerulosclerosis in vivo. Kidney International. 2000; **58**(3):1219-1227

[12] Iglarz M et al. Involvement of oxidative stress in the profibrotic action of aldosterone. Interaction with the renin-angiotension system. American Journal of Hypertension. 2004;**17**(7): 597-603

[13] Sun Y et al. Aldosterone-induced inflammation in the rat heart: Role of oxidative stress. The American Journal of Pathology. 2002;**161**(5):1773-1781

[14] Gromotowicz A et al. Study of the mechanisms of aldosterone prothrombotic effect in rats. Journal of the Renin-Angiotensin-Aldosterone System. 2011;**12**(4):430-439

[15] Gromotowicz-Poplawska A et al. The acute prothrombotic effect of aldosterone in rats is partially mediated via angiotensin II receptor type 1. Thrombosis Research. 2016;**138**:114-120

[16] Dooley R, Harvey BJ, Thomas W. Non-genomic actions of aldosterone: From receptors and signals to membrane targets. Molecular and Cellular Endocrinology. 2012;**350**(2): 223-234

[17] Krug AW et al. Cell membrane-associated mineralocorticoid receptors?

New evidence. Hypertension. 2011; **57**(6):1019-1025

[18] Rossier MF, Python M, Maturana AD. Contribution of mineralocorticoid and glucocorticoid receptors to the chronotropic and hypertrophic actions of aldosterone in neonatal rat ventricular myocytes. Endocrinology. 2010;**151**(6):2777-2787

[19] Gros R et al. Aldosterone mediates its rapid effects in vascular endothelial cells through GPER activation. American Journal of Physiology. Cell Physiology. 2013;**304**(6):C532-C540

[20] Pitt B et al. The effect of spironolactone on morbidity and mortality in patients with severe heart failure. Randomized Aldactone evaluation study investigators. The New England Journal of Medicine. 1999; **341**(10):709-717

[21] Vukadinovic D et al. True rate of mineralocorticoid receptor antagonists-related hyperkalemia in placebo-controlled trials: A meta-analysis. American Heart Journal. 2017;**188**:99-108

[22] Kolkhof P, Borden SA. Molecular pharmacology of the mineralocorticoid receptor: Prospects for novel therapeutics. Molecular and Cellular Endocrinology. 2012;**350**(2):310-317

[23] Barfacker L et al. Discovery of BAY 94-8862: A nonsteroidal antagonist of the mineralocorticoid receptor for the treatment of cardiorenal diseases. ChemMedChem. 2012;7(8):1385-1403

[24] Bauersachs J. The ARTS of third-generation mineralocorticoid receptor antagonists: Achieving cardiovascular benefit with minimized renal side effects? European Heart Journal. 2013; **34**(31):2426-2428

[25] Kolkhof P, Barfacker L. 30 years of the mineralocorticoid receptor: Mineralocorticoid receptor antagonists: 60 years of research and development. The Journal of Endocrinology. 2017; **234**(1):T125-T140

[26] McMurray JJ et al. ESC guidelines for the diagnosis and treatment of acute and chronic heart failure 2012: The task force for the diagnosis and treatment of acute and chronic heart failure 2012 of the European Society of Cardiology. Developed in collaboration with the heart failure association (HFA) of the ESC. European Heart Journal. 2012; **33**(14):1787-1847

[27] Zannad F et al. Eplerenone in patients with systolic heart failure and mild symptoms. The New England Journal of Medicine. 2011;**364**(1):11-21

[28] Chan AK et al. Aldosterone receptor antagonism induces reverse remodeling when added to angiotensin receptor blockade in chronic heart failure. Journal of the American College of Cardiology. 2007;**50**(7):591-596

[29] Kolkhof P et al. Finerenone, a novel selective nonsteroidal mineralocorticoid receptor antagonist protects from rat cardiorenal injury. Journal of Cardiovascular Pharmacology. 2014; **64**(1):69-78

[30] Grune J et al. Steroidal and nonsteroidal mineralocorticoid receptor antagonists cause differential cardiac gene expression in pressure overload-induced cardiac hypertrophy. Journal of Cardiovascular Pharmacology. 2016; **67**(5):402-411

[31] Pitt B et al. Safety and tolerability of the novel non-steroidal mineralocorticoid receptor antagonist BAY 94-8862 in patients with chronic heart failure and mild or moderate chronic kidney disease: A randomized, double-blind trial. European Heart Journal. 2013;**34**(31): 2453-2463

[32] Pitt B et al. Rationale and design of ARTS: A randomized, double-blind

study of BAY 94-8862 in patients with chronic heart failure and mild or moderate chronic kidney disease. European Journal of Heart Failure. 2012; **14**(6):668-675

[33] Filippatos G et al. A randomized controlled study of finerenone vs. eplerenone in patients with worsening chronic heart failure and diabetes mellitus and/or chronic kidney disease. European Heart Journal. 2016;**37**(27): 2105-2114

[34] Sato N et al. A randomized controlled study of Finerenone vs. eplerenone in Japanese patients with worsening chronic heart failure and diabetes and/or chronic kidney disease. Circulation Journal. 2016;**80**(5): 1113-1122

[35] Bauersachs J, Fraccarollo D. Mineralocorticoid receptor-dependent adverse Remodeling after myocardial infarction mediated by uNGALant activation of NFkappaB. Hypertension. 2017;**70**(6):1080-1081

[36] Silvestre JS et al. Activation of cardiac aldosterone production in rat myocardial infarction: Effect of angiotensin II receptor blockade and role in cardiac fibrosis. Circulation. 1999;**99**(20):2694-2701

[37] Fraccarollo D et al. Immediate mineralocorticoid receptor blockade improves myocardial infarct healing by modulation of the inflammatory response. Hypertension. 2008;**51**(4): 905-914

[38] Fraccarollo D et al. Efficacy of mineralocorticoid receptor antagonism in the acute myocardial infarction phase: Eplerenone versus spironolactone. ESC Heart Failure. 2015;**2**(3):150-158

[39] Hayashi M et al. Immediate administration of mineralocorticoid receptor antagonist spironolactone prevents post-infarct left ventricular remodeling associated with suppression of a marker of myocardial collagen synthesis in patients with first anterior acute myocardial infarction. Circulation. 2003;**107**(20):2559-2565

[40] Pitt B et al. Eplerenone, a selective aldosterone blocker, in patients with left ventricular dysfunction after myocardial infarction. The New England Journal of Medicine. 2003; **348**(14):1309-1321

[41] Adamopoulos C et al. Timing of eplerenone initiation and outcomes in patients with heart failure after acute myocardial infarction complicated by left ventricular systolic dysfunction: Insights from the EPHESUS trial. European Journal of Heart Failure. 2009;**11**(11):1099-1105

[42] Montalescot G et al. Early eplerenone treatment in patients with acute ST-elevation myocardial infarction without heart failure: The randomized double-blind Reminder study. European Heart Journal. 2014; **35**(34):2295-2302

[43] Beygui F et al. Early aldosterone blockade in acute myocardial infarction: The ALBATROSS randomized clinical trial. Journal of the American College of Cardiology. 2016;**67**(16):1917-1927

[44] Pitt B. MRAs in patients with AMI without early evidence of heart failure: Time for reappraisal? Journal of the American College of Cardiology. 2016; **67**(16):1928-1930

[45] Beygui F et al. Individual participant data analysis of two trials on aldosterone blockade in myocardial infarction. Heart. Nov 2018;**104**(22):1843-1849. DOI: 10.1136/heartjnl-2018-312950. Epub 2018 Apr 25

[46] Rajagopalan S et al. Mineralocorticoid receptor antagonism in experimental atherosclerosis. Circulation. 2002;**105**(18):2212-2216

[47] Keidar S et al. Effect of eplerenone, a selective aldosterone blocker, on blood pressure, serum and macrophage oxidative stress, and atherosclerosis in apolipoprotein E-deficient mice. Journal of Cardiovascular Pharmacology. 2003; **41**(6):955-963

[48] Suzuki J et al. Eplerenone with valsartan effectively reduces atherosclerotic lesion by attenuation of oxidative stress and inflammation. Arteriosclerosis, Thrombosis, and Vascular Biology. 2006;**26**(4):917-921

[49] Dutzmann J, Bauersachs J, Sedding DG. Evidence for the use of mineralocorticoid receptor antagonists in the treatment of coronary artery disease and post-angioplasty restenosis. Vascular Pharmacology. 2017

[50] Dutzmann J et al. The novel mineralocorticoid receptor antagonist finerenone attenuates neointima formation after vascular injury. PLoS One. 2017;**12**(9):e0184888

[51] Tomaschitz A et al. Plasma aldosterone levels are associated with increased cardiovascular mortality: The Ludwigshafen risk and cardiovascular health (LURIC) study. European Heart Journal. 2010;**31**(10):1237-1247

[52] Ivanes F et al. Aldosterone, mortality, and acute ischaemic events in coronary artery disease patients outside the setting of acute myocardial infarction or heart failure. European Heart Journal. 2012;**33**(2):191-202

[53] de Rita O, Hackam DG, Spence JD. Effects of aldosterone on human atherosclerosis: Plasma aldosterone and progression of carotid plaque. The Canadian Journal of Cardiology. 2012; **28**(6):706-711

[54] Vukusich A et al. A randomized, double-blind, placebo-controlled trial of spironolactone on carotid intima-media thickness in nondiabetic hemodialysis patients. Clinical Journal of the American Society of Nephrology. 2010; **5**(8):1380-1387

[55] Garg R et al. Mineralocorticoid receptor blockade improves coronary microvascular function in individuals with type 2 diabetes. Diabetes. 2015; **64**(1):236-242

[56] Gutierrez E et al. Endothelial dysfunction over the course of coronary artery disease. European Heart Journal. 2013;**34**(41):3175-3181

[57] Farquharson CA, Struthers AD. Spironolactone increases nitric oxide bioactivity, improves endothelial vasodilator dysfunction, and suppresses vascular angiotensin I/angiotensin II conversion in patients with chronic heart failure. Circulation. 2000;**101**(6): 594-597

[58] Bavry AA et al. Aldosterone inhibition and coronary endothelial function in women without obstructive coronary artery disease: An ancillary study of the national heart, lung, and blood institute-sponsored women's ischemia syndrome evaluation. American Heart Journal. 2014;**167**(6): 826-832

[59] Sudano I et al. Vascular effects of eplerenone in coronary artery disease with preserved ejection fraction: A double-blind, randomized, placebo-controlled trial. Clinical Cardiology. 2016;**39**(5):285-290

Chapter 2

# Mineralocorticoid Receptor and Leptin: A Dangerous Liaison in the Obese Heart

*Gema Marin-Royo, María Luaces, Victoria Cachofeiro and Ernesto Martínez-Martínez*

## Abstract

Multiple factors have been proposed as being responsible for cardiac damage in the context of obesity, including aldosterone/mineralocorticoid receptor and leptin. Aldosterone exerts proinflammatory, prooxidant and profibrotic actions, which can play a key role in the development of cardiac damage associated with different pathologies, through binding of mineralocorticoid receptor (MR). Moreover, its pharmacological blockade has demonstrated to improve these situations. Different studies have demonstrated that aldosterone is inappropriately elevated in obesity and MR antagonism improves left ventricle function and reduces circulating procollagen levels in patients with obesity without other comorbidities. Leptin is locally produced in the myocardium and its production is up-regulated in obesity. This adipokine is a proinflammatory, prooxidant and profibrotic factor that can participate in the cardiac damage associated with obesity. Interactions among leptin and aldosterone have previously been reported in different scenarios and at different levels, supporting a link between leptin and MR and that could result in the potentiation of the cardiac damage associated with obesity. Therefore, the aim of this review is to discuss whether MR activation can mediate the deleterious effects of leptin in the heart in the context of obesity, as well as the potential mechanisms involved in this process.

**Keywords:** leptin, mineralocorticoid receptor, fibrosis, heart, oxidative stress

## 1. Cardiac effects of obesity

Obesity has become a global problem of the first magnitude worldwide and is associated with an increase in total mortality, especially that of cardiovascular origin [1]. Obesity is an exaggeration of normal adiposity and plays a central role in the pathophysiology of various diseases such as type 2 diabetes mellitus, cardiovascular disease, stroke, hypertension, and dyslipidemia [2]. Obesity is associated with several structural and function alterations in the heart which are characterized by cardiac hypertrophy and left ventricle systolic and diastolic dysfunction that contribute to the development of heart failure [3]. There have been reported changes in left ventricle geometry in obese individuals, with these being more prevalent in an eccentric pattern defined by an increase in left ventricle mass but not in relative parietal thickness [4]. This cardiac hypertrophy could be a consequence of higher metabolic demand required by obese individuals, as well as increased cardiac output which is associated with higher ventricular filling and which promotes ventricular dilatation and, in consequence, an enlargement of myocardial mass [5]. It is well known that left ventricular hypertrophy is a risk factor for heart failure development [6]. Diastolic dysfunction is the main functional alteration observed in obese patients [7]. Ventricular hypertrophy along with an increase in blood flow and circulating volume predisposes to diastolic dysfunction observed in obese patients [4]. Pascual et al. reported subclinical left ventricular diastolic dysfunction in all degrees of obesity (mildly, moderate, and severely obese patients) [8]. Another study reported that the severity of the diastolic dysfunction observed in obesity increases proportionally with the body mass index [9]. Conflicting results have been found [8, 10–14] with regard to systolic function in obese individuals. These contradictory effects on systolic function could be consequence of the presence or not of comorbidities frequently associated with obesity (hypertension, metabolic disorders, and coronary artery disease) which can also have an impact on cardiac function. Several studies have postulated that perivascular and interstitial fibrosis could contribute to the cardiac dysfunction, especially diastolic one, observed in obesity [15]. Cardiac fibrosis is characterized by increased deposit of extracellular matrix (ECM) proteins in the myocardium. This is a dynamic process regulated by the balance between the synthesis and degradation of the ECM proteins within the heart. Collagen, especially collagen type I, is the main protein involved in fibrotic process, and metalloproteinases (MMPs) are the enzymes involved in ECM protein degradation. It has been described that obese patients present elevated serum levels of collagen peptides and are associated with indices of insulin resistance and with diastolic dysfunction [16, 17]. Moreover, the reduction in body mass index after bariatric surgery is not always accompanied by the normalization of diastolic function suggesting myocardial damage probably due to the accumulation of ECM [4].

Several mechanisms and factors have been proposed for the structural and functional changes that occur in the obese heart, such as, the effects of aldosterone, through mineralocorticoid receptor (MR) binding, and leptin, two hormones whose levels are increased in the context of obesity. Aldosterone/MR and leptin promote cardiac damage through its prooxidant and proinflammatory effects which can trigger an excessive ECM accumulation, promoting fibrogenic and hypertrophic responses and functional alterations [18–20]. We herein review the MR and leptin effects at cardiac level with special focus on the context of obesity as well as the interaction of aldosterone and leptin and its role in the development of cardiac remodeling.

## 2. Cardiac effects of mineralocorticoid receptor

Aldosterone is the main mineralocorticoid hormone, which plays an important role in the pathophysiology of cardiovascular disease through its binding to MR, which resides in the cytosol and is translocated to the nucleus after ligand binding, thereby promoting gene transcription [21]. Besides the hypertensive and the renal effects of aldosterone, chronic hyperaldosteronism promotes cardiovascular complications, including left ventricular hypertrophy, myocardial infarction, and atrial fibrillation [22]. The deleterious effects of aldosterone have traditionally been considered over the years due to its effects on sodium/water retention and its effects on blood pressure. However, its extrarenal effects through MR activation in non-epithelial cells of the cardiovascular system have been confirmed in recent years [23]. Several clinical studies have demonstrated that the activation of MR plays an important role in mild to severe heart failure [24–26]. MR blockade through MR antagonists (MRA) reduces morbidity and mortality in heart failure patients. MRA treatment has demonstrated beneficial effects at cardiac level even in the absence of aldosterone level modifications [24–26]. In accordance with these observations, the effects of MR by genetic modulation in different cell types have been demonstrated. Specifically, MR overexpression in cardiomyocytes leads to cardiac arrhythmias in mice in the absence of changes in aldosterone levels [27], and this effect is accompanied by severe coronary endothelial dysfunction due at least in part to an increase in oxidative stress [28]. In addition, mice with MR genetic deletion in cardiomyocytes are resistant to developing cardiac fibrosis induced by deoxycorticosterone/salt (DOCA-salt) and do not show inflammatory cell infiltration after 8 weeks of treatment [29]. In another animal model of cardiac disease, Fraccarollo et al. have demonstrated that MR deletion in cardiomyocytes improved infarct healing, cardiac function, cardiac fibrosis, and mitochondrial superoxide anion production after myocardial infarction, which confirms the role of MR activation in cardiac cells in cardiac pathophysiology [30]. Similar beneficial effects on cardiac remodeling, hypertrophy, and profibrotic and proinflammatory markers have been observed in endothelial [31, 32] or macrophage [33] MR inactivation after DOCA-salt mineralocorticoid challenge and also in vascular smooth muscle MR inactivation in myocardial infarction [34].

In the context of obesity, clinical and experimental studies have demonstrated that aldosterone production is increased in obesity and is correlated with white adipose tissue mass [35–37]. In addition, weight loss in obese individuals is accompanied by a reduction in aldosterone levels [38]. Aldosterone is primarily synthesized in the outer layer of the adrenal cortex. However, it has been demonstrated that adipose tissue possesses the machinery necessary to produce aldosterone, which can act in an autocrine or paracrine manner [39]. Activation of renin-angiotensin-aldosterone system has been reported in animal models of obesity [20, 40, 41]. Endothelial-specific MR deletion in female mice was able to prevent the diastolic dysfunction induced by high-fat diet [42]. This improvement was accompanied by a reduction in cardiac fibrosis, ECM protein deposition, cardiac inflammation, and oxidative stress as well as an improvement in insulin metabolic signaling [42]. These results were confirmed by the same research group where the administration of the MRA spironolactone reproduced the same results [43] in female mice fed with a high-fat diet as well as prevented the development of arterial stiffening in the animals [44]. In agreement with these findings, a randomized controlled clinical study has shown that aldosterone blockade with spironolactone for 6 months improved left ventricular function and reduced circulating procollagen peptide levels in obese patients without other comorbidities [45]. The addition of spironolactone to the standard treatment (angiotensin II inhibitors) was also able to improve left ventricle dysfunction and collagen turnover in patients with metabolic syndrome [46]. In a recent study, we have demonstrated that galectin-3, a lectin upregulated by MR activation, is increased in obese patients and its levels were associated with diastolic function [17]. In addition, pharmacological blockade of galectin-3 with an activity inhibitor blunted the cardiovascular remodeling and inflammation in obese male rats [17]. Another study in obese rats showed that the administration of spironolactone normalized cardiac diastolic function and reduced cardiac fibrosis [47]. The studies performed in the context of obesity overall show the implication of MR in cardiac damage and the beneficial consequences of the use of MRA in the treatment of obesity-related cardiovascular dysfunction.

## 3. Cardiac effects of leptin

Leptin is the product of the *ob* gene that circulates in proportion to body fat [48]. This hormone is considered critical for informing the central nervous system about the status of energy reserves and control satiety [49]. It is thought that obese people are leptin-resistant due to the lack of satiation observed. However, this leptin resistance does not occur in peripheral tissues, including the cardiovascular system, where leptin promotes several actions in obesity [50]. Leptin is mainly produced by adipose tissue, but it is also produced in different tissues, including the heart [48]. Plasma leptin levels have been considered to be an independent predictor of coronary heart disease [51] and a risk factor for myocardial infarction [52] and coronary atherosclerosis [53]. During obesity there is an increase in systemic leptin levels, as well as in the heart where it is locally produced [54]. Leptin acts via transmembrane receptors which are the product of *db* gene [55]. Genetic deletion of *ob* or *db* genes promotes obese animals, which have been used in conjunction with diet-induced obese animals in order to study the role of leptin in the cardiovascular system [56–58]. Several mechanisms have demonstrated the pathogenic role of leptin at cardiac level. Leptin receptor-deficient obese Zucker rats have been a studied animal model of hyperglycemia and diabetes [59], cardiac lipotoxicity [60], and diastolic cardiac dysfunction [61] as well. In accordance with this metabolic alterations, it has been demonstrated that leptin increased fatty acid uptake in HL-1 cells leading to intracellular lipid accumulation [62] being one possible mechanism involved in cardiac lipotoxicity that can facilitate the development of heart failure [63].

Concerning structural modifications observed in obesity, clinical data have shown a positive correlation between plasma leptin levels with left ventricular hypertrophy [64]. Infusion of leptin in myocardial infarction mice increased left ventricle diameter as compared with animals without leptin infusion [65]. In vitro data show the direct hypertrophic effects of leptin inducing elongation of cardiac myocytes via the activation of JAK/STAT pathway [65]. Despite the well-established hypertrophic effects of leptin, there is one report that documented contradictory effects. *Ob/ob* mice have shown cardiac hypertrophy which is reverted after leptin repletion [66]. It is documented that oxidative stress plays an important role in the development of cardiac hypertrophy [67]. Leptin levels are correlated with superoxide anion levels in peripheral blood mononuclear cells from obese patients after adjusting for age and sex [68]. In this context, leptin produced an increase in reactive oxygen species (ROS) accumulation in a dose- and time-dependent manner in endothelial cells, accompanied by an activation of the JNK pathway [69]. Similar results have been observed in vascular smooth muscle cells [70] and in cardiac fibroblasts [54]. In addition, an antioxidant treatment in vascular and cardiac cells was able to prevent the increase in collagen production induced by leptin [54, 70], showing the role of oxidative stress in fibrogenic responses. Experimental studies have shown that leptin administration in *ob/ob* mice increased myocardial collagen deposition, thus confirming its profibrotic effects [71]. Complementary techniques revealed cardiac interstitial fibrosis in *db/db* mice [72] and in Zucker rats [73], and it is associated with diastolic dysfunction. Multiple mechanisms have been suggested as being responsible for the interstitial fibrosis observed in these animals, including metabolic alterations and the activation of renin-angiotensin-aldosterone system. However, the potential role of leptin in the aldosterone/MR activation observed in these animals is likely acting through mechanisms other than leptin, since both *db/db* mice and Zucker rats have impaired leptin signaling. These potential mechanisms could include angiotensin II, oxidative stress, or metabolic alterations [47, 74–76].

In a recent study, we have demonstrated that leptin enhances lysyl oxidase (LOX) protein levels in cardiac fibroblasts [77]. LOX is an ECM enzyme that catalyzes the cross-linking of collagen fibers [78]. The pharmacological inhibition of LOX is able to prevent the increase in collagen production induced by leptin in cardiac and vascular cells as well as the cardiovascular fibrosis associated with obesity [77]. In addition, we have observed that leptin increased the aldosterone downstream product, galectin-3, protein levels in cardiac fibroblasts, which at the same time mediates the fibrotic effect of leptin [54] supporting the possible relationship between leptin and MR.

Another mechanism involved in cardiac injury in obesity is the inflammation [79]. Leptin can be considered to be an inflammatory cytokine itself [80] but also promotes monocyte recruitment [81] and macrophage foam cell formation [82] and promotes the secretion of another inflammatory cytokines [83]. The present knowledge of the mechanisms triggered by leptin has established the implication of this adipokine in the deleterious consequences of obesity in the cardiovascular system.

## 4. Leptin-aldosterone/MR axis

Leptin is a major stimulus to the production of aldosterone in obesity [41, 84] and may be responsible for the excessive MR signaling that is the hallmark of obesity-related heart failure [85, 86]. This thus supports a cross talk between leptin and MR, which can have deleterious consequences in the context of obesity including sodium balance. In this regard, visceral adiposity leads to positive sodium balance through the leptin receptor, which can cause sodium retention [87] through different mechanisms which include a direct action on the renal tubules, an increase in renal sympathetic nerve traffic [88, 89], and a direct stimulation of renin-angiotensin-aldosterone system [90, 91].

Obesity is associated with dysfunctional adipose tissue, which is characterized by the increase in the synthesis of different cytokines as well as leptin. In addition to leptin which is able to stimulate aldosterone synthesis and therefore active MR, whether other adipokines, such as, tumor necrosis factor-α, are able to increase aldosterone is not totally established in the literature since a variety of results have been reported [41, 92].

Leptin infusion in obese and lean mice promotes an increase in aldosterone plasma levels suggesting a relationship between both hormones [93]. Confirming these results, Huby et al. have demonstrated that there is an increase in aldosterone production in an animal model of leptin hypersensitivity due to an increase in *CYP11B2* (aldosterone synthase) expression [90]. The authors showed in the same study that this increase in aldosterone and CYP11B2 is absent in three different transgenic models of leptin activity deletion [90]. In fact, leptin receptors are colocalized with *CYP11B2* in human adrenal cells. In addition, the administration of the leptin receptor antagonist prevented the rise in aldosterone plasma levels observed in the leptin hypersensitivity animal model as well as in obese mice [94]. These data taken together demonstrate that aldosterone production induced by leptin is dependent on leptin signaling rather than on the increase in body weight. However, there are several discrepancies in this suggestion [95]. The mechanisms involved in aldosterone production induced by leptin are still unclear, although it has been proposed to be a calcium-dependent process. In human adrenocortical carcinoma cells, leptin increased calcium activity as well as *CYP11B2* aldosterone production. When intracellular calcium is chelated, leptin-treated cells do not show the increase in *CYP11B2* promoter activity [90].

Female mice infused with leptin presented reduced endothelium-dependent relaxation, which was prevented by spironolactone treatment—this demonstrates that leptin induces endothelial dysfunction via MR [90]. In the same study, the authors showed that leptin administration for 7 days induced an increase in mRNA levels in profibrotic markers at cardiac level, which was blunted by treatment with spironolactone. This effect is independent of body weight since obese transgenic mice (*ob/ob*) only presented the increase in the profibrotic markers when they were treated with leptin [90]. The transgenic background could explain this effect since *ob/ob* mice are deficient in leptin, suggesting that leptin induced cardiac fibrosis through MR.

As it has been mentioned above, circulating leptin levels are increased in obesity but also are increased locally at cardiac level [54]. In previous studies, we have demonstrated that leptin participates in collagen I production through its prooxidant effects and suggests its possible role in the cardiac fibrosis associated with obesity [54]. Considering that mitochondria is the main source of ROS production, we explored in a recent study the possible role of mitochondrial oxidative stress in cardiac alterations in obesity [40]. For this purpose, we used a normotensive model of diet-induced obesity in rats treated with either MitoTEMPO (a mitochondrial ROS scavenger) or vehicle. The mitochondrial antioxidant was able to prevent the increase in superoxide anion production, as well as the cardiac hypertrophy and fibrosis in obese rats, thus showing the role of mitochondrial ROS in these alterations [40]. Interestingly, these effects of MitoTEMPO were accompanied by a reduction in leptin and aldosterone plasma levels in obese rats, suggesting a possible cross talk between both hormones. For this reason, we explored this possible interaction in cardiac myofibroblasts. In these cells, leptin increased *CYP11B2* mRNA levels (**Figure 1A**) which was accompanied by an increase in the production of aldosterone in a dose- and time-dependent manner (**Figure 1B** and **C**).

In addition, leptin increased ECM proteins, profibrotic mediators, and the production of superoxide anion at total and mitochondrial level through the activation of Akt and ERK1/ERK2 pathways [40]. The pharmacological blockade of MR through pretreatment of the cells with eplerenone was able to prevent all these alterations induced by leptin in the cardiac cells, thus showing the cross talk between MR and leptin. The results taken together show the possible role of leptin in cardiac fibrosis in the context of obesity through MR-dependent mechanisms (**Figure 2**) [40].

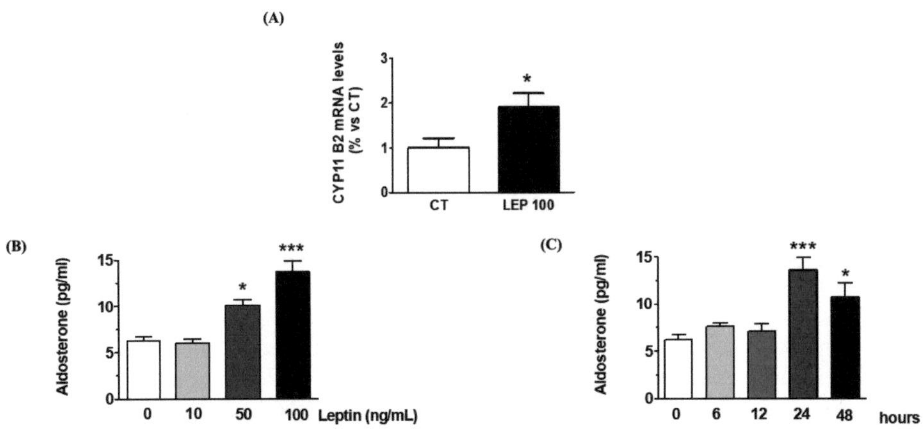


**Figure 1.**
*(A) Effects of leptin (100 ng/mL) on CYP11B2 mRNA levels at 24 hours of stimulation. (B) Dose-response and (C) time-course of leptin on aldosterone secretion in human cardiac fibroblasts.* *$p < 0.05$; ***$p < 0.001$ *vs. control.*

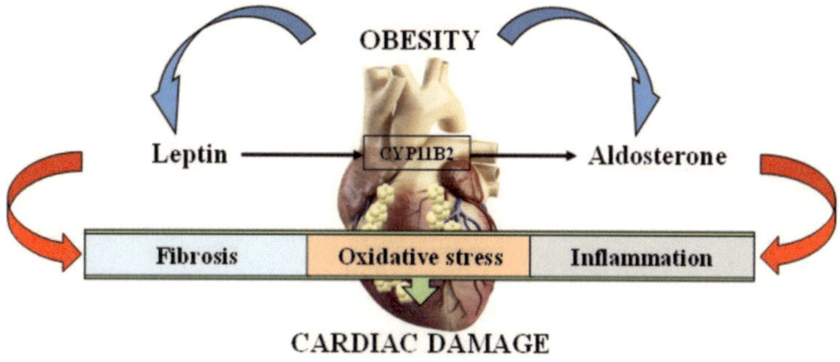


**Figure 2.**
*Scheme illustrating the cross talk between leptin and aldosterone and different mechanisms involved in the cardiac damage associated with obesity.*

## Acknowledgements

This publication is based upon work from the EU COST Action ADMIRE BM1301 in aldosterone and mineralocorticoid receptor (MR) physiology and pathophysiology. This work was supported by Instituto de Salud Carlos III-Fondo Europeo de Desarrollo Regional (FEDER) (PI15/01060; CIBERCV), a way to build Europe. EM-M was supported by a contract from CAM (Atracción de talento).

## Author details

Gema Marin-Royo[1], María Luaces[2], Victoria Cachofeiro[1]* and Ernesto Martínez-Martínez[1]

1 Departamento de Fisiología, Facultad de Medicina, Universidad Complutense de Madrid and Instituto de Investigación Sanitaria Gregorio Marañón (IiSGM), Madrid, Spain

2 Servicio de Cardiología, Instituto Cardiovascular, Hospital Clínico San Carlos, Madrid, Spain

*Address all correspondence to: vcara@med.ucm.es

## References


[1] Kenchaiah S et al. Obesity and the risk of heart failure. The New England Journal of Medicine. 2002;**347**(5):305-313

[2] Pischon T et al. General and abdominal adiposity and risk of death in Europe. The New England Journal of Medicine. 2008;**359**(20):2105-2120

[3] Alpert MA, Karthikeyan K, Abdullah O, Ghadban R. Obesity and cardiac remodeling in adults: Mechanisms and clinical implications. Progress in Cardiovascular Diseases. 2018;**61**(2):114-123

[4] Luaces M et al. Anatomical and functional alterations of the heart in morbid obesity. Changes after bariatric surgery. Revista Española de Cardiología (English Edition). 2012;**65**(1):14-21

[5] Ku CS, Lin SL, Wang DJ, Chang SK, Lee WJ. Left ventricular filling in young normotensive obese adults. The American Journal of Cardiology. 1994;**73**(8):613-615

[6] Kannel WB et al. Profile for estimating risk of heart failure. Archives of Internal Medicine. 1999;**159**(11):1197-1204

[7] Alpert MA, Omran J, Bostick BP. Effects of obesity on cardiovascular hemodynamics, cardiac morphology, and ventricular function. Current Obesity Reports. 2016;**5**(4):424-434

[8] Pascual M et al. Effects of isolated obesity on systolic and diastolic left ventricular function. Heart. 2003;**89**(10):1152-1156

[9] Alpert MA et al. Cardiac morphology and left ventricular function in normotensive morbidly obese patients with and without congestive heart failure, and effect of weight loss. The American Journal of Cardiology. 1997;**80**(6):736-740

[10] Herszkowicz N et al. Contribution of Doppler echocardiography to the evaluation of systolic and diastolic function of obese women versus a control group. Arquivos Brasileiros de Cardiologia. 2001;**76**(3):189-196

[11] Willens HJ et al. Tissue Doppler imaging of the right and left ventricle in severe obesity (body mass index >35 kg/m$^2$). The American Journal of Cardiology. 2004;**94**(8):1087-1090

[12] Otto ME et al. Comparison of right and left ventricular function in obese and nonobese men. The American Journal of Cardiology. 2004;**93**(12):1569-1572

[13] Tumuklu MM, Etikan I, Kisacik B, Kayikcioglu M. Effect of obesity on left ventricular structure and myocardial systolic function: Assessment by tissue Doppler imaging and strain/strain rate imaging. Echocardiography. 2007;**24**(8):802-809

[14] Orhan AL et al. Effects of isolated obesity on left and right ventricular function: A tissue Doppler and strain rate imaging study. Echocardiography. 2010;**27**(3):236-243

[15] Wong C, Marwick TH. Obesity cardiomyopathy: Pathogenesis and pathophysiology. Nature Clinical Practice. Cardiovascular Medicine. 2007;**4**(8):436-443

[16] Quilliot D et al. Myocardial collagen turnover in normotensive obese patients: Relation to insulin resistance. International Journal of Obesity. 2005;**29**(11):1321-1328

[17] Martinez-Martinez E et al. Galectin-3 participates in cardiovascular remodeling associated with obesity. Hypertension. 2015;**66**(5):961-969

[18] Abel ED, Litwin SE, Sweeney G. Cardiac remodeling in obesity. Physiological Reviews. 2008;**88**(2):389-419

[19] Lumeng CN, Saltiel AR. Inflammatory links between obesity and metabolic disease. The Journal of Clinical Investigation. 2011;**121**(6):2111-2117

[20] Cavalera M, Wang J, Frangogiannis NG. Obesity, metabolic dysfunction, and cardiac fibrosis: Pathophysiological pathways, molecular mechanisms, and therapeutic opportunities. Translational Research. 2014;**164**(4):323-335

[21] Jaisser F, Farman N. Emerging roles of the mineralocorticoid receptor in pathology: Toward new paradigms in clinical pharmacology. Pharmacological Reviews. 2016;**68**(1):49-75

[22] Briet M, Schiffrin EL. Aldosterone: Effects on the kidney and cardiovascular system. Nature Reviews. Nephrology. 2010;**6**(5):261-273

[23] Fiebeler A, Muller DN, Shagdarsuren E, Luft FC. Aldosterone, mineralocorticoid receptors, and vascular inflammation. Current Opinion in Nephrology and Hypertension. 2007;**16**(2):134-142

[24] Pitt B et al. The effect of spironolactone on morbidity and mortality in patients with severe heart failure. Randomized Aldactone Evaluation Study Investigators. New England Journal of Medicine. 1999;**341**(10):709-717

[25] Pitt B et al. Eplerenone, a selective aldosterone blocker, in patients with left ventricular dysfunction after myocardial infarction. The New England Journal of Medicine. 2003;**348**(14):1309-1321

[26] Zannad F et al. Eplerenone in patients with systolic heart failure and mild symptoms. The New England Journal of Medicine. 2011;**364**(1):11-21

[27] Ouvrard-Pascaud A et al. Conditional mineralocorticoid receptor expression in the heart leads to life-threatening arrhythmias. Circulation. 2005;**111**(23):3025-3033

[28] Favre J et al. Coronary endothelial dysfunction after cardiomyocyte-specific mineralocorticoid receptor overexpression. American Journal of Physiology. Heart and Circulatory Physiology. 2011;**300**(6):H2035-H2043

[29] Rickard AJ et al. Cardiomyocyte mineralocorticoid receptors are essential for deoxycorticosterone/salt-mediated inflammation and cardiac fibrosis. Hypertension. 2012;**60**(6):1443-1450

[30] Fraccarollo D et al. Deletion of cardiomyocyte mineralocorticoid receptor ameliorates adverse remodeling after myocardial infarction. Circulation. 2011;**123**(4):400-408

[31] Rickard AJ et al. Endothelial cell mineralocorticoid receptors regulate deoxycorticosterone/salt-mediated cardiac remodeling and vascular reactivity but not blood pressure. Hypertension. 2014;**63**(5):1033-1040

[32] Lother A et al. Deoxycorticosterone acetate/salt-induced cardiac but not renal injury is mediated by endothelial mineralocorticoid receptors independently from blood pressure. Hypertension. 2016;**67**(1):130-138

[33] Rickard AJ et al. Deletion of mineralocorticoid receptors from macrophages protects against deoxycorticosterone/salt-induced cardiac fibrosis and increased blood pressure. Hypertension. 2009;**54**(3):537-543

[34] Gueret A et al. Vascular smooth muscle mineralocorticoid receptor contributes to coronary and left

ventricular dysfunction after myocardial infarction. Hypertension. 2016;**67**(4):717-723

[35] Goodfriend TL, Egan BM, Kelley DE. Plasma aldosterone, plasma lipoproteins, obesity and insulin resistance in humans. Prostaglandins, Leukotrienes, and Essential Fatty Acids. 1999;**60**(5-6):401-405

[36] Harada E et al. Increased urinary aldosterone excretion is associated with subcutaneous not visceral, adipose tissue area in obese individuals: A possible manifestation of dysfunctional subcutaneous adipose tissue. Clinical Endocrinology. 2013;**79**(4):510-516

[37] Silva MA et al. Mineralocorticoid receptor blockade prevents vascular remodelling in a rodent model of type 2 diabetes mellitus. Clinical Science (London, England). 2015;**129**(7):533-545

[38] Calhoun DA, Sharma K. The role of aldosteronism in causing obesity-related cardiovascular risk. Cardiology Clinics. 2010;**28**(3):517-527

[39] Briones AM et al. Adipocytes produce aldosterone through calcineurin-dependent signaling pathways: Implications in diabetes mellitus-associated obesity and vascular dysfunction. Hypertension. 2012;**59**(5):1069-1078

[40] Gutierrez-Tenorio J et al. The role of oxidative stress in the crosstalk between leptin and mineralocorticoid receptor in the cardiac fibrosis associated with obesity. Scientific Reports. 2017;7(1):16802

[41] Xie D, Bollag WB. Obesity, hypertension and aldosterone: Is leptin the link? The Journal of Endocrinology. 2016;**230**(1):F7-F11

[42] Jia G et al. Endothelial mineralocorticoid receptor deletion prevents diet-induced cardiac diastolic dysfunction in females. Hypertension. 2015;**66**(6):1159-1167

[43] Bostick B et al. Mineralocorticoid receptor blockade prevents Western diet-induced diastolic dysfunction in female mice. American Journal of Physiology. Heart and Circulatory Physiology. 2015;**308**(9):H1126-H1135

[44] DeMarco VG et al. Low-dose mineralocorticoid receptor blockade prevents western diet-induced arterial stiffening in female mice. Hypertension. 2015;**66**(1):99-107

[45] Kosmala W, Przewlocka-Kosmala M, Szczepanik-Osadnik H, Mysiak A, Marwick TH. Fibrosis and cardiac function in obesity: A randomised controlled trial of aldosterone blockade. Heart. 2013;**99**(5):320-326

[46] Kosmala W et al. A randomized study of the beneficial effects of aldosterone antagonism on LV function, structure, and fibrosis markers in metabolic syndrome. JACC: Cardiovascular Imaging. 2011;**4**(12):1239-1249

[47] Bender SB et al. Mineralocorticoid receptor antagonism treats obesity-associated cardiac diastolic dysfunction. Hypertension. 2015;**65**(5):1082-1088

[48] Pan WW, Myers MG Jr. Leptin and the maintenance of elevated body weight. Nature Reviews. Neuroscience. 2018;**19**(2):95-105

[49] Rahmouni K. Leptin-induced sympathetic nerve activation: Signaling mechanisms and cardiovascular consequences in obesity. Current Hypertension Reviews. 2010;**6**(2):104-209

[50] Enriori PJ, Evans AE, Sinnayah P, Cowley MA. Leptin resistance and obesity. Obesity (Silver Spring). 2006;**14**(Suppl 5):254S-258S

[51] Wallace AM et al. Plasma leptin and the risk of cardiovascular disease in the west of Scotland coronary prevention study (WOSCOPS). Circulation. 2001;**104**(25):3052-3056

[52] Soderberg S et al. Leptin is associated with increased risk of myocardial infarction. Journal of Internal Medicine. 1999;**246**(4):409-418

[53] Wolk R et al. Plasma leptin and prognosis in patients with established coronary atherosclerosis. Journal of the American College of Cardiology. 2004;**44**(9):1819-1824

[54] Martinez-Martinez E et al. Leptin induces cardiac fibrosis through galectin-3, mTOR and oxidative stress: Potential role in obesity. Journal of Hypertension. 2014;**32**(5):1104-1114, discussion 1114

[55] Sweeney G. Leptin signalling. Cellular Signalling. 2002;**14**(8):655-663

[56] do Carmo JM et al. Neuronal suppressor of cytokine signaling 3: Role in modulating chronic metabolic and cardiovascular effects of leptin. Hypertension. 2018;**71**(6):1248-1257

[57] Abel ED, Sweeney G. Modulation of the cardiovascular system by leptin. Biochimie. 2012;**94**(10):2097-2103

[58] Sweeney G. Cardiovascular effects of leptin. Nature Reviews. Cardiology. 2010;**7**(1):22-29

[59] Chatham JC, Seymour AM. Cardiac carbohydrate metabolism in Zucker diabetic fatty rats. Cardiovascular Research. 2002;**55**(1):104-112

[60] Wende AR, Abel ED. Lipotoxicity in the heart. Biochimica et Biophysica Acta. 2010;**1801**(3):311-319

[61] Barbeau PA et al. Alpha-Linolenic acid and exercise training independently, and additively, decrease blood pressure and prevent diastolic dysfunction in obese Zucker rats. The Journal of Physiology. 2017;**595**(13):4351-4364

[62] Palanivel R, Eguchi M, Shuralyova I, Coe I, Sweeney G. Distinct effects of short- and long-term leptin treatment on glucose and fatty acid uptake and metabolism in HL-1 cardiomyocytes. Metabolism. 2006;**55**(8):1067-1075

[63] Stanley WC, Recchia FA. Lipotoxicity and the development of heart failure: Moving from mouse to man. Cell Metabolism. 2010;**12**(6):555-556

[64] Hall ME, Harmancey R, Stec DE. Lean heart: Role of leptin in cardiac hypertrophy and metabolism. World Journal of Cardiology. 2015;**7**(9):511-524

[65] Abe Y et al. Leptin induces elongation of cardiac myocytes and causes eccentric left ventricular dilatation with compensation. American Journal of Physiology. Heart and Circulatory Physiology. 2007;**292**(5):H2387-H2396

[66] Barouch LA, Berkowitz DE, Harrison RW, O'Donnell CP, Hare JM. Disruption of leptin signaling contributes to cardiac hypertrophy independently of body weight in mice. Circulation. 2003;**108**(6):754-759

[67] Sawyer DB et al. Role of oxidative stress in myocardial hypertrophy and failure. Journal of Molecular and Cellular Cardiology. 2002;**34**(4):379-388

[68] Fortuno A et al. Is leptin involved in phagocytic NADPH oxidase overactivity in obesity? Potential clinical implications. Journal of Hypertension. 2010;**28**(9):1944-1950

[69] Bouloumie A, Marumo T, Lafontan M, Busse R. Leptin induces oxidative stress in human endothelial cells. The FASEB Journal. 1999;**13**(10):1231-1238

[70] Martinez-Martinez E et al. The potential role of leptin in the vascular remodeling associated with obesity. International Journal of Obesity. 2014;**38**(12):1565-1572

[71] Zibadi S, Cordova F, Slack EH, Watson RR, Larson DF. Leptin's regulation of obesity-induced cardiac extracellular matrix remodeling. Cardiovascular Toxicology. 2011;**11**(4):325-333

[72] Khaidar A, Marx M, Lubec B, Lubec G. L-arginine reduces heart collagen accumulation in the diabetic db/db mouse. Circulation. 1994;**90**(1):479-483

[73] Fredersdorf S et al. Myocardial hypertrophy and enhanced left ventricular contractility in Zucker diabetic fatty rats. Cardiovascular Pathology. 2004;**13**(1):11-19

[74] Aroor AR et al. Dipeptidyl peptidase-4 (DPP-4) inhibition with linagliptin reduces western diet-induced myocardial TRAF3IP2 expression, inflammation and fibrosis in female mice. Cardiovascular Diabetology. 2017;**16**(1):61

[75] Wang X et al. Pharmacogenomic, physiological, and biochemical investigations on safety and efficacy biomarkers associated with the peroxisome proliferator-activated receptor-gamma activator rosiglitazone in rodents: A translational medicine investigation. The Journal of Pharmacology and Experimental Therapeutics. 2010;**334**(3):820-829

[76] Takahashi K et al. Roles of oxidative stress and the mineralocorticoid receptor in cardiac pathology in a rat model of metabolic syndrome. Nagoya Journal of Medical Science. 2015;**77**(1-2):275-289

[77] Martinez-Martinez E et al. The lysyl oxidase inhibitor (beta-aminopropionitrile) reduces leptin profibrotic effects and ameliorates cardiovascular remodeling in diet-induced obesity in rats. Journal of Molecular and Cellular Cardiology. 2016;**92**:96-104

[78] Rodriguez C et al. Regulation of lysyl oxidase in vascular cells: Lysyl oxidase as a new player in cardiovascular diseases. Cardiovascular Research. 2008;**79**(1):7-13

[79] Li H et al. Inflammatory biomarkers of coronary heart disease. Frontiers in Bioscience (Scholar Edition). 2018;**10**:185-196

[80] Martin SS, Qasim A, Reilly MP. Leptin resistance: A possible interface of inflammation and metabolism in obesity-related cardiovascular disease. Journal of the American College of Cardiology. 2008;**52**(15):1201-1210

[81] Yamagishi SI et al. Leptin induces mitochondrial superoxide production and monocyte chemoattractant protein-1 expression in aortic endothelial cells by increasing fatty acid oxidation via protein kinase a. The Journal of Biological Chemistry. 2001;**276**(27):25096-25100

[82] O'Rourke L, Gronning LM, Yeaman SJ, Shepherd PR. Glucose-dependent regulation of cholesterol ester metabolism in macrophages by insulin and leptin. The Journal of Biological Chemistry. 2002;**277**(45):42557-42562

[83] Lam QL, Lu L. Role of leptin in immunity. Cellular & Molecular Immunology. 2007;**4**(1):1-13

[84] Faulkner JL, Bruder-Nascimento T, Belin de Chantemele EJ. The regulation of aldosterone secretion by leptin: Implications in obesity-related cardiovascular disease. Current Opinion in Nephrology and Hypertension. 2018;**27**(2):63-69

[85] Vatutin NT, Shevelok AN. Relationship between blood aldosterone

and somatometric parameters in patients with chronic heart failure and preserved ejection fraction of left ventricle. Klinicheskaia Meditsina. 2016;**94**(4):265-269

[86] Olivier A et al. Effect of eplerenone in patients with heart failure and reduced ejection fraction: Potential effect modification by abdominal obesity. Insight from the EMPHASIS-HF trial. European Journal of Heart Failure. 2017;**19**(9):1186-1197

[87] Beltowski J. Leptin and the regulation of renal sodium handling and renal Na-transporting ATPases: Role in the pathogenesis of arterial hypertension. Current Cardiology Reviews. 2010;**6**(1):31-40

[88] Hall JE, do Carmo JM, da Silva AA, Wang Z, Hall ME. Obesity-induced hypertension: Interaction of neurohumoral and renal mechanisms. Circulation Research. 2015;**116**(6):991-1006

[89] Hall JE, Hildebrandt DA, Kuo J. Obesity hypertension: Role of leptin and sympathetic nervous system. American Journal of Hypertension. 2001;**14** (6 Pt 2):103S-115S

[90] Huby AC et al. Adipocyte-derived hormone leptin is a direct regulator of aldosterone secretion, which promotes endothelial dysfunction and cardiac fibrosis. Circulation. 2015;**132**(22):2134-2145

[91] Xue B et al. Leptin mediates high-fat diet sensitization of angiotensin II-elicited hypertension by upregulating the brain renin-angiotensin system and inflammation. Hypertension. 2016;**67**(5):970-976

[92] Natarajan R, Ploszaj S, Horton R, Nadler J. Tumor necrosis factor and interleukin-1 are potent inhibitors of angiotensin-II-induced aldosterone synthesis. Endocrinology. 1989;**125**(6):3084-3089

[93] Belin de Chantemele EJ, Mintz JD, Rainey WE, Stepp DW. Impact of leptin-mediated sympatho-activation on cardiovascular function in obese mice. Hypertension. 2011;**58**(2):271-279

[94] Huby AC, Otvos L Jr, Belin de Chantemele EJ. Leptin induces hypertension and endothelial dysfunction via aldosterone-dependent mechanisms in obese female mice. Hypertension. 2016;**67**(5):1020-1028

[95] Hofmann A et al. Elevated steroid hormone production in the db/db mouse model of obesity and type 2 diabetes. Hormone and Metabolic Research. 2017;**49**(1):43-49

Chapter 3

# Aldosterone/Mineralocorticoid Receptor Downstream Targets as Novel Therapeutic Targets to Prevent Cardiovascular Remodeling

*Jaime Ibarrola, Frederic Jaisser and Natalia López-Andrés*

## Abstract

The incidence of heart failure (HF) is increasing because of aging of the population. Despite optimal therapy, patients with HF experience disease progression associated with high mortality rates. HF is still the first cause of hospital admission in subjects aged >65 years. The obvious solution for HF epidemics is to prevent new-onset HF with therapies directed specifically to mechanistic targets that are involved in the transition to HF. The mineralocorticoid receptor (MR) and its natural ligand, the hormone aldosterone (Aldo), play important roles during cardiac and arterial remodeling, but the underlying effects are still not understood. MR antagonists are highly recommended for treatment of systolic symptomatic HF. However, adverse effects limit their use in clinical practice. Galectin-3 (Gal-3), neutrophil gelatinase-associated lipocalin (NGAL), and cardiotrophin-1 (CT-1) have been identified as highly focused targets controlling downstream key MR-mediated HF mechanisms. Therefore, interfering with mechanistic pathways involved in downstream MR activation may provide therapeutic alternatives to MR antagonists. The aim of this review is to focus on the role of the MR biotargets in cardiovascular remodeling.

**Keywords:** biotarget, galectin-3, neutrophil gelatinase-associated lipocalin, cardiotrophin-1

## 1. Introduction

Inappropriate mineralocorticoid signaling has been shown to play an important role in the progression of cardiovascular disease. Aldosterone (Aldo) is a main regulator of renal sodium reabsorption with an overall effect on volemia and blood pressure. Aldo binds to the mineralocorticoid receptor (MR), which works as a transcription factor of the nuclear receptor family present in the kidney and also in various other non-epithelial cells including the heart and the vasculature [1]. Indeed, new extrarenal pathophysiological effects of this hormone have been characterized, extending its actions to the cardiovascular system [2]. A growing body of clinical and preclinical evidence suggests that Aldo and MR play an important pathophysiological role in cardiovascular remodeling by promoting changes involving cardiac hypertrophy, fibrosis, arterial stiffness, as well as in inflammation and oxidative stress [3]. In line with these findings, inappropriate MR activation has been shown to promote cardiovascular remodeling in experimental models [4]. The RALES, EPHESUS, and the EMPHASIS-HF clinical trials demonstrated that the addition of MR antagonists (MRAs) to standard care markedly reduced the overall and cardiovascular mortality in patients with systolic heart failure (HF) [5–7]. The beneficial effects were mainly associated with a reduction of cardiovascular fibrosis, as assessed by circulating biomarkers of cardiovascular extracellular matrix [8]. Moreover, results of the recently completed REMINDER (impact of eplerenone on CV outcomes in patients post myocardial infarction, clinical trial number NCT01176968) trial and TOPCAT (NCT00094302) trial suggest that MR blockade might be clinically beneficial, respectively, for acute myocardial infarction healing and progression of HF with preserved ejection fraction.

The molecular targets involved in the remodeling processes modulated by Aldo/MR activation in the cardiovascular system need to be more precisely analyzed. Inflammatory processes are tightly linked with fibrosis during cardiovascular remodeling. In addition to profibrotic targets, there is evidence that Aldo/MR may trigger inflammatory processes negatively impacting on cardiovascular remodeling processes. Thus, MR activation and inhibition modulate the expression of several pro-inflammatory molecules that may contribute to the pathogenesis of cardiovascular remodeling: Aldo/MR activation increases monocyte chemoattractant protein-1 (CCL-2), transforming growth factor-β1 (TGF-β1), connective tissue growth factor (CTGF), plasminogen activator inhibitor type-1 (PAI-1), as well as collagen and metalloproteases through MR-dependent mechanisms. The identification of the Aldo/MR-modulated targets in cardiovascular remodeling associated with HF development is actually a medical need. Their inhibition could add therapeutic benefits in patients at high risk for the development of HF and cardiovascular remodeling. In the last years, new candidates to be Aldo/MR biotargets emerged in preclinical and clinical studies, such as galectin-3 (Gal-3), neutrophil gelatinase-associated lipocalin (NGAL), and cardiotrophin-1 (CT-1) (**Figure 1**).

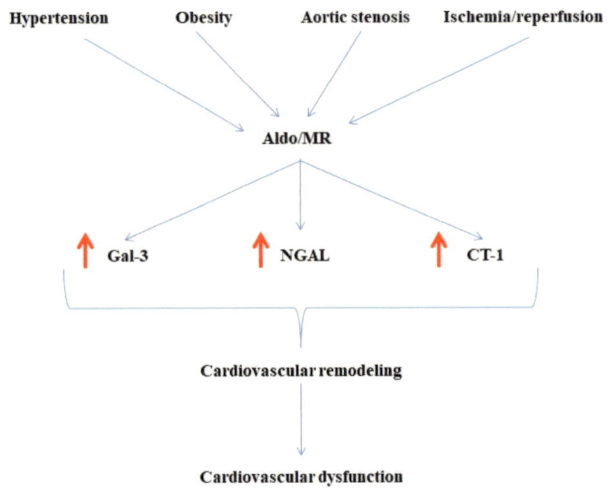


**Figure 1.**
*Aldo/MR biotargets Gal-3, NGAL, and CT-1 contribute to cardiovascular remodeling and dysfunction in various pathological and clinical conditions.*

## 2. Galectin-3

### 2.1 Galectin-3 induces fibrosis, inflammation, and oxidative stress

Galectin-3 (Gal-3) is a 29–35 kDa protein, member of a β-galactoside-binding lectin family, localized in the nucleus, cytoplasm, cell surface, and extracellular space [9]. It is composed of a highly conserved N-terminal domain and a C-terminal carbohydrate recognition domain, which interacts with glycoproteins [10]. The damaging effects of Gal-3 have been associated with its capacity to bind matrix proteins such as cell surface receptors (integrins), collagen, elastin, or fibronectin [11]. The expression of this lectin has been reported in many tissues, including the heart, vessels, and kidney [12]. Moreover, Gal-3 is expressed in many cell types of the cardiovascular system such as cardiac fibroblasts [13], vascular smooth muscle cells [14], endothelial cells [15], and inflammatory cells [16]. Gal-3 is involved in numerous physiological and pathological processes, some of which, inflammation and fibrosis, are pivotal contributing to pathophysiological mechanisms in the development and progression of HF. Indeed, it has been demonstrated in cell culture that Gal-3 turns quiescent fibroblasts into myofibroblasts that produce and secrete matrix proteins, including collagens [13, 17]. Gal-3 exerts its effects during several other stages of fibrogenesis besides collagen production, such as collagen maturation, externalization, and cross-linking, which underscores the pivotal importance of Gal-3 in cardiovascular fibrosis. Moreover, Gal-3 has emerged as a potential mediator of cardiac damage in different pathological situations through its ability to stimulate key pro-inflammatory molecules [16]. Thus, it has been demonstrated that in human cardiac fibroblasts, Gal-3 enhances the production and the secretion of pro-inflammatory and profibrotic mediators such as interleukin (IL)-1β, IL-6, CCL-2, collagen type I, collagen type III, and fibronectin as well as the activity of MMP-1, MMP-2, and MMP-9 [18]. The in vitro findings have been corroborated by animal studies. Thus, Gal-3 administration induces cardiac fibrosis leading to cardiac dysfunction in rats [13]. Additionally, a new line of evidence points out that Gal-3 is involved in reactive oxygen species (ROS) production, although the mechanisms have not been elucidated. Gal-3 increases the expression of Nox4 in cardiac cells and could regulate Nox4-derived ROS levels during cardiac fibrosis [19]. Moreover, Gal-3 downregulates peroxiredoxin-4 inducing a decrease in total antioxidant capacity and a consequent increase in peroxide production and in oxidative stress markers in cardiac fibroblasts [20]. Additionally, Gal-3 downregulates the protective fumarate hydratase increasing fumarate production in human cardiac fibroblasts, leading to increased ROS levels and increased collagen production [21].

### 2.2 Galectin-3 as a mediator of Aldo/MR activation

Preclinical studies have demonstrated that Gal-3 is a key mediator of cardiovascular and renal fibrosis and dysfunction in pathological conditions associated with high Aldo levels [14, 18, 22–24]. In addition, hyperaldosteronism worsens hypertension-induced cardiovascular fibrosis through an increase of Gal-3 [25]. A summary of Gal-3 mediating Aldo/MR effects is shown in **Figure 2**.

#### *2.2.1 Aldosterone/MR regulates galectin-3 expression in vitro*

In vitro, in primary cultured vascular smooth muscle cells (VSMCs), Calvier and co-workers described that Aldo increases Gal-3 expression in a dose- and

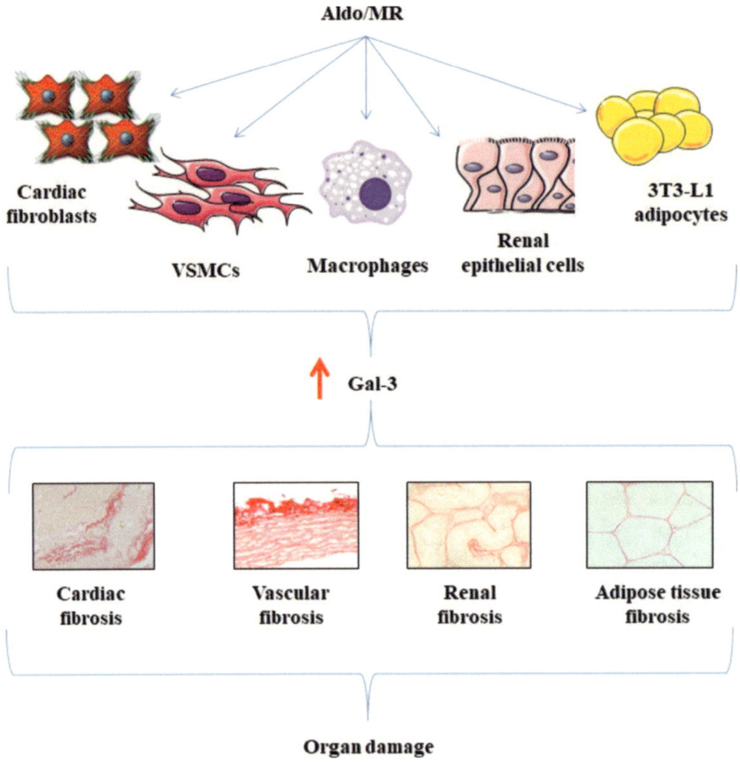


**Figure 2.**
*Gal-3 as a mediator of Aldo/MR effects on fibrosis in several cells and tissues.*

time-dependent manner via its MR [14]. Gal-3, via its lectin activity, is a necessary mediator allowing Aldo-induced collagen type I synthesis, because the blockade of Gal-3 with carbohydrates such as modified citrus pectin (MCP, a complex water-soluble indigestible polysaccharide rich in β-galactose) or N-Acetyl-D-lactosamine abolishes Aldo-induced collagen type I deposition. In confirmation of the pharmacological data, Gal-3-depleted VSMCs are resistant to Aldo profibrotic effects, especially collagen type I deposition [14].

In human cardiac fibroblasts, Aldo also increased Gal-3 expression via its MR, and Gal-3 and Aldo enhance pro-inflammatory and profibrotic markers, as well as metalloproteinase activities, those effects being not observed in Gal-3-silenced cells treated with Aldo [18].

In line with these observations, it has been described that Aldo induces Gal-3 secretion in inflammatory cells (macrophage cell lines THP-1 and RAW 264.7 cells) through MR and via PI3K/Akt and NF-kB transcription signaling pathways [26], amplifying the inflammatory response.

Finally, unpublished data from our group confirmed Gal-3 induction by Aldo via MR in other cell types such and renal cells and 3T3-L1 adipocytes.

### *2.2.2 Beneficial effects of galectin-3 blockade in experimental models with high aldosterone*

In vivo, it has been shown that rats treated with Aldo-salt for 3 weeks present hypertension and display vascular hypertrophy, inflammation, fibrosis, and increased aortic Gal-3 expression. Spironolactone or MCP treatment reverses all the above effects. Interestingly, MCP also blunts Aldo-induced hypertension. In wild-type (WT) and Gal-3 knockout (KO) mice treated with Aldo for 6 hours or 3 weeks—a normotensive model—Aldo increases aortic Gal-3 expression, inflammation, and collagen type I in WT mice at both the short- and the long-term, whereas no changes occur in Gal-3 KO mice. Altogether, these data show that Gal-3 is required for the inflammatory and fibrotic responses to Aldo in VSMCs in vivo, suggesting a key role for Gal-3 in vascular fibrosis [14]. While using the same experimental models, downstream in vitro experiments in human cardiac fibroblasts and the influence of Gal-3 on Aldo-mediated cardiac and renal effects have been also explored. Hypertensive Aldo-salt-treated rats present cardiac and renal hypertrophy (at morphometric, cellular, and molecular levels) and dysfunction. Cardiac and renal expressions of Gal-3 as well as levels of molecular markers attesting fibrosis are also augmented by Aldo-salt treatment. Spironolactone or MCP treatment reverses all of these effects. In WT mice, Aldo does not alter blood pressure levels but increases cardiac and renal Gal-3 expression, fibrosis, and renal epithelial-mesenchymal transition (i.e., renal epithelial cells differentiate onto extracellular matrix secreting and profibrotic myofibroblasts). Gal-3 KO mice are resistant to Aldo-induced deleterious cardiorenal effects [22].

Aldo levels are increased in spontaneously hypertensive rats (SHR) [27], as well as in hypertensive patients [28], being considered as an inducer of hypertensive organ damage [29]. MR activation and high salt intake cause hypertension as well as inflammation, leading to cardiac inflammation and fibrosis [30]. Gal-3 levels, as well as cardiorenal inflammation and fibrosis, are also increased in the myocardium and kidney from SHR as compared to normotensive controls. Gal-3 pharmacological inhibition using MCP exerts beneficial effects, diminishing cardiorenal inflammation and fibrosis in the absence of blood pressure modifications [18, 23, 31].

Obesity is frequently associated with increased Aldo concentrations in humans [32] and is considered as HF stage A [33]. Obesity upregulates Gal-3 production in the cardiovascular and in the renal system in a normotensive animal model of diet-induced obesity by feeding for 6 weeks a high-fat diet, while Gal-3 inhibition with MCP reduces cardiovascular and renal levels of Gal-3, fibrosis, and inflammation in obese animals without changes in body weight or blood pressure [34]. In adipose tissue, obese male Wistar rats fed with a high-fat diet for 6 weeks present an increase in Gal-3 levels that are accompanied by an increase in pericellular collagen. Obese rats exhibit higher adipose tissue inflammation, as well as enhanced differentiation degree of the adipocytes. Treatment with MCP prevents all the above effects [24]. In summary, Gal-3 emerges as a potential therapeutic target in adipose tissue remodeling associated with obesity—a condition associated with hyperaldosteronemia—and could have an important role in the development of metabolic, cardiovascular, and renal alterations associated with obesity.

In theory, MR activation can promote aortic sclerosis and aortic stenosis (AS), due to its effect on inflammation and fibrosis. Once aortic valve disease has been established, the pressure or volume overload may induce left ventricular dysfunction. In a normotensive animal model of pressure overload (AS), cardiac, vascular, and renal Gal-3 is augmented, and its pharmacological inhibition with MCP prevents cardiovascular and renal functional alterations as well as cardiovascular and renal fibrosis and inflammation [21, 34, 35].

The acute administration of MRAs, either before the onset of ischemia or at the moment of reperfusion, profoundly reduces infarct size (reviewed in [36]). In an animal model of ischemia–reperfusion, cardiac Gal-3 is augmented, and its pharmacological inhibition with MCP prevented cardiac functional, histological, and molecular alterations (unpublished data from our group).

*2.2.3 Aldosterone-galectin-3 in clinical populations*

As mentioned above, Aldo increases Gal-3 expression in the cardiovascular and renal system as well as in adipose tissue in experimental models.

In a cohort of patients with Aldo-producing adenoma, the authors demonstrated that Gal-3 levels are enhanced. Interestingly, 1 year after adrenalectomy, plasma Gal-3 levels decrease, reinforcing the relation of Aldo-Gal-3 and confirming the results obtained using preclinical models [26]. In contrast with these observations, another group recently described that Gal-3 levels are not increased in patients with primary hyperaldosteronism (as compared to hypertensive patients) and levels do not decrease after adrenalectomy [37].

In untreated congestive HF, Aldo plasma concentrations are elevated in proportion to the severity of the disease and are further increased by the use of diuretic treatment [38]. Interestingly, the serum Gal-3 level has been correlated with serum markers of cardiac extracellular matrix turnover in HF patients, and, therefore, Gal-3 emerges as a biomarker associated with HF onset, morbidity, and mortality [39].

In morbidly obese patients presenting high Aldo levels, insulin resistance, and left ventricular hypertrophy, high Gal-3 levels are associated with a worsening of diastolic function [23]. Moreover, in patients with AS, cardiac Gal-3 is increased and associates with markers of myocardial fibrosis and inflammation [35]. Interestingly, both Aldo and Gal-3 are increased in pulmonary arterial hypertension patients. The axis Aldo/Gal-3 is relevant in pulmonary arterial hypertension because plasma levels of both molecules are associated with pulmonary arterial hypertension severity [40]. Furthermore, Gal-3 positively correlated with Nox4 (related to oxidative stress production) in pulmonary arterial hypertension patients [41].

Given the intimate relation between Aldo, Gal-3, and cardiovascular fibrosis, the predictive value of Gal-3 in patients treated with MRAs has been analyzed. In a cohort of HF patients, MRA treatment does not alter the prognostic value of Gal-3 [42]. An analysis examining the interaction between baseline Gal-3 levels and MRA therapy on outcomes shows no difference in patients who were receiving MRA [43]. Moreover, among patients with chronic HF and elevated Gal-3 concentrations, there is no specific benefit from addition or intensification of MRA therapy [44].

## 3. NGAL

### 3.1 NGAL induces fibrosis and inflammation

NGAL, also known as lipocalin-2, 24p3, siderocalin, or uterocalin, is a small glycoprotein of 25 kDa member of the lipocalin family. NGAL is expressed by different cell types including renal, endothelial, VSMCs, macrophages, dendritic cells, cardiomyocytes or cardiac fibroblasts (reviewed in [45]).

NGAL is involved in a wide variety of pathological situations as cardiovascular and renal diseases. Indeed, it has been demonstrated in cell culture that NGAL enhances the production and the secretion of pro-inflammatory and profibrotic mediators such as interleukin (IL)-1β, IL-6, CCL-2, osteopontin, collagen type I, and collagen type III in human cardiac fibroblasts [46, 47]. NGAL also increases collagen type I production as well as CT-1 and Gal-3 expression and secretion in VSMCs [48]. In cardiac cells, NGAL can also activate the inflammatory pathway NF-kB [47]. Moreover, NGAL treatment induces migration of neutrophils [49], and NGAL KO mice have been shown to present reduced chemotaxis and adhesion

[50]. Moreover, NGAL KO mice subjected to ischemia/reperfusion do not present immune cell recruitment [51].

### 3.2 NGAL as a mediator of Aldo/MR activation

In vitro, in HL-1 cardiomyocytes, Aldo induces NGAL expression via its MR [52]. These results have been also expanded to other cell types such as cardiac fibroblasts, where Aldo also enhances NGAL expression [47].

Preclinical studies have demonstrated that NGAL is a key mediator of cardiovascular and renal fibrosis, inflammation, and dysfunction in pathological conditions associated with high Aldo levels. Firstly, NGAL has been found to be increased in mice overexpressing MR in cardiomyocytes [52]. Moreover, NGAL KO mice have been found to be resistant to Aldo-salt-induced hypertension and vascular fibrosis [48]. Interestingly, NGAL KO mice subjected to myocardial infarction show lower cardiac fibrosis and inflammation as well as improved cardiac function [47]. Recently it has been described using mice depleted for NGAL in their immune cells by bone marrow transplantation that NGAL from immune cells is mandatory for Aldo-induced cardiac fibrosis and inflammation [53].

In hypertensive patients, NGAL plasma concentrations are elevated and correlate with blood pressure levels [54]. NGAL serum levels are also increased in myocardial infarction patients and in HF patients [55, 56], as well as in obese patients [57]. Importantly, the rise of the complex NGAL/MMP-9 in obese subjects (stage A HF) and its association with plasma Aldo levels suggest that NGAL may serve as a biomarker of MR activation [48].

## 4. Cardiotrophin-1

### 4.1 Cardiotrophin-1 induces fibrosis and inflammation

CT-1 is a member of the interleukin-6 superfamily, which is expressed in different tissues including the heart, vessels, skeletal muscle, liver, lung, adipose tissue, and kidney [58, 59]. In the myocardium, CT-1 is produced by both cardiomyocytes and fibroblasts, exerting its action through the glycoprotein 130 (gp130)/leukemia inhibitory factor receptor (LIFR) heterodimer. Whereas CT-1 was initially described as a stress-response factor promoting cardiomyocyte survival [60], chronic exposure to this cytokine induces cardiomyocyte hypertrophy and dysfunction [61, 62]. In addition, experimental in vitro findings in rodent and canine fibroblasts [63–66] as well as in VSMCs [67] suggest that CT-1 behaves also as a profibrotic factor. In particular, CT-1 induces fibroblast growth and proliferation and collagen production. Moreover, in human cardiac fibroblasts, CT-1 has been shown to stimulate myofibroblast differentiation and collagen type I and III production [68]. Coherently, rats chronically exposed to CT-1 present increased fibrosis in the cardiovascular and in the renal system characterized by increased collagen deposition [62]. Finally, data in chronic HF patients indicate that an association exists between CT-1 and collagen type I and III production in the myocardium [68].

### 4.2 Cardiotrophin-1 as a mediator of Aldo/MR activation

In vitro, in HL-1 cardiomyocytes, Aldo induces CT-1 in a dose- and time-dependent manner via its MR and through the activation of p38MAPK signaling pathway [69]. Moreover, Aldo also enhances CT-1 expression in VSMCs [67]. Interestingly, CT-1 blockade with specific antibodies avoids Aldo-induced hypertrophy of cardiomyocytes. According to the in vitro data, CT-1-null mice subjected to acute Aldo treatment are resistant to Aldo-induced expression of hypertrophic markers [69]. These results were confirmed in other studies demonstrating that in experimental hyperaldosteronism, the increase of cardiac CT-1 expression is associated with parameters showing left ventricular hypertrophy and fibrosis. Moreover, CT-1-null mice are resistant to Aldo-induced left ventricular hypertrophy and fibrosis [70].

CT-1 expression has been found to be increased in the myocardium of HF patients of different etiologies [68, 71]. Importantly, and according to the results obtained in experimental models, in HF patients high Aldo levels are associated with high CT-1 levels [72].

## Acknowledgements

This publication is based upon work from the EU COST Action ADMIRE BM1301 in Aldosterone and Mineralocorticoid Receptor Physiology and Pathophysiology (www.admirecosteu.com).

## Author details

Jaime Ibarrola[1], Frederic Jaisser[2] and Natalia López-Andrés[1]*

1 Cardiovascular Translational Research, Navarrabiomed, Complejo Hospitalario de Navarra (CHN), Universidad Pública de Navarra (UPNA), IdiSNA, Pamplona, Spain

2 INSERM UMRS 1138 Team 1, Centre de Recherche des Cordeliers, University Pierre and Marie Curie, Paris, France

*Address all correspondence to: natalia.lopez.andres@navarra.es

## References

[1] Viengchareun S, Le Menuet D, Martinerie L, Munier M, Pascual-Le Tallec L, Lombès M. The mineralocorticoid receptor: Insights into its molecular and (patho)physiological biology. Nuclear Receptor Signaling. 2007;**5**:e012. Available from: https://www.nursa.org/NRS/nrs05012.pdf

[2] Messaoudi S, Azibani F, Delcayre C, Jaisser F. Aldosterone, mineralocorticoid receptor, and heart failure. Molecular and Cellular Endocrinology. 2012;**350**(2):266-272. Available from: http://www.ncbi.nlm.nih.gov/pubmed/21784127

[3] Bauersachs J, Jaisser F, Toto R. Mineralocorticoid receptor activation and mineralocorticoid receptor antagonist treatment in cardiac and renal diseases. Hypertension. 2015;**65**(2):257-263. Available from: http://www.ncbi.nlm.nih.gov/pubmed/25368026

[4] Brilla CG. Aldosterone and myocardial fibrosis in heart failure. Herz. 2000;**25**(3):299-306. Available from: http://www.ncbi.nlm.nih.gov/pubmed/10904856

[5] Pitt B, Remme W, Zannad F, Neaton J, Martinez F, Roniker B, et al. Eplerenone, a selective aldosterone blocker, in patients with left ventricular dysfunction after myocardial infarction. The New England Journal of Medicine. 2003;**348**(14):1309-1321. Available from: http://www.nejm.org/doi/abs/10.1056/NEJMoa030207

[6] Pitt B, Zannad F, Remme WJ, Cody R, Castaigne A, Perez A, et al. The effect of spironolactone on morbidity and mortality in patients with severe heart failure. Randomized Aldactone evaluation study investigators. The New England Journal of Medicine. 1999;**341**(10):709-717. Available from: http://www.nejm.org/doi/abs/10.1056/NEJM199909023411001

[7] Zannad F, McMurray JJV, Krum H, van Veldhuisen DJ, Swedberg K, Shi H, et al. Eplerenone in patients with systolic heart failure and mild symptoms. The New England Journal of Medicine. 2011;**364**(1):11-21. Available from: http://www.ncbi.nlm.nih.gov/pubmed/21073363

[8] Zannad F, Alla F, Dousset B, Perez A, Pitt B. Limitation of excessive extracellular matrix turnover may contribute to survival benefit of spironolactone therapy in patients with congestive heart failure: Insights from the randomized aldactone evaluation study (RALES) . Rales investigators. Circulation. 2000;**102**(22):2700-2706. Available from: http://www.ncbi.nlm.nih.gov/pubmed/11094035

[9] Dumic J, Dabelic S, Flögel M. Galectin-3: An open-ended story. Biochimica et Biophysica Acta. 2006;**1760**(4):616-635. Available from: http://linkinghub.elsevier.com/retrieve/pii/S0304416505004083

[10] Dennis JW, Pawling J, Cheung P, Partridge E, Demetriou M. UDP-N-acetylglucosamine:alpha-6-D-mannoside beta1,6 N-acetylglucosaminyltransferase V (Mgat5) deficient mice. Biochimica et Biophysica Acta. 2002;**1573**(3):414-422. Available from: http://www.ncbi.nlm.nih.gov/pubmed/12417426

[11] Ochieng J, Furtak V, Lukyanov P. Extracellular functions of galectin-3. Glycoconjugate Journal. 2002;**19** (7-9):527-535. Available from: http://www.ncbi.nlm.nih.gov/pubmed/14758076

[12] Kim H, Lee J, Hyun JW, Park JW, Joo H, Shin T. Expression and immunohistochemical localization of

galectin-3 in various mouse tissues. Cell Biology International. 2007;**31**(7): 655-662. Available from: http://doi.wiley.com/10.1016/j.cellbi.2006.11.036

[13] Sharma UC, Pokharel S, van Brakel TJ, van Berlo JH, Cleutjens JPM, Schroen B, et al. Galectin-3 marks activated macrophages in failure-prone hypertrophied hearts and contributes to cardiac dysfunction. Circulation. 2004;**110**(19):3121-3128. Available from: http://www.ncbi.nlm.nih.gov/pubmed/15520318

[14] Calvier L, Miana M, Reboul P, Cachofeiro V, Martinez-Martinez E, de Boer RA, et al. Galectin-3 mediates aldosterone-induced vascular fibrosis. Arteriosclerosis, Thrombosis, and Vascular Biology. 2013;**33**(1): 67-75. Available from: http://atvb.ahajournals.org/cgi/doi/10.1161/ATVBAHA.112.300569

[15] Wan SY, Zhang TF, Ding Y. Galectin-3 enhances proliferation and angiogenesis of endothelial cells differentiated from bone marrow mesenchymal stem cells. Transplantation Proceedings. 2011;**43**(10):3933-3938. Available from: http://linkinghub.elsevier.com/retrieve/pii/S0041134511015272

[16] Papaspyridonos M, McNeill E, de Bono JP, Smith A, Burnand KG, Channon KM, et al. Galectin-3 is an amplifier of inflammation in atherosclerotic plaque progression through macrophage activation and monocyte chemoattraction. Arteriosclerosis, Thrombosis, and Vascular Biology. 2008;**28**(3):433-440. Available from: http://atvb.ahajournals.org/cgi/doi/10.1161/ATVBAHA.107.159160

[17] Yu L, Ruifrok WPT, Meissner M, Bos EM, van Goor H, Sanjabi B, et al. Genetic and pharmacological inhibition of galectin-3 prevents cardiac remodeling by interfering with myocardial fibrogenesis. Circulation. Heart Failure. 2013;**6**(1):107-117. Available from: http://circheartfailure.ahajournals.org/cgi/doi/10.1161/CIRCHEARTFAILURE.112.971168

[18] Martínez-Martínez E, Calvier L, Fernández-Celis A, Rousseau E, Jurado-López R, Rossoni LV, et al. Galectin-3 blockade inhibits cardiac inflammation and fibrosis in experimental Hyperaldosteronism and hypertension novelty and significance. Hypertension. 2015;**66**(4):767-775. Available from: http://www.ncbi.nlm.nih.gov/pubmed/26238446

[19] He J, Li X, Luo H, Li T, Zhao L, Qi Q, et al. Galectin-3 mediates the pulmonary arterial hypertension-induced right ventricular remodeling through interacting with NADPH oxidase 4. Journal of the American Society of Hypertension. 2017;**11**(5):275-289.e2. Available from: http://linkinghub.elsevier.com/retrieve/pii/S1933171117300980

[20] Ibarrola J, Arrieta V, Sádaba R, Martinez-Martinez E, Garcia-Peña A, Alvarez V, et al. Galectin-3 down-regulates antioxidant peroxiredoxin-4 in human cardiac fibroblasts: A new pathway to induce cardiac damage. Clinical Science (London, England). 2018;**132**(13):1471-1485. Available from: http://clinsci.org/lookup/doi/10.1042/CS20171389

[21] Ibarrola J, Martínez-Martínez E, Sádaba J, Arrieta V, García-Peña A, Álvarez V, et al. Beneficial effects of Galectin-3 blockade in vascular and aortic valve alterations in an experimental pressure overload model. International Journal of Molecular Sciences. 2017;**18**(8):1664. Available from: http://www.ncbi.nlm.nih.gov/pubmed/28758988

[22] Calvier L, Martinez-Martinez E, Miana M, Cachofeiro V, Rousseau E, Sádaba JR, et al. The impact of galectin-3 inhibition on

aldosterone-induced cardiac and renal injuries. JACC: Heart Failure. 2015;**3**(1):59-67. Available from: http://linkinghub.elsevier.com/retrieve/pii/S2213177914003886

[23] Martínez-Martínez E, López-Ándres N, Jurado-López R, Rousseau E, Bartolomé MV, Fernández-Celis A, et al. Galectin-3 participates in cardiovascular Remodeling associated with ObesityNovelty and significance. Hypertension. 2015;**66**(5):961-969. Available from: http://www.ncbi.nlm.nih.gov/pubmed/26351031

[24] Martínez-Martínez E, Calvier L, Rossignol P, Rousseau E, Fernández-Celis A, Jurado-López R, et al. Galectin-3 inhibition prevents adipose tissue remodelling in obesity. International Journal of Obesity. 2016;**40**(6):1034-1038. Available from: http://www.nature.com/doifinder/10.1038/ijo.2016.19

[25] Azibani F, Benard L, Schlossarek S, Merval R, Tournoux F, Fazal L, et al. Aldosterone inhibits antifibrotic factors in mouse hypertensive heart. Hypertension (Dallas, Texas 1979). 2012;**59**(6):1179-1187. Available from: http://hyper.ahajournals.org/cgi/doi/10.1161/HYPERTENSIONAHA.111.190512

[26] Lin Y-H, Chou C-H, Wu X-M, Chang Y-Y, Hung C-S, Chen Y-H, et al. Aldosterone induced galectin-3 secretion in vitro and in vivo: From cells to humans. Syn W-K, editor. PLoS One. 2014;**9**(9):e95254. Available from: http://dx.plos.org/10.1371/journal.pone.0095254

[27] Sowers J, Tuck M, Asp ND, Sollars E. Plasma aldosterone and corticosterone responses to adrenocorticotropin, angiotensin, potassium, and stress in spontaneously hypertensive rats. Endocrinology. 1981;**108**(4):1216-1221. Available from: https://academic.oup.com/endo/article-lookup/doi/10.1210/endo-108-4-1216

[28] Tsybouleva N, Zhang L, Chen S, Patel R, Lutucuta S, Nemoto S, et al. Aldosterone, through novel signaling proteins, is a fundamental molecular bridge between the genetic defect and the cardiac phenotype of hypertrophic cardiomyopathy. Circulation. 2004;**109**(10):1284-1291. Available from: http://circ.ahajournals.org/cgi/doi/10.1161/01.CIR.0000121426.43044.2B

[29] Zia AA, Kamalov G, Newman KP, McGee JE, Bhattacharya SK, Ahokas RA, et al. From aldosteronism to oxidative stress: The role of excessive intracellular calcium accumulation. Hypertension Research. 2010;**33**(11):1091-1101. Available from: http://www.nature.com/articles/hr2010159

[30] Amador CA, Barrientos V, Peña J, Herrada AA, González M, Valdés S, et al. Spironolactone decreases DOCA-salt-induced organ damage by blocking the activation of T helper 17 and the downregulation of regulatory T lymphocytes. Hypertension (Dallas, Texas 1979). 2014;**63**(4):797-803. Available from: http://hyper.ahajournals.org/lookup/doi/10.1161/HYPERTENSIONAHA.113.02883

[31] Martinez-Martinez E, Jurado-Lopez R, Valero-Munoz M, Bartolome MV, Ballesteros S, Luaces M, et al. Leptin induces cardiac fibrosis through galectin-3, mTOR and oxidative stress: Potential role in obesity. Journal of Hypertension. 2014;**32**(5):1104-1114. discussion 1114

[32] Engeli S, Bohnke J, Gorzelniak K, Janke J, Schling P, Bader M, et al. Weight loss and the renin-angiotensin-aldosterone system. Hypertension. 2005;**45**(3):356-362. Available from: http://www.ncbi.nlm.nih.gov/pubmed/15630041

[33] Hunt SA, Abraham WT, Chin MH, Feldman AM, Francis GS, Ganiats TG, et al. ACC/AHA 2005 guideline update for the diagnosis and Management of Chronic Heart Failure in the adult: A report of the American College of Cardiology/American Heart Association task force on practice guidelines (writing committee to update the 2001 guidelines for the evaluation and Management of Heart Failure): Developed in collaboration with the American College of Chest Physicians and the International Society for Heart and Lung Transplantation: Endorsed by the Heart Rhythm Society. Circulation. 2005;**112**(12):e154-e235. Available from: http://www.ncbi.nlm.nih.gov/pubmed/16160202

[34] Martinez-Martinez E, Ibarrola J, Calvier L, Fernandez-Celis A, Leroy C, Cachofeiro V, et al. Galectin-3 blockade reduces renal fibrosis in two normotensive experimental models of renal damage. Rouet P, editor. PLoS One. 2016;**11**(11):e0166272. Available from: http://dx.plos.org/10.1371/journal.pone.0166272

[35] Arrieta V, Martinez-Martinez E, Ibarrola J, Alvarez V, Sádaba R, Garcia-Peña A, et al. A role for galectin-3 in the development of early molecular alterations in short-term aortic stenosis. Clinical Science (London, England). 2017;**131**(10):935-949. Available from: http://clinsci.org/lookup/doi/10.1042/CS20170145

[36] van den Berg TNA, Rongen GA, Fröhlich GM, Deinum J, Hausenloy DJ, Riksen NP. The cardioprotective effects of mineralocorticoid receptor antagonists. Pharmacology & Therapeutics. 2014;**142**(1):72-87. Available from: http://www.ncbi.nlm.nih.gov/pubmed/24275323

[37] van den Berg TNAD, Meijers WC, Donders ART, Van Herwaarden AE, Rongen GA, de Boer RA, et al. Plasma galectin-3 concentrations in patients with primary aldosteronism. Journal of Hypertension. 2017;**35**(9):1849-1856. Available from: http://insights.ovid.com/crossref?an=00004872-201709000-00019

[38] Zannad F. Aldosterone and heart failure. European Heart Journal. 1995;**16**(Suppl N):98-102. Available from: http://www.ncbi.nlm.nih.gov/pubmed/8682070

[39] Lopez-Andrès N, Rossignol P, Iraqi W, Fay R, Nuée J, Ghio S, et al. Association of galectin-3 and fibrosis markers with long-term cardiovascular outcomes in patients with heart failure, left ventricular dysfunction, and dyssynchrony: Insights from the CARE-HF (cardiac resynchronization in heart failure) trial. European Journal of Heart Failure. 2012;**14**(1):74-81. Available from: http://doi.wiley.com/10.1093/eurjhf/hfr151

[40] Calvier L, Legchenko E, Grimm L, Sallmon H, Hatch A, Plouffe BD, et al. Galectin-3 and aldosterone as potential tandem biomarkers in pulmonary arterial hypertension. Heart. 2016;**102**(5):390-396. Available from: http://heart.bmj.com/lookup/doi/10.1136/heartjnl-2015-308365

[41] He J, Li X, Luo H, Li T, Zhao L, Qi Q, et al. Galectin-3 mediates the pulmonary arterial hypertension–induced right ventricular remodeling through interacting with NADPH oxidase 4. Journal of the American Society of Hypertension. 2017;**11**(5):275-289.e2. Available from: http://www.ncbi.nlm.nih.gov/pubmed/28431936

[42] Koukoui F, Desmoulin F, Galinier M, Barutaut M, Caubère C, Evaristi MF, et al. The prognostic value of plasma galectin-3 in chronic heart failure patients is maintained when treated with mineralocorticoid receptor antagonists. Mischak H, editor. PLoS One. 2015;**10**(3):e0119160. Available

from: http://dx.plos.org/10.1371/journal.pone.0119160

[43] Fiuzat M, Schulte PJ, Felker M, Ahmad T, Neely M, Adams KF, et al. Relationship between galectin-3 levels and mineralocorticoid receptor antagonist use in heart failure: Analysis from HF-ACTION. Journal of Cardiac Failure. 2014;**20**(1):38-44. Available from: http://linkinghub.elsevier.com/retrieve/pii/S107191641301261X

[44] Gandhi PU, Motiwala SR, Belcher AM, Gaggin HK, Weiner RB, Baggish AL, et al. Galectin-3 and mineralocorticoid receptor antagonist use in patients with chronic heart failure due to left ventricular systolic dysfunction. American Heart Journal. 2015;**169**(3):404-411.e3. Available from: http://www.ncbi.nlm.nih.gov/pubmed/25728731

[45] Buonafine M, Martinez-Martinez E, Jaisser F. More than a simple biomarker: The role of NGAL in cardiovascular and renal diseases. Clinical Science (London, England). 2018;**132**(9):909-923. Available from: http://clinsci.org/lookup/doi/10.1042/CS20171592

[46] Buonafine M, Martínez-Martínez E, Amador C, Gravez B, Ibarrola J, Fernández-Celis A, et al. Neutrophil Gelatinase-associated Lipocalin from immune cells is mandatory for aldosterone-induced cardiac remodeling and inflammation. Journal of Molecular and Cellular Cardiology. 2018;**115**:32-38. Available from: http://www.ncbi.nlm.nih.gov/pubmed/29289651

[47] Martinez-Martinez E, Buonafine M, Boukhalfa I, Ibarrola J, Fernandez-Celis A, Kolkhof P, et al. Aldosterone target NGAL (neutrophil Gelatinase-associated Lipocalin) is involved in cardiac Remodeling after myocardial infarction through NFkappaB pathway. Hypertension (Dallas, Texas 1979). 2017;**70**(6):1148-1156

[48] Tarjus A, Martínez-Martínez E, Amador C, Latouche C, El Moghrabi S, Berger T, et al. Neutrophil Gelatinase-associated Lipocalin, a novel mineralocorticoid biotarget, mediates vascular Profibrotic effects of mineralocorticoids. Hypertension (Dallas, Texas 1979). 2015;**66**(1):158-166. Available from: http://hyper.ahajournals.org/lookup/doi/10.1161/HYPERTENSIONAHA.115.05431

[49] Schroll A, Eller K, Feistritzer C, Nairz M, Sonnweber T, Moser PA, et al. Lipocalin-2 ameliorates granulocyte functionality. European Journal of Immunology. 2012;**42**(12):3346-3357. Available from: http://doi.wiley.com/10.1002/eji.201142351

[50] Shao S, Cao T, Jin L, Li B, Fang H, Zhang J, et al. Increased Lipocalin-2 contributes to the pathogenesis of psoriasis by modulating neutrophil Chemotaxis and cytokine secretion. The Journal of Investigative Dermatology. 2016;**136**(7):1418-1428. Available from: http://linkinghub.elsevier.com/retrieve/pii/S0022202X16308703

[51] Aigner F, Maier HT, Schwelberger HG, Wallnöfer EA, Amberger A, Obrist P, et al. Lipocalin-2 regulates the inflammatory response during ischemia and reperfusion of the transplanted heart. American Journal of Transplantation. 2007;**7**(4):779-788. Available from: http://www.ncbi.nlm.nih.gov/pubmed/17391123

[52] Latouche C, El Moghrabi S, Messaoudi S, Nguyen Dinh Cat A, Hernandez-Diaz I, Alvarez de la Rosa D, et al. Neutrophil gelatinase-associated lipocalin is a novel mineralocorticoid target in the cardiovascular system. Hypertension (Dallas, Texas 1979). 2012;**59**(5):966-972. Available from: http://hyper.ahajournals.org/cgi/doi/10.1161/HYPERTENSIONAHA.111.187872

[53] Buonafine M, Martinez-Martinez E, Amador C, Gravez B, Ibarrola J, Fernandez-Celis A, et al. Neutrophil

Gelatinase-associated Lipocalin from immune cells is mandatory for aldosterone-induced cardiac remodeling and inflammation. Journal of Molecular and Cellular Cardiology. 2017;**115**:32-38

[54] Ong K-L, Tso AWK, Cherny SS, Sham P-C, Lam T-H, Lam KSL, et al. Role of genetic variants in the gene encoding lipocalin-2 in the development of elevated blood pressure. Clinical and Experimental Hypertension. 2011;**33**(7):484-491. Available from: http://www.tandfonline.com/doi/full/10.3109/10641963.2010.549276

[55] Damman K, van Veldhuisen DJ, Navis G, Voors AA, Hillege HL. Urinary neutrophil gelatinase associated lipocalin (NGAL), a marker of tubular damage, is increased in patients with chronic heart failure. European Journal of Heart Failure. 2008;**10**(10):997-1000. Available from: http://www.ncbi.nlm.nih.gov/pubmed/18804416

[56] Yndestad A, Landrø L, Ueland T, Dahl CP, Flo TH, Vinge LE, et al. Increased systemic and myocardial expression of neutrophil gelatinase-associated lipocalin in clinical and experimental heart failure. European Heart Journal. 2009;**30**(10):1229-1236. Available from: https://academic.oup.com/eurheartj/article-lookup/doi/10.1093/eurheartj/ehp088

[57] Wang Y. Small lipid-binding proteins in regulating endothelial and vascular functions: Focusing on adipocyte fatty acid binding protein and lipocalin-2. British Journal of Pharmacology. 2012;**165**(3):603-621. Available from: http://www.ncbi.nlm.nih.gov/pubmed/21658023

[58] Escoté X, Gómez-Zorita S, López-Yoldi M, Milton-Laskibar I, Fernández-Quintela A, Martínez JA, et al. Role of Omentin, Vaspin, Cardiotrophin-1, TWEAK and NOV/CCN3 in obesity and diabetes development. International Journal of Molecular Sciences. 2017;**18**(8):1770. Available from: http://www.mdpi.com/1422-0067/18/8/1770

[59] López-Andrés N, Calvier L, Labat C, Fay R, Díez J, Benetos A, et al. Absence of cardiotrophin 1 is associated with decreased age-dependent arterial stiffness and increased longevity in mice. Hypertension (Dallas, Texas 1979). 2013;**61**(1):120-129. Available from: http://hyper.ahajournals.org/cgi/doi/10.1161/HYPERTENSIONAHA.112.201699

[60] López N, Díez J, Fortuño MA. Characterization of the protective effects of cardiotrophin-1 against non-ischemic death stimuli in adult cardiomyocytes. Cytokine. 2005;**30**(5):282-292. Available from: http://www.ncbi.nlm.nih.gov/pubmed/15927854

[61] López N, Díez J, Fortuño MA. Differential hypertrophic effects of cardiotrophin-1 on adult cardiomyocytes from normotensive and spontaneously hypertensive rats. Journal of Molecular and Cellular Cardiology. 2006;**41**(5):902-913. Available from: http://www.ncbi.nlm.nih.gov/pubmed/17014864

[62] López-Andrés N, Rousseau A, Akhtar R, Calvier L, Iñigo C, Labat C, et al. Cardiotrophin 1 is involved in cardiac, vascular, and renal fibrosis and dysfunction. Hypertension (Dallas, Texas 1979). 2012;**60**(2):563-573. Available from: http://hyper.ahajournals.org/cgi/doi/10.1161/HYPERTENSIONAHA.112.194407

[63] Tsuruda T, Jougasaki M, Boerrigter G, Huntley BK, Chen HH, D'Assoro AB, et al. Cardiotrophin-1 stimulation of cardiac fibroblast growth: Roles for glycoprotein 130/leukemia inhibitory factor receptor and the endothelin type a receptor. Circulation Research. 2002;**90**(2):128-134. Available from:

http://www.ncbi.nlm.nih.gov/pubmed/11834704

[64] Freed DH, Moon MC, Borowiec AM, Jones SC, Zahradka P, IMC D. Cardiotrophin-1: Expression in experimental myocardial infarction and potential role in post-MI wound healing. Molecular and Cellular Biochemistry. 2003;**254**(1-2):247-256. Available from: http://www.ncbi.nlm.nih.gov/pubmed/14674704

[65] Freed DH, Borowiec AM, Angelovska T, IMC D. Induction of protein synthesis in cardiac fibroblasts by cardiotrophin-1: Integration of multiple signaling pathways. Cardiovascular Research. 2003;**60**(2):365-375. Available from: http://www.ncbi.nlm.nih.gov/pubmed/14613866

[66] Drobic V, Cunnington RH, Bedosky KM, Raizman JE, Elimban VV, Rattan SG, et al. Differential and combined effects of cardiotrophin-1 and TGF-$\beta_1$ on cardiac myofibroblast proliferation and contraction. American Journal of Physiology-Heart and Circulatory Physiology. 2007;**293**(2):H1053-H1064. Available from: http://www.physiology.org/doi/10.1152/ajpheart.00935.2006

[67] Lopez-Andres N, Fortuno MA, Diez J, Zannad F, Lacolley P, Rossignol P. Vascular effects of cardiotrophin-1: A role in hypertension? Journal of Hypertension. 2010;**28**(6):1261-1272. Available from http://www.ncbi.nlm.nih.gov/pubmed/20216087

[68] López B, González A, Querejeta R, Larman M, Rábago G, Díez J. Association of cardiotrophin-1 with myocardial fibrosis in hypertensive patients with heart failure. Hypertension (Dallas, Texas 1979). 2014;**63**(3):483-489. Available from: http://hyper.ahajournals.org/cgi/doi/10.1161/HYPERTENSIONAHA.113.02654

[69] López-Andrés N, Iñigo C, Gallego I, Díez J, Fortuño MA. Aldosterone induces cardiotrophin-1 expression in HL-1 adult cardiomyocytes. Endocrinology. 2008;**149**(10):4970-4978. Available from: https://academic.oup.com/endo/article-lookup/doi/10.1210/en.2008-0120

[70] López-Andrés N, Martin-Fernandez B, Rossignol P, Zannad F, Lahera V, Fortuno MA, et al. A role for cardiotrophin-1 in myocardial remodeling induced by aldosterone. American Journal of Physiology-Heart and Circulatory Physiology. 2011;**301**(6):H2372-H2382. Available from: http://www.ncbi.nlm.nih.gov/pubmed/21926338

[71] Zolk O, Ng LL, O'Brien RJ, Weyand M, Eschenhagen T. Augmented expression of cardiotrophin-1 in failing human hearts is accompanied by diminished glycoprotein 130 receptor protein abundance. Circulation. 2002;**106**(12):1442-1446. Available from: http://www.ncbi.nlm.nih.gov/pubmed/12234945

[72] López B, González A, Querejeta R, Barba J, Díez J. Association of plasma cardiotrophin-1 with stage C heart failure in hypertensive patients: Potential diagnostic implications. Journal of Hypertension. 2009;**27**(2):418-424. Available from: http://www.ncbi.nlm.nih.gov/pubmed/19155793

Chapter 4

# Aldosterone/MR Signaling, Oxidative Stress, and Vascular Dysfunction

*Ana M. Briones and Rhian M. Touyz*


## Abstract

The mineralocorticoid receptor (MR) is a transcription factor of the family of steroid receptors that classically binds the hormone aldosterone. The contribution of MR in the regulation of sodium retention and blood pressure is well known. However, MR is expressed in extrarenal tissues including endothelial and vascular smooth muscle cells, and its activation leads to vascular remodeling, vascular stiffness, and endothelial dysfunction leading to vascular damage, an important pathophysiological process in hypertension and other cardiovascular diseases. Moreover, MR is expressed in nonvascular cells in close contact with the vascular wall including immune cells and adipocytes that might influence vascular function and structure. MR activation involves its translocation to the nucleus and regulation of gene transcription. In addition, aldosterone exerts rapid non-genomic effects mediated by MR-dependent and MR-independent mechanisms. Both genomic and non-genomic effects facilitate reactive oxygen species (ROS) production (particularly by the enzyme NADPH oxidase), inflammation, and fibrosis, which, in turn, promote tissue remodeling, vascular stiffening, and endothelial dysfunction. Studies with MR antagonists and experimental models with cell-specific knockout or overexpression of MR further support a role for aldosterone/MR-mediated oxidative stress-dependent processes in vascular damage. This review focuses on the relationship between aldosterone/MR signaling and oxidative stress and the implications in vascular regulation in health and disease.


**Keywords:** aldosterone, mineralocorticoid receptor, oxidative stress, NADPH oxidase

## 1. Introduction

The mineralocorticoid receptor (MR) classically binds the hormone aldosterone and in the kidney regulates sodium retention, volume homeostasis, and blood pressure. The MR, originally thought to be expressed only in the kidney, is now known to have an extensive extrarenal distribution and is functionally active in the cardiovascular and immune systems. MR activation is involved in various cardiovascular diseases [1, 2] and has also been implicated in metabolic disorders and insulin resistance. At the vascular level, MR is expressed in endothelial and vascular smooth muscle cells (VSMC), and its activation leads to vascular remodeling, vascular fibrosis, and endothelial dysfunction leading to vascular damage, arterial stiffness, and hypertension [1–3]. However, MR is also expressed in nonvascular

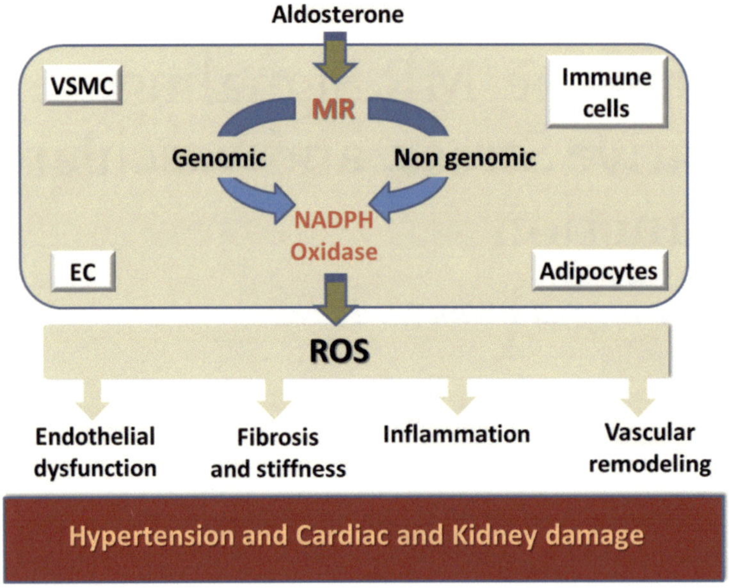


**Figure 1.**
*At the vascular level, MR is expressed in endothelial (EC) and vascular smooth muscle cells (VSMC). Its activation by genomic and rapid non-genomic effects mediated by MR-dependent and MR-independent mechanisms leads to activation of NADPH oxidase that produced reactive oxygen species (ROS) leading to vascular remodeling, fibrosis, inflammation, and endothelial dysfunction that produces vascular damage and arterial stiffness and might participate in hypertension and cardiac and kidney damage.*

cells in close contact with the vascular wall including immune cells and adipocytes where it influences inflammatory and metabolic processes [4, 5].

The MR is an intracellular receptor that has three domains: (i) an N-terminal domain that controls transcriptional activity of the receptor, (ii) the DNA-binding domain that influences binding of the specific response element on the promoter of MR target genes, and (iii) the ligand-binding domain for aldosterone. Upon activation, the MR is translocated to the nucleus and further regulates gene transcription and translation of proteins by binding to DNA hormone/steroid stimulatory or negative response elements [1, 2]. In addition, aldosterone exerts rapid non-genomic effects mediated by MR-dependent and MR-independent mechanisms [6], and recent studies uncovered an MR-dependent suppression of miRNA expression resulting in upregulation of vascular miRNA targets [7]. Both genomic and non-genomic effects promote reactive oxygen species (ROS) production particularly by the enzyme NADPH oxidase, as well as inflammation and fibrosis, which, in turn, leads to tissue remodeling and vascular stiffening and endothelial dysfunction. This review focuses on the relationship between aldosterone/MR signaling and oxidative stress and its vascular effects (**Figure 1**).

## 2. MR and oxidative stress in vascular cells

Extensive evidence has demonstrated a relationship between MR and redox signaling in vascular cells. Animal models including the deoxycorticosterone acetate (DOCA)/salt model and the aldosterone/salt model with or without nephrectomy exhibit vascular oxidative stress. The significance of ROS in these models is supported by studies that demonstrated that MR blockers reduce ROS levels in cardiovascular pathologies including hypertension, obesity, atherosclerosis, or heart failure. In many of the experimental and human studies, evidence of altered oxidative stress was often based on a single method to determine oxidative stress, i.e., altered gene or protein expression of NADPH oxidase subunits, NADPH oxidase activity, lipid peroxidation determinations, fluorescence-based studies, etc., and this might explain, at least in part, some divergent findings. Because of the complexity of redox biology and difficulties in accurately measuring ROS, expert recommendations have been published suggesting that multiple different assays need to be used to accurately assess redox status in biological systems and experimental models [8]. Here we will not discuss specific methods to measure ROS in the context of aldosterone/MR, and the reader is referred to comprehensive reviews [8, 9].

Aldosterone increases ROS production in cultured VSMC [10–15] and endothelial cells [16–21]. Moreover, aldosterone infusion into mice or rats increases plasma and vascular oxidative stress, and MR blockade reduces ROS production in the setting of hypertension, obesity, and other cardiovascular diseases [21–29]. Earlier studies identified NADPH oxidase as responsible for increased production of vascular ROS, specifically superoxide ($O_2^-$), in the aorta from mineralocorticoid (DOCA-salt) hypertensive rats excluding other ROS sources (i.e., uncoupled eNOS or xanthine oxidase) as potential contributors [30]. NADPH oxidase is considered the major source of ROS in response to aldosterone/MR stimulation in vessels.

The NADPH oxidase (Nox) family is composed of seven Nox isoforms (Nox1–Nox5 and Duox1 and Duox2); several regulatory subunits p22phox, p47phox, Noxo1, p67phox, Noxa1, and p40phox; and the major binding partner Rac. The main catalytic function of NADPH oxidases is the generation of ROS. NADPH oxidase reduces oxygen to $O_2^-$, with NADPH being the electron donor. Nox-2 is the classical Nox that was characterized initially in leukocytes. Nox-1, Nox-2, Nox-4, and Nox-5 are expressed in the cardiovascular system with Nox5 not being present in rodents. Nox-1, Nox-2, Nox-3, and Nox-5 produce $O_2^-$, while Nox-4, Duox-1, and Duox-2 produce $H_2O_2$ [31, 32]. In vessels, in addition to vascular cells possessing functional Noxes, resident macrophages, neutrophils, and platelets express NADPH oxidase, particularly in pathological states. Accordingly, these cells can also contribute to vascular oxidative stress in disease [32, 33].

### 2.1 Genomic and non-genomic effects of aldosterone/MR on ROS production

At the vascular level, a combination of aldosterone and high salt caused $O_2^-$ production in VSMC through upregulation of Nox1 without affecting expression of mRNA Nox4, p22phox, and p47phox [11]. In human vein endothelial cells (HUVEC), aldosterone increased p47phox transcription, but no effect on transcription levels of Nox1, Nox2, Nox4, p22phox, p40phox, or p67phox was observed [16]. However, other studies showed that incubation with aldosterone for 24 h dose-dependently increased Nox4 mRNA expression in HUVEC [17]. In human pulmonary artery endothelial cells, aldosterone increased protein levels of Nox4 and p22phox as well as $H_2O_2$ production [20]. Similarly, in bovine retinal endothelial cells, aldosterone increased mRNA for Nox4 [19], and other studies showed that aldosterone administration modulated exclusively p22phox mRNA expression in freshly isolated aortic endothelial cells [21]. Aldosterone plus salt infusion into rats increased vascular NADPH oxidase activity and expression of p47phox, gp91phox, and p22phox [34], and recently, Jia et al. [29] found vascular upregulation of Nox2 expression and nitrotyrosine (a marker of nitrosative stress) formation after 3 weeks of aldosterone infusion in mice. Together, these findings clearly show a pattern of vascular NADPH oxidase upregulation by aldosterone at the vascular level. This is also supported by the fact that MR antagonists decrease NADPH oxidase subunit expression [9]. For example, eplerenone treatment decreased the expression of p22phox, p47phox, and p40phox in a model of high-fat diet [21]. Moreover, deletion of MR in specific vascular cell types also downregulates NADPH oxidase isoforms (discussed below).

For the rapid MR-dependent aldosterone effects, the MR seems to be localized near the plasma membrane, but not directly inserted into it. It is located at the cytosolic site associated with scaffolding proteins that are associated with or inserted in the cell membrane such as striatin or caveolin-1 [6]. In this location, aldosterone can also interact with receptors such as receptor tyrosine kinases including epidermal growth factor receptor (EGFR), platelet-derived growth factor receptor (PDGFR), and insulin-like growth factor 1 receptor (IGF1R) or G protein-coupled receptors (GPCR) such as angiotensin type 1 receptor (AT1) or G protein-coupled estrogen receptor 1 (GPER1) [6].

The Src family of non-receptor tyrosine kinases seems to be involved in non-genomic ROS generation by aldosterone [9]. In cultured VSMC, NADPH oxidase-dependent ROS generation through non-genomic effects of aldosterone is increased in spontaneously hypertensive rats and is dependent on c-Src [10]. A role for c-Src and Rac-1 in NADPH oxidase activation in endothelial cells has also been described although this effect might be mediated via genomic actions because long incubation times were tested [18]. In VSMC, EGFR and PDGFR, but not IGFR, transactivation by MR and AT1 activates c-Src that in turn facilitates activation of NADPH oxidase and ROS production leading to VSMC migration [35].

Besides receptor tyrosine kinases, GPCR are important partners involved in the non-genomic actions of aldosterone. Thus, MR/AT1 receptor interaction has been implicated, because MR blockade can inhibit angiotensin II-induced ROS production in vascular tissue [22], and more recently, it has been shown that AT1a is required for MR-induced endothelial dysfunction and vascular remodeling, oxidative stress, and inflammation [27], although a genomic effect cannot be excluded in these studies. In cardiac myocytes, an interaction between MR and AT1 participates in aldosterone-induced ROS generation by Nox4 via G protein-coupled receptor kinase (GRK) 2 likely via non-genomic actions [36], but whether this GRK2-dependent mechanism also occurs in vascular cells is unknown. Similarly, there is a paucity of information regarding the novel putative aldosterone receptor GPER1 (also known as GPR30) in aldosterone-induced ROS production in vascular cells, and the evidence supporting this possibility comes from cardiac cells [37, 38].

Non-genomic MR signaling can modulate MR genomic effects [6], thus further perpetuating ROS generation in vascular cells.

### 2.2 Aldosterone/MR/oxidative stress pathway and endothelial and smooth muscle cells

Extensive experimental evidence has demonstrated a beneficial effect of aldosterone/MR blockade in vascular damage (i.e., endothelial dysfunction, vascular remodeling, and stiffness) and oxidative stress [1–3, 21, 22, 39–42]. As such, it has been suggested that many of the beneficial effects of MR antagonist rely, at least in part, on its ability to decrease oxidative stress. This is supported by direct evidence emerging from studies using models of aldosterone or mineralocorticoid infusion together with antioxidant treatments and by the use of transgenic mouse models of MR overexpression or deletion.

MR expressed in cerebral artery endothelial cells mediates increased capacity for $O_2^-$ production in response to chronically increased systemic levels of aldosterone [26]. Moreover, mRNA expression of p22phox, but not gp91phox, was upregulated by aldosterone, and this effect was abolished in endothelial cell-specific MR knockout mice (EC-MR-KO) [21], concomitant with improved endothelial function. However, in the absence of stimuli, conditional overexpression of the MR in endothelial cells is not sufficient to increase local vascular or systemic oxidative stress [43], suggesting that upregulation of the MR alone is not enough to produce increased oxidative stress generation. This is consistent with the idea that EC-MR might be vasoprotective in healthy states and that this protection is lost when cardiovascular risk factors such as hypertension, obesity, or increased aldosterone levels are present, as suggested recently [2, 44] (**Figure 2**). In support of this hypothesis, EC-MR deficiency prevented western diet-induced Nox2, Nox4, p22phox, and 3-nitrotyrosine expression, and this was concomitant with reduced aortic fibrosis and stiffness and restoration of endothelial nitric oxide synthase activation [28]. Similarly, EC-MR deletion prevented resistance vessel endothelial dysfunction associated with hyperlipidemia in females, but not in males, and this was associated with decreased $O_2^-$ generation [45].

Although adult SMC-MR-KO mice show no difference in basal vascular ROS, aged SMC-MR-KO mice vessels produce significantly less vascular ROS [7, 46]. Moreover, both young and aged SMC-MR-KO mice show attenuated angiotensin II-stimulated ROS production [46] which might have contributed to the lower blood pressure observed in these mice via improved vascular contraction. More recently, an inverse relationship between SMC-MR and miR-155 has been described in aging [7], whereby this miRNA would repress the SMC-MR-associated oxidative stress also having an impact in vascular function [7]. However, the specific ROS source that is modulated by miR-155 is unknown. VSMC-MR was also shown to be involved in the progression of heart failure post myocardial infarction, through its direct role in oxidative stress-induced coronary endothelial dysfunction and in decreased coronary reserve [47]. In this study the antioxidants apocynin and superoxide dismutase (SOD) improved endothelium-dependent relaxation of

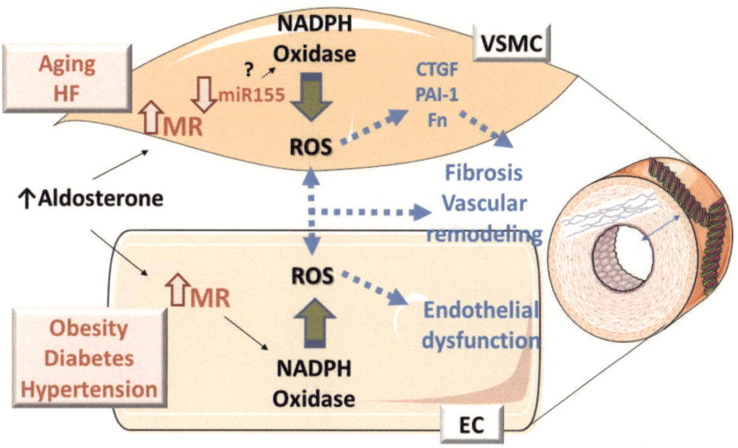


**Figure 2.**
*MR expressed in endothelial cells mediates increased capacity for $O_2^-$ production in response to chronically increased systemic levels of aldosterone such as those occurring in hypertension, obesity, or diabetes. In aging or heart failure after myocardial infarction (HF), SMC-MR facilitates increased ROS production. In addition, an inverse relationship between SMC-MR and miR-155 has been described in aging, whereby this miRNA would repress the SMC-MR-associated oxidative stress. Whether this is via NADPH oxidase is unknown. In these pathologies, both EC and SMC-MR activation facilitate ROS formation that participates in endothelial dysfunction, vasoconstriction, vascular remodeling, and fibrosis, the latter being mediated by the increased expression of different extracellular matrix proteins and profibrotic factors (CTFG, connective tissue growth factor; PAI-1, plasminogen activator inhibitor 1; Fn, fibronectin).*

coronary arteries from myocardial infarction mice without affecting relaxation of arteries from myocardial infarction-MR-SMC-knockout or treated with finerenone, indicating a lower effect of oxidative stress when MR is absent in VSMCs or after general MR blockade [47]. Together, these findings point to both endothelial cells and VSMC as potential sources of ROS in response to aldosterone or pathological conditions that impact vascular function (**Figure 2**).

Regarding the role of oxidative stress in vascular remodeling and stiffness, it has been demonstrated that a combination of aldosterone and high salt caused $O_2^-$ production and VSMC hypertrophy through the upregulation of Nox1 [11] and antioxidants attenuated aldosterone-induced VSMC senescence and Ki-ras2A expression [48]. In addition, it has been suggested that aldosterone augments vascular hypertrophic effects of insulin via an MR- and oxidative stress-mediated pathways [49]. Aldosterone-induced hypertrophy and perivascular fibrosis were significantly ameliorated by long-term treatment with spironolactone or antioxidants [50, 51]. However, the profibrotic, but not the hypertrophic, action of aldosterone in resistance arteries was blocked by the antioxidant tempol treatment [23]. Mechanisms responsible for these effects likely rely on the ability of aldosterone-derived ROS to modulate a number of genes involved in vascular injury including placental growth factor, metallothioneins 1 and 2, or connective tissue growth factor [52]. In addition, aldosterone increased expression of profibrotic factors fibronectin and plasminogen activator inhibitor (PAI)-1 in wild type but not in Nox-1 knockout mice [53, 62] (**Figure 2**). Moreover, tempol treatment inhibited other proinflammatory and profibrotic markers such as osteopontin, intracellular adhesion molecule 1, vascular cell adhesion molecule 1, or PAI-1 mRNA expressions that were induced by aldosterone infusion in rats [54].

Among the mechanisms responsible for endothelial dysfunction, it is generally assumed that the interaction between NO and $O_2^-$, usually from NADPH oxidase, leads to $ONOO^-$ formation or eNOS uncoupling, thus decreasing NO availability, among other mechanisms (for detailed reviews, see [31–33, 55, 56]) (**Figure 3**). In this scenario, aldosterone-induced inhibition of NO production in endothelial cells was partially restored by p47phox knockdown using siRNA [16]. Other potential mechanisms responsible for aldosterone/MR/ROS-induced endothelial dysfunction include (i) oxidative posttranslational modification(s) of guanylyl cyclase activity that impair sensing of this enzyme by NO [12], (ii) downregulation of the antioxidant enzyme glucose-6-phosphate dehydrogenase [57], or (iii) oxidative modification of the redox sensitive, functional cysteinyl thiol(s) in the endothelin receptor (ETBR) (Cys405) by Nox-4-dependent $H_2O_2$, to impair ETB-dependent activation of eNOS and decrease synthesis of NO [20]. In this sense, during renal ischemia, activation of MR signals Rac1 to increase ROS production in the SMCs that diffuse to ECs to induce posttranslational sulfenic acid modification in ETBR that impairs eNOS activation and diminishes NO production leading to sustained vasoconstriction and reduced kidney perfusion [58]. In addition, cardiomyocyte-specific overexpression of human MR induces severe coronary endothelial dysfunction with decreased NO-mediated relaxing responses to acetylcholine in coronary arteries (but not in peripheral arteries), effects prevented by 1-month treatment with an MR antagonist, vitamin E/vitamin C, or a NADPH oxidase inhibitor [59]. Finally, a role for the epithelial sodium channel in aldosterone-induced oxidative stress and in endothelium stiffness and endothelial dysfunction and fibrosis has also been described [29] (**Figure 3**). Interestingly, Rac1 is not only one of the NADPH oxidase components but also serves as the upregulator of MR signaling in the kidney [60]. This Rac1-MR pathway is activated by ROS in cardiomyocytes [61] and also plays a crucial role in ROS production and cardiac dysfunction [62].

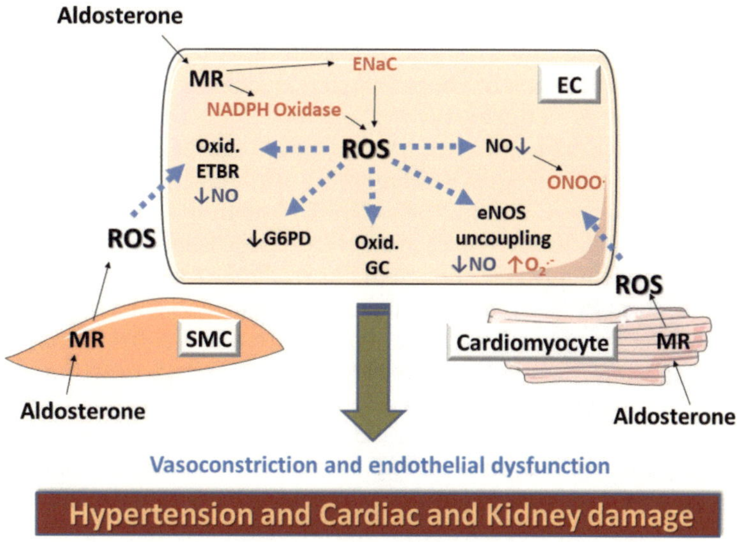


**Figure 3.**
*Mechanisms responsible for aldosterone/MR-induced endothelial dysfunction. The interaction between NO and $O_2^-$, usually from NADPH oxidase, leads to $ONOO^-$ formation or eNOS uncoupling, thus decreasing NO availability. Other potential mechanisms include oxidative posttranslational modification(s) of guanylyl cyclase (GC) activity that impair sensing of this enzyme by NO, downregulation of the antioxidant enzyme glucose-6-phosphate dehydrogenase (G6PD), or oxidative modification of the endothelin receptor (ETBR) to impair ETB-dependent activation of eNOS and decrease synthesis of NO. In renal ischemia, ROS production in the SMCs diffuses to ECs to induce modifications in ETBR that diminishes NO production leading to sustained vasoconstriction and reduced kidney perfusion. Also, cardiomyocyte-specific overexpression of human MR induces severe coronary endothelial dysfunction with decreased NO-mediated relaxing responses via NADPH oxidase-dependent ROS. Epithelial sodium channel (ENac) also participates in aldosterone-induced oxidative stress and endothelial dysfunction.*

## 3. MR and oxidative stress in immune cells

Growing evidence suggests that aldosterone induces vascular monocyte/macrophage and T-cell infiltration in different pathological states [24, 63, 64]. MR is expressed in both macrophages and T cells, where it functions as an important transcriptional regulator of cellular phenotype and function and can be activated even with normal or low aldosterone levels in pathological conditions [5, 65].

The relationship between immune cells, MR, and oxidative stress was demonstrated in uninephrectomized rats treated for 4 weeks with dietary 1% NaCl and aldosterone, where there was an increased $H_2O_2$ production by monocytes and lymphocytes, upregulation of oxidative stress-inducible tyrosine phosphatase and Mn-SOD genes in peripheral blood mononuclear cells, and the presence of 3-nitrotyrosine in CD4+ inflammatory cells invading intramural coronary arteries [66]. Guzik et al. [67] showed that DOCA/salt-induced hypertension and $O_2^-$ production in the aorta were blunted in rag$^{-/-}$ mice deficient in T and B lymphocytes. Notably, enhanced suppressor regulatory T lymphocytes, which are suppressors of the innate and adaptive immune responses, prevented aldosterone-induced endothelial dysfunction, vascular remodeling, and oxidative stress [25]. More recently, the key role of immune cell MR in oxidative stress generation was demonstrated by Sun and coworkers [68] that showed that blood vessels from T-cell MR knockout mice had suppressed $O_2^-$ production, and this was paralleled by attenuated target organ damage including better endothelial function and less vascular hypertrophy and fibrosis after angiotensin II infusion. This may be due to a lower proportion of IFN-γ-producing T cells in the arteries [68]. In fact, T-cell MR facilitates activation of T cells modulating the production of inflammatory cytokines such as IFNγ and IL-6 [69] that can induce ROS production at vascular level.

Regarding macrophages, it has been shown that aldosterone stimulation of macrophages induces a proinflammatory M1 phenotype [5]. Macrophages from mice lacking MR in myeloid cells exhibited a transcription profile of alternative activation from a M1 phenotype toward a M2 more anti-inflammatory phenotype [70]. This might modulate vascular function as NLRP3 inflammasome in macrophages explains aldosterone-induced hypercontractility, endothelial dysfunction, and hypertrophic remodeling [71], although in this study the specific contribution of macrophage-derived ROS was not evaluated. Interestingly, a shift in polarization to a M2 phenotype in the EC-MR-KO mice exposed to a western diet was also observed [28], suggesting a role for endothelial cells-MR in macrophage function. Regarding oxidative stress, aldosterone increases $O_2^-$ production and NADPH oxidase activation in macrophages both in vivo and in vitro [72] and also mitochondrial ROS generation [71] that might contribute to the activation of inflammasome in this cell type as suggested previously [73]. Notably, aldosterone-induced endothelial dysfunction and vascular oxidative stress were decreased in mcsfOp/+, which have a low monocyte/macrophage number in the vessel wall [24], suggesting that MR activation in macrophages modulates vascular oxidative stress. Interestingly, oxidative stress assessed as Nox2 and p22phox gene expression is equivalently increased in the heart of wild-type and mac-MR-KO with L-NAME/salt treatment [74], and MR deficiency in macrophages did not influence their oxidative status in the context of atherosclerosis [75], suggesting a different contribution of MR-derived ROS in different tissues and pathologies. In vivo, MR deficiency in macrophages mimicked the effects of MR antagonists and protected against vascular damage

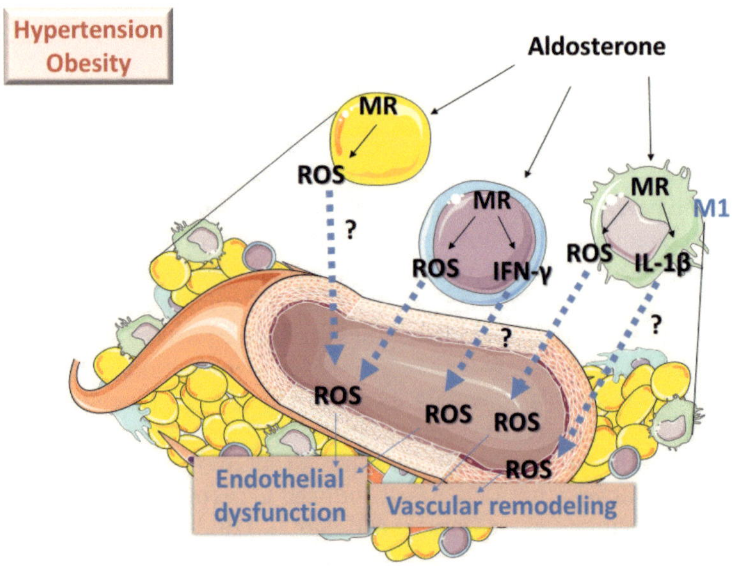


**Figure 4.**
*Aldosterone induces vascular monocyte/macrophage and T-cell infiltration in different pathological states such as hypertension and obesity. MR is expressed in both macrophages and T cells. T-cell MR facilitates activation of T cells modulating the production of inflammatory cytokines such as IFNγ and IL-6 that can induce ROS production at vascular level. MR activation in macrophages induces a proinflammatory M1 phenotype leading to the production of IL-1β. Either directly or through the production of these proinflammatory cytokines, immune cell-derived ROS seems to facilitate vascular remodeling and endothelial dysfunction. MR expression is increased in the adipose tissue in obesity. MR in the different cell types included in the adipose tissue (i.e., adipocytes, preadipocytes, macrophages) might facilitate oxidative stress and vascular alterations associated with obesity.*

caused by L-NAME/angiotensin II [70], and selective deletion of MR in myeloid cells limits macrophage accumulation that leads to less VSMC activation and vascular inflammation and inhibits neointimal hyperplasia and vascular remodeling [76]. In both studies, again the specific contribution of macrophage-derived ROS was not evaluated.

Together, these findings highlight a key contribution of MR-dependent ROS from immune cells in vascular damage. Whether this is due to locally produced ROS by infiltrated cells or through the release of proinflammatory cytokines affecting the underlying VSMC or endothelial cells to induce oxidative stress, or both, remains unclear (**Figure 4**).

## 4. MR and oxidative stress in adipose tissue

Other extrarenal tissue that express MR is the adipose tissue where MR is involved in essential processes such as differentiation, autophagy, and adipokine secretion [4, 77]. MR expression is increased in adipose tissue of murine models of obesity and in obese human subjects, and different studies using MR antagonists and also adipocyte-specific MR transgenic mice have demonstrated a key role of MR in insulin signaling and inflammation, as reviewed previously [4, 77, 78].

It is well accepted that adipose tissue, particularly perivascular adipose tissue (PVAT), modulates vascular health and disease through the release of a number of adipokines that affect contractile and relaxant properties, vascular smooth muscle cell proliferation and hypertrophy, fibrosis, and inflammation [79]. Among the many substances released, ROS such as $H_2O_2$ seems to have a pivotal role both in physiological and pathological conditions; however, in some disease states such as obesity or hypertension, proinflammatory cytokines such as IL-1, IL-6, or TNF-α released from PVAT clearly affect vascular tone [79], probably in part through increased oxidative stress generation. Thus, in healthy rat mesenteric arteries, the anticontractile effect of PVAT was lost following incubation with aldosterone (10 minutes and 3 hours), and this was restored by a combination of SOD and catalase and by eplerenone, and this is likely dependent on macrophage infiltration in the PVAT [80]. Moreover, MR blockade reduced ROS production in 3 T3-L1 adipocytes [81, 82].

Earlier studies showed that the NADPH oxidase subunits p22 and p47phox were significantly increased in adipose tissue from ob/ob and db/db obese mice compared with lean control mice and that eplerenone treatment suppressed this increase [81]. The increase in ROS levels observed in adipose tissue of these models of obesity could also be due to the decreased gene expression of the ROS-eliminating enzymes, catalase, and Cu/Zn-SOD, which were reduced in both ob/ob and db/db mice and which were also restored by administration of eplerenone [81]. Other studies also reported upregulation of antioxidant enzymes (SOD-1 and catalase) at vascular level by MR blockade in obesity/diabetes [41]. Finally, in the adipose tissue of nephrectomized rats, oxidative stress increased, and this was reversed by spironolactone [83].

In vivo conditional upregulation of MR in mouse adipocytes led to increased production of $H_2O_2$ from epididymal adipose tissue likely due to the decrease in catalase mRNA levels and the increased Nox-4 mRNA levels without changes in Nox-1 and Nox-2 expressions which likely explain changes in vascular contractility [84]. Interestingly, adipocyte-specific MR knockout mice (AdipoMR-KO) fed with high-fat/high-sucrose diet showed similar levels of 8-isoprostane, p22phox, SOD-1, or catalase mRNA levels, and they did not show differences in body weight, fat weight, glucose tolerance, insulin sensitivity, or inflammation [85]. Similar results were reported by Feraco and coworkers [86] using inducible adipocyte-specific deletion of MR fed a 45% high-fat diet although in this study oxidative stress was not evaluated. Further studies are warranted to identify the specific contribution of MR in the different cell types included in the adipose tissue (i.e., adipocytes, preadipocytes, macrophages) as responsible for the MR-dependent inflammation, oxidative stress, and metabolic alterations associated with obesity (**Figure 4**).

## 5. Clinical relevance

While there is extensive preclinical data indicating that aldosterone-MR signals through redox-dependent pathways, there is a paucity of information in humans. However, a few clinical studies have suggested that hyperaldosteronism is associated with increased concentration of circulating markers of oxidative stress. In patients with stable heart failure and in patients with hypertension, higher aldosterone levels were associated with systemic evidence of oxidative stress, inflammation, and matrix turnover [87]. In heart failure patients, aldosterone-associated cardiovascular damage and renal fibrosis were linked to decreased production of NO, increased oxidative stress, and activation of proinflammatory transcription factors, including NF-κB [9]. At the cellular level, there is also some suggestion that aldosterone stimulates ROS production in humans. In human endothelial cells, spironolactone inhibited Nox-induced oxidative stress and increased eNOS activity [88], indicating a role for MR-mediated regulation of ROS in human vessels. In patients with hyperaldosteronism and adrenal adenomas, a number of studies have reported increased expression of redox-related genes and proteins including Nrf2, p22phox, HO-1, and proinflammatory transcription factors [89–91]. In human cardiomyocytes, aldosterone impairs mitochondrial function, important in redox regulation [91]. Despite suggestions that hyperaldosteronism promotes oxidative stress in human cardiovascular disease, studies using MR antagonists have not shown significant improvement in oxidative stress markers. Thus, Hwang and coworkers [92] demonstrated that eplerenone-related improvement in flow-mediated dilation (a marker of endothelial function) was not associated with oxidative stress markers, plasma F2-isoprostanes, and vascular endothelial cell protein expression of nitrotyrosine and p47phox. In a small group of older adults with metabolic syndrome, flow-mediated dilation, levels of oxidized low-density lipoproteins, or F2-isoprostanes did not improve in response to MR blockade, despite a large reduction (10 mmHg) in systolic blood pressure [93]. In addition, there was no effect of 1-month treatment with eplerenone on oxidative stress (oxidized LDL) and arterial stiffness in healthy older adults [94]. However, Chen et al. [95] recently demonstrated that increased NADPH oxidase-dependent oxidative stress, oxidative BH4 degradation, eNOS uncoupling, and reduced NO generation were responsible for the impaired in vivo endothelial repair capacity of early endothelial progenitor cells from hypertensive patients with primary hyperaldosteronism [95]. Further clinical studies are needed to confirm the role of ROS in aldosterone-mediated cardiovascular injury. Moreover, trials that assess effects of MR antagonists on ROS levels rather than markers of oxidative stress (oxidized LDL, F2-isoprostanes) are warranted.

## 6. Conclusions

Experimental evidence clearly shows that MR/aldosterone blockade decreases vascular oxidative stress and improves vascular function, structure, and mechanical properties in different experimental models. Among the cell types involved in aldosterone/MR/oxidative-associated vascular damage are endothelial cells and vascular smooth muscle cells. However, growing evidence suggests that these vascular effects can also be modulated by MR expressed in infiltrating immune cells, i.e., lymphocytes and macrophages, and in the surrounding perivascular adipose tissue that might release ROS directly impacting the endothelium and vascular wall. Alternatively, these cells can generate MR-dependent inflammatory cytokines (or adipokines) that act in a paracrine manner in the underlying vessels to induce oxidative stress and hence vascular damage. Thus, MR-associated oxidative stress in different cell types emerges as an important pathway contributing to vascular dysfunction and injury associated with conditions of high aldosterone/MR activation. Accordingly, it is suggested that some of the vasoprotective effects of MR antagonists used clinically may be mediated by inhibiting ROS-induced vascular damage.

## Acknowledgements

This publication is based upon work from the EU COST Action ADMIRE BM1301 in Aldosterone and Mineralocorticoid Receptor (MR) Physiology and Pathophysiology www.admirecosteu.com. AMB is supported by the Spanish Ministerio de Economía, Industria y Competitividad (SAF2016-80305P), Instituto de Salud Carlos III (PI13/01488; CIBER de Enfermedades Cardiovasculares, CB16/11/00286), Comunidad de Madrid (AORTASANA-CM B2017/BMD-3676), Fondo Social Europeo (FSE), Fondo Europeo de Desarrollo Regional (FEDER) a way to build Europe, and Roche-IdiPaz. RMT is supported by grants from the British Heart Foundation (CH/4/29762, RE/13/5/30177).

## Conflicts of interest/disclosures

The authors declare no conflict of interest.

## Author details

Ana M. Briones[1,2*] and Rhian M. Touyz[3*]

1 Departmento de Farmacología, Instituto de Investigación Hospital La Paz, Universidad Autónoma de Madrid, Madrid, Spain

2 Ciber de Enfermedades Cardiovasculares, Spain

3 Institute of Cardiovascular and Medical Sciences, University of Glasgow, UK

*Address all correspondence to: ana.briones@uam.es and Rhian.Touyz@glasgow.ac.uk

## References

[1] Jaisser F, Farman N. Emerging roles of the mineralocorticoid receptor in pathology: Toward new paradigms in clinical pharmacology. Pharmacological Reviews. 2016;**68**(1):49-75

[2] DuPont JJ, Jaffe IZ. 30 Years of the mineralocorticoid receptor: The role of the mineralocorticoid receptor in the vasculature. The Journal of Endocrinology. 2017;**234**(1):T67-T82

[3] Briet M, Schiffrin EL. Vascular actions of aldosterone. Journal of Vascular Research. 2013;**50**(2):89-99

[4] Armani A, Marzolla V, Fabbri A, Caprio M. Cellular mechanisms of MR regulation of adipose tissue physiology and pathophysiology. Journal of Molecular Endocrinology. 2015;**55**(2):R1-R10

[5] van der Heijden CDCC et al. The mineralocorticoid receptor as a modulator of innate immunity and atherosclerosis. Cardiovascular Research. 2018;**114**(7):944-953

[6] Ruhs S, Nolze A, Hübschmann R, Grossmann C. 30 Years of the mineralocorticoid receptor: Nongenomic effects via the mineralocorticoid receptor. The Journal of Endocrinology. 2017;**234**(1):T107-T124

[7] DuPont JJ et al. Vascular mineralocorticoid receptor regulates microRNA-155 to promote vasoconstriction and rising blood pressure with aging. JCI Insight. 2016;**1**(14):e88942

[8] Griendling KK et al. American Heart Association Council on basic cardiovascular sciences. Measurement of reactive oxygen species, reactive nitrogen species, and redox-dependent signaling in the cardiovascular system: A scientific statement from the American Heart Association. Circulation Research. 2016;**119**(5):e39-e75

[9] Queisser N, Schupp N. Aldosterone, oxidative stress, and NF-κB activation in hypertension-related cardiovascular and renal diseases. Free Radical Biology & Medicine. 2012;**53**(2):314-327

[10] Callera GE et al. c-Src-dependent nongenomic signaling responses to aldosterone are increased in vascular myocytes from spontaneously hypertensive rats. Hypertension. 2005;**46**(4):1032-1038

[11] Fan C et al. Synergy of aldosterone and high salt induces vascular smooth muscle hypertrophy through up-regulation of NOX1. The Journal of Steroid Biochemistry and Molecular Biology. 2008;**111**(1-2):29-36

[12] Maron BA et al. Aldosterone increases oxidant stress to impair guanylyl cyclase activity by cysteinyl thiol oxidation in vascular smooth muscle cells. The Journal of Biological Chemistry. 2009;**284**(12):7665-7672

[13] Fu Y et al. The mitochondria mediate the induction of NOX1 gene expression by aldosterone in an ATF-1-dependent manner. Cellular & Molecular Biology Letters. 2011;**16**(2):226-235

[14] Muehlfelder M, Arias-Loza PA, Fritzemeier KH, Pelzer T. Both estrogen receptor subtypes, ERα and ERβ, prevent aldosterone-induced oxidative stress in VSMC via increased NADPH bioavailability. Biochemical and Biophysical Research Communications. 2012;**423**(4):850-856

[15] Zhang X et al. Aldosterone induces C-reactive protein expression via MR-ROS-MAPK-NF-κB signal pathway in rat vascular smooth muscle cells.

Molecular and Cellular Endocrinology. 2014;**395**(1-2):61-68

[16] Nagata D et al. Molecular mechanism of the inhibitory effect of aldosterone on endothelial NO synthase activity. Hypertension. 2006;**48**(1):165-171

[17] Hashikabe Y, Suzuki K, Jojima T, Uchida K, Hattori Y. Aldosterone impairs vascular endothelial cell function. Journal of Cardiovascular Pharmacology. 2006;**47**(4):609-613

[18] Iwashima F et al. Aldosterone induces superoxide generation via Rac1 activation in endothelial cells. Endocrinology. 2008;**149**(3):1009-1014

[19] Wilkinson-Berka JL, Tan G, Jaworski K, Miller AG. Identification of a retinal aldosterone system and the protective effects of mineralocorticoid receptor antagonism on retinal vascular pathology. Circulation Research. 2009;**104**(1):124-133

[20] Maron BA et al. Aldosterone inactivates the endothelin-B receptor via a cysteinyl thiol redox switch to decrease pulmonary endothelial nitric oxide levels and modulate pulmonary arterial hypertension. Circulation. 2012;**126**(8):963-974

[21] Schäfer N et al. Endothelial mineralocorticoid receptor activation mediates endothelial dysfunction in diet-induced obesity. European Heart Journal. 2013;**34**(45):3515-3524

[22] Virdis A et al. Spironolactone improves angiotensin-induced vascular changes and oxidative stress. Hypertension. 2002;**40**(4):504-510

[23] Iglarz M, Touyz RM, Viel EC, Amiri F, Schiffrin EL. Involvement of oxidative stress in the profibrotic action of aldosterone. Interaction with the renin-angiotensin system. American Journal of Hypertension. 2004;**17**(7):597-603

[24] Leibovitz E, Ebrahimian T, Paradis P, Schiffrin EL. Aldosterone induces arterial stiffness in absence of oxidative stress and endothelial dysfunction. Journal of Hypertension. 2009;**27**(11):2192-2200

[25] Kasal DA et al. T regulatory lymphocytes prevent aldosterone-induced vascular injury. Hypertension. 2012;**59**(2):324-330

[26] Dinh QN et al. Aldosterone-induced oxidative stress and inflammation in the brain are mediated by the endothelial cell mineralocorticoid receptor. Brain Research. 2016;**1637**:146-153

[27] Briet M et al. Aldosterone-induced vascular remodeling and endothelial dysfunction require functional angiotensin type 1a receptors. Hypertension. 2016;**67**(5):897-905

[28] Jia G et al. Endothelial mineralocorticoid receptor mediates diet-induced aortic stiffness in females. Circulation Research. 2016;**118**(6):935-943

[29] Jia G et al. Epithelial Sodium Channel in aldosterone-induced endothelium stiffness and aortic dysfunction. Hypertension. 2018;**72**(3):731-738

[30] Beswick RA, Dorrance AM, Leite R, Webb RC. NADH/NADPH oxidase and enhanced superoxide production in the mineralocorticoid hypertensive rat. Hypertension. 2001;**38**(5):1107-1111

[31] Lassègue B, San Martín A, Griendling KK. Biochemistry, physiology, and pathophysiology of NADPH oxidases in the cardiovascular system. Circulation Research. 2012;**110**(10):1364-1390

[32] Nguyen Dinh Cat A, Montezano AC, Burger D, Touyz RM. Angiotensin II, NADPH oxidase, and redox signaling in

the vasculature. Antioxidants & Redox Signaling. 2013;**19**(10):1110-1120

[33] Martin-Ventura JL et al. Oxidative stress in human Atherothrombosis: Sources, markers and therapeutic targets. International Journal of Molecular Sciences. 2017;**18**(11):2315

[34] Park YM, Lim BH, Touyz RM, Park JB. Expression of NAD(P)H oxidase subunits and their contribution to cardiovascular damage in aldosterone/salt-induced hypertensive rat. Journal of Korean Medical Science. 2008;**23**(6):1039-1045

[35] Montezano AC et al. Aldosterone and angiotensin II synergistically stimulate migration in vascular smooth muscle cells through c-Src-regulated redox-sensitive RhoA pathways. Arteriosclerosis, Thrombosis, and Vascular Biology. 2008;**28**(8):1511-1518

[36] Cannavo A et al. Myocardial pathology induced by aldosterone is dependent on non-canonical activities of G protein-coupled receptor kinases. Nature Communications. 2017;**7**:10877

[37] De Giusti VC et al. Aldosterone stimulates the cardiac sodium/bicarbonate cotransporter via activation of the g protein-coupled receptor gpr30. Journal of Molecular and Cellular Cardiology. 2015;**89**(Pt B):260-267

[38] Ashton AW et al. Role of nongenomic signaling pathways activated by aldosterone during cardiac reperfusion injury. Molecular Endocrinology. 2015;**29**(8):1144-1155

[39] Sanz-Rosa D et al. Eplerenone reduces oxidative stress and enhances eNOS in SHR: Vascular functional and structural consequences. Antioxidants & Redox Signaling. 2005;**7**(9-10):1294-1301

[40] Mulder P et al. Aldosterone synthase inhibition improves cardiovascular function and structure in rats with heart failure: A comparison with spironolactone. European Heart Journal. 2008;**29**(17):2171-2179

[41] Silva MA et al. Spironolactone treatment attenuates vascular dysfunction in type 2 diabetic mice by decreasing oxidative stress and restoring NO/GC signaling. Frontiers in Physiology. 2015a;**6**:269

[42] Silva MA et al. Mineralocorticoid receptor blockade prevents vascular remodelling in a rodent model of type 2 diabetes mellitus. Clin Sci. 2015b;**129**(7):533-545

[43] Nguyen Dinh Cat A et al. The endothelial mineralocorticoid receptor regulates vasoconstrictor tone and blood pressure. The FASEB Journal. 2010;**24**(7):2454-2463

[44] Davel AP, Anwar IJ, Jaffe IZ. The endothelial mineralocorticoid receptor: Mediator of the switch from vascular health to disease. Current Opinion in Nephrology and Hypertension. 2017;**26**(2):97-104

[45] Davel AP et al. Sex-specific mechanisms of resistance vessel endothelial dysfunction induced by cardiometabolic risk factors. Journal of the American Heart Association. 2018;**7**(4):e007675. DOI: 10.1161/JAHA.117.007675

[46] McCurley A et al. Direct regulation of blood pressure by smooth muscle cell mineralocorticoid receptors. Nature Medicine. 2012;**18**(9):1429-1433

[47] Gueret A et al. Vascular smooth muscle mineralocorticoid receptor contributes to coronary and left ventricular dysfunction after myocardial infarction. Hypertension. 2016;**67**(4):717-723

[48] Min LJ et al. Cross-talk between aldosterone and angiotensin II in vascular smooth muscle cell senescence. Cardiovascular Research. 2007;**76**(3):506-516

[49] Sherajee SJ et al. Aldosterone induces vascular insulin resistance by increasing insulin-like growth factor-1 receptor and hybrid receptor. Arteriosclerosis, Thrombosis, and Vascular Biology. 2012;**32**(2):257-263

[50] Sun Y et al. Aldosterone-induced inflammation in the rat heart: Role of oxidative stress. The American Journal of Pathology. 2002;**161**(5):1773-1781

[51] Nakano S, Kobayashi N, Yoshida K, Ohno T, Matsuoka H. Cardioprotective mechanisms of spironolactone associated with the angiotensin-converting enzyme/epidermal growth factor receptor/extracellular signal-regulated kinases, NAD(P)H oxidase/lectin-like oxidized low-density lipoprotein receptor-1, and rho-kinase pathways in aldosterone/salt-induced hypertensive rats. Hypertension Research. 2005;**28**(11):925-936

[52] Newfell BG et al. Aldosterone regulates vascular gene transcription via oxidative stress-dependent and -independent pathways. Arteriosclerosis, Thrombosis, and Vascular Biology. 2011;**31**(8):1871-1880

[53] Harvey AP et al. Vascular dysfunction and fibrosis in stroke-prone spontaneously hypertensive rats: The aldosterone-mineralocorticoid receptor-Nox1 axis. Life Sciences. 2017;**179**:110-119

[54] Hirono Y et al. Angiotensin II receptor type 1-mediated vascular oxidative stress and proinflammatory gene expression in aldosterone-induced hypertension: The possible role of local renin-angiotensin system. Endocrinology. 2007;**148**(4):1688-1696

[55] Vanhoutte PM, Zhao Y, Xu A, Leung SW. Thirty Years of saying NO: Sources, fate, actions, and misfortunes of the endothelium-derived vasodilator mediator. Circulation Research. 2016;**119**(2):375-396

[56] Förstermann U, Xia N, Li H. Roles of vascular oxidative stress and nitric oxide in the pathogenesis of atherosclerosis. Circulation Research. 2017;**120**(4):713-735

[57] Leopold JA et al. Aldosterone impairs vascular reactivity by decreasing glucose-6-phosphate dehydrogenase activity. Nature Medicine. 2007;**13**(2):189-197

[58] Barrera-Chimal J et al. Sulfenic acid modification of endothelin B receptor is responsible for the benefit of a nonsteroidal mineralocorticoid receptor antagonist in renal ischemia. J Am Soc Nephrol. 2016;**27**(2):398-404

[59] Favre J et al. Coronary endothelial dysfunction after cardiomyocyte-specific mineralocorticoid receptor overexpression. American Journal of Physiology. Heart and Circulatory Physiology. 2011;**300**(6):H2035-H2043

[60] Shibata S et al. Modification of mineralocorticoid receptor function by Rac1 GTPase: Implication in proteinuric kidney disease. Nature Medicine. 2008;**14**(12):1370-1376

[61] Nagase M et al. Oxidative stress causes mineralocorticoid receptor activation in rat cardiomyocytes: Role of small GTPase Rac1. Hypertension. 2012;**59**(2):500-506

[62] Ayuzawa N et al. Rac1-mediated activation of mineralocorticoid receptor in pressure overload-induced cardiac injury. Hypertension. 2016;**67**(1):99-106

[63] McGraw AP et al. Aldosterone increases early atherosclerosis and

promotes plaque inflammation through a placental growth factor-dependent mechanism. Journal of the American Heart Association. 2013;**2**(1):e000018

[64] Marzolla V et al. Essential role of ICAM-1 in aldosterone-induced atherosclerosis. International Journal of Cardiology. 2017;**232**:233-242

[65] Belden Z, Deiuliis JA, Dobre M, Rajagopalan S. The role of the mineralocorticoid receptor in inflammation: Focus on kidney and vasculature. American Journal of Nephrology. 2017;**46**(4):298-314

[66] Ahokas RA et al. Aldosteronism and peripheral blood mononuclear cell activation: A neuroendocrine-immune interface. Circulation Research. 2003;**93**(10):e124-e135

[67] Guzik TJ et al. Role of the T cell in the genesis of angiotensin II induced hypertension and vascular dysfunction. The Journal of Experimental Medicine. 2007;**204**(10):2449-2460

[68] Sun XN et al. T-cell mineralocorticoid receptor controls blood pressure by regulating interferon-gamma. Circulation Research. 2017;**120**(10):1584-1597

[69] Li C et al. Mineralocorticoid receptor deficiency in T cells attenuates pressure overload-induced cardiac hypertrophy and dysfunction through modulating T-cell activation. Hypertension. 2017;**70**(1):137-147

[70] Usher MG et al. Myeloid mineralocorticoid receptor controls macrophage polarization and cardiovascular hypertrophy and remodeling in mice. The Journal of Clinical Investigation. 2010;**120**(9):3350-3364

[71] Bruder-Nascimento T et al. NLRP3 Inflammasome mediates aldosterone-induced vascular damage. Circulation. 2016;**134**(23):1866-1880

[72] Keidar S et al. Aldosterone administration to mice stimulates macrophage NADPH oxidase and increases atherosclerosis development: A possible role for angiotensin-converting enzyme and the receptors for angiotensin II and aldosterone. Circulation. 2004;**109**(18):2213-2220

[73] Kadoya H et al. Excess aldosterone is a critical danger signal for inflammasome activation in the development of renal fibrosis in mice. The FASEB Journal. 2015;**29**(9):3899-3910

[74] Bienvenu LA et al. Macrophage mineralocorticoid receptor signaling plays a key role in aldosterone-independent cardiac fibrosis. Endocrinology. 2012;**153**(7):3416-3425

[75] Shen ZX et al. Mineralocorticoid receptor deficiency in macrophages inhibits atherosclerosis by affecting foam cell formation and efferocytosis. The Journal of Biological Chemistry. 2017;**292**(3):925-935

[76] Sun JY et al. Mineralocorticoid receptor deficiency in macrophages inhibits neointimal hyperplasia and suppresses macrophage inflammation through SGK1-AP1/NF-κB pathways. Arteriosclerosis, Thrombosis, and Vascular Biology. 2016;**36**(5):874-885

[77] Jia G, Aroor AR, Sowers JR. The role of mineralocorticoid receptor signaling in the cross-talk between adipose tissue and the vascular wall. Cardiovascular Research. 2017;**113**(9):1055-1063

[78] Garg R, Adler GK. Aldosterone and the mineralocorticoid receptor: Risk factors for cardiometabolic disorders. Current Hypertension Reports. 2015;**17**(7):52

[79] Fernández-Alfonso MS et al. Role of perivascular adipose tissue in health and disease. Comprehensive Physiology. 2017;**8**(1):23-59

[80] Withers SB et al. Macrophage activation is responsible for loss of anticontractile function in inflamed perivascular fat. Arteriosclerosis, Thrombosis, and Vascular Biology. 2011;**31**(4):908-913

[81] Hirata A et al. Blockade of mineralocorticoid receptor reverses adipocyte dysfunction and insulin resistance in obese mice. Cardiovascular Research. 2009;**84**(1):164-172

[82] Hirata A et al. Contribution of glucocorticoid-mineralocorticoid receptor pathway on the obesity-related adipocyte dysfunction. Biochemical and Biophysical Research Communications. 2012;**419**(2):182-187

[83] Hosoya K et al. Insulin resistance in chronic kidney disease is ameliorated by spironolactone in rats and humans. Kidney International. 2015;**87**(4):749-760

[84] Nguyen Dinh Cat A et al. Adipocyte-specific mineralocorticoid receptor overexpression in mice is associated with metabolic syndrome and vascular dysfunction: Role of redox-sensitive PKG-1 and rho kinase. Diabetes. 2016;**65**(8):2392-2403

[85] Hayakawa T et al. Impact of MR on mature adipocytes in high-fat/high-sucrose diet-induced obesity. The Journal of Endocrinology. 2018;**239**(1):63-71

[86] Feraco A et al. Minor role of mature adipocyte mineralocorticoid receptor in high fat induced obesity. The Journal of Endocrinology. 2018;**239**(2):229-240. DOI: 10.1530/JOE-18-0314 [Epub ahead of print]

[87] Kotlyar E et al. The relationship between aldosterone, oxidative stress, and inflammation in chronic, stable human heart failure. Journal of Cardiac Failure. 2006;**12**(2):122-127

[88] Taye A, Morawietz H. Spironolactone inhibits NADPH oxidase-induced oxidative stress and enhances eNOS in human endothelial cells. Iran J Pharm Res. 2011;**10**(2):329-337

[89] Calò LA et al. Oxidative stress-related proteins in a Conn's adenoma tissue. Relevance for aldosterone's prooxidative and proinflammatory activity. Journal of Endocrinological Investigation. 2010;**33**(1):48-53

[90] Zhou J et al. Transcriptome pathway analysis of pathological and physiological aldosterone-producing human tissues. Hypertension. 2016;**68**(6):1424-1431

[91] Ibarrola J et al. Aldosterone impairs mitochondrial function in human cardiac fibroblasts via A-kinase anchor protein 12. Scientific Reports. 2018;**8**(1):6801

[92] Hwang MH et al. Mineralocorticoid receptors modulate vascular endothelial function in human obesity. Clinical Science. 2013a;**125**(11):513-520

[93] Hwang MH et al. Effect of selective mineralocorticoid receptor blockade on flow-mediated dilation and insulin resistance in older adults with metabolic syndrome. Metabolic Syndrome and Related Disorders. 2015;**13**(8):356-361

[94] Hwang MH et al. Role of mineralocorticoid receptors in arterial stiffness in human aging. Experimental Gerontology. 2013b;**48**(8):701-704

[95] Chen L et al. Impaired endothelial repair capacity of early endothelial progenitor cells in hypertensive patients with primary hyperaldosteronemia: Role of 5,6,7,8-tetrahydrobiopterin oxidation and endothelial nitric oxide synthase uncoupling. Hypertension. 2016;**67**(2):430-439

Chapter 5

# Renin-Angiotensin-Aldosterone System in Heart Failure: Focus on Nonclassical Angiotensin Pathways as Novel Upstream Targets Regulating Aldosterone

*Urszula Tyrankiewicz, Agnieszka Kij, Tasnim Mohaissen, Mariola Olkowicz, Ryszard T. Smolenski and Stefan Chlopicki*

## Abstract

Aldosterone plays an important role in the regulation of blood pressure, body fluid, and electrolyte homeostasis. Overactivation of aldosterone/mineralocorticoid receptor (MR) pathway leads to hypertension, atherosclerosis, vascular damage, heart failure, and chronic kidney disease and is involved in many other diseases associated with endothelial dysfunction, inflammation, fibrosis, and metabolic disorders. Aldosterone is a final product of the renin-angiotensin-aldosterone system (RAAS), and its production is activated by angiotensin II, while angiotensin-(1–7) negatively regulates angiotensin II-mediated aldosterone production and in some experimental models inhibits aldosterone-induced damage in target tissues. In fact, the aldosterone/mineralocorticoid receptor-dependent pathway is regulated upstream by at least two major axes of RAAS: classical axis (ACE/Ang II) and nonclassical axis (ACE2/Ang-(1–7)). The relative balance between these two axes determines aldosterone production and activity. To better understand the regulation of aldosterone activity in physiology and diseases, it is important to analyze the role of aldosterone/mineralocorticoid receptor-dependent pathways in the context of upstream angiotensin pathways as some of the recently described mechanisms of RAAS represent possible novel upstream targets to inhibit aldosterone/mineralocorticoid receptor-dependent responses. In this review, we highlight the complexity of angiotensin pathways focusing on their role in various tissues in heart failure, with particular emphasis on nonclassical pathways including protective ACE2/Ang-(1–7) axis and detrimental Ang-(1–12)/chymase/Ang II axis.

**Keywords:** angiotensin pathways, angiotensin-converting enzyme (ACE), angiotensin-converting enzyme 2 (ACE2), chymase, aldosterone, heart failure

## 1. Introduction

The renin-angiotensin-aldosterone system (RAAS) includes angiotensin (poly) peptides such as angiotensinogen, angiotensin I, angiotensin II, angiotensin III,



IntechOpen

angiotensin IV, angiotensin-(1–9), angiotensin-(1–7), alamandine and angiotensin A [1], and a number of enzymes regulating the production of particular angiotensins (renin, angiotensin-converting enzyme (ACE) and angiotensin-converting enzyme 2 (ACE2), chymase, neutral endopeptidase (NEP), prolyl endopeptidase (PEP), and others) [2–5], as well as specific receptors such as $AT_1R$, $AT_2R$, $AT_4R$, MasR, or MrgDR, activated in response to a given angiotensin sub-type [5]. All these elements contribute to the incredible complexity of the RAAS that is not perceived any more like a simple linear system with two major enzymes (renin and ACE) generating Ang II but rather as a network of tightly regulated peptides and enzymes endowed not only with endocrine (tissue to tissue) but also paracrine (cell-to-cell) and an intracrine (intercellular/nuclear) activities. There is also abundant evidence for the importance of tissue-based angiotensin pathways that seems to be heterogeneously organized in various organs which act independently of the RAAS in plasma. The major role of the protective ACE2/Ang-(1–7) axis counteracting classic ACE/Ang II axis has also been well documented. A simplified scheme of the angiotensin pathways with major angiotensins, enzymes, and receptors is shown in **Figure 1**.

The final RAAS product, aldosterone, plays an important role in the regulation of blood pressure, body fluid, and electrolyte homeostasis, but overactivation of aldosterone/mineralocorticoid receptor (MR) pathway leads to hypertension, atherosclerosis, vascular damage, heart failure, and chronic kidney disease and is involved in many other diseases associated with endothelial dysfunction, inflammation, fibrosis, metabolic disorders, and organ damage [6–9]. The overstimulation of $AT_1R$ (by Ang II and its metabolites) and increased aldosterone production result among others in increased ROS production and NADPH oxidase activation [9, 10] that contribute to cardiac and vascular pathology [11].

The importance of RAAS in cardiovascular, hypertensive, and kidney diseases has been firmly established by therapeutic effects of renin inhibitors,

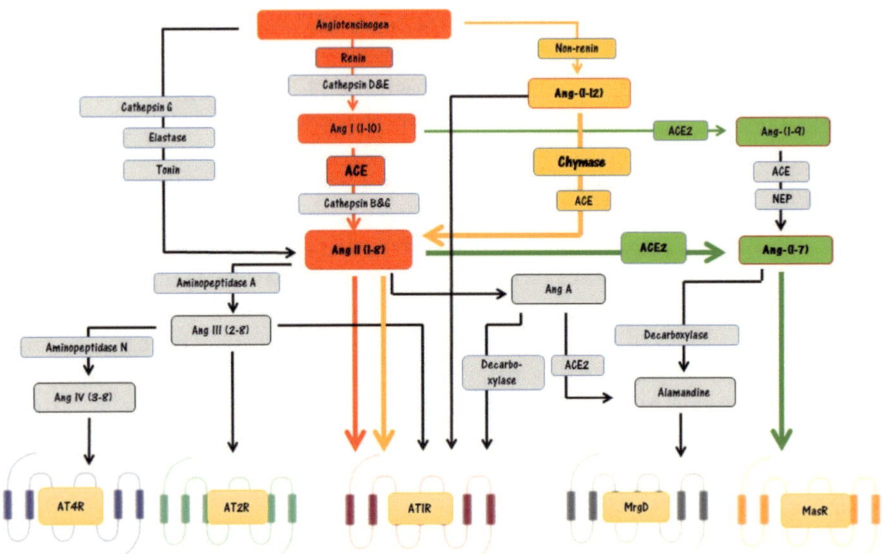


**Figure 1.**
*Simplified scheme of major angiotensin pathways with respective enzymes and receptors. Abbreviations: Ang, angiotensin; ACE, angiotensin-converting enzyme; ACE2, angiotensin-converting enzyme 2; NEP, neutral endopeptidase; AT1R, angiotensin receptor type 1; AT2R, angiotensin receptor type 2; AT4R, angiotensin receptor type 4; MasR, Mas receptor; MrgD, MAS-related G protein-coupled receptor member D. Colors: Red, classical axis (renin/ACE/Ang II); green, nonclassical protective axis (ACE2/Ang-(1–7); orange, non-renin non-ACE, chymase-dependent axis Ang-(1–12)/chymase/Ang II axis; gray, other elements.*

angiotensin-converting enzyme inhibitors (ACE-I), angiotensin receptor blockers (ARBs), and finally mineralocorticoid receptor antagonists (MRA). Importantly, these drugs influence not only the downstream but also the upstream activity of the RAAS. This phenomenon is rather overlooked but needs to be taken into account in designing the optimal RAAS-targeted therapy for the treatment of a variety of diseases. In particular, evidence accumulated showing reciprocal regulation of major angiotensins and aldosterone/mineralocorticoid pathway (**Figure 2**).

Indeed, MRA modify upstream pathways. MRA decrease ACE activity and increase ACE2 activity, suggesting a protective role for MRA is not only mediated by the direct inhibition of MR-dependent pathways but also by increasing the expression of ACE2 and generating angiotensin-(1–7) and decreasing the formation of angiotensin II as documented in heart failure (HF) patients and in the rat model of renal dysfunction [12–14]. Noteworthy, plasma levels of Ang-(1–7) increase after treatment with ACE-I or ARB [15–20]. On the other hand, aldosterone upregulates the expression and activity of upstream ACE [21]. Furthermore, aldosterone-induced accelerated production of an angiotensin II is negatively regulated by angiotensin-(1–7) via the Mas receptor and JAK/STAT signaling in human adrenal cells [22]. Angiotensin-(1–7) may also suppress aldosterone-induced damage in target tissues. For example, angiotensin-(1–7) inhibits hypertensive kidney damage induced by infusion of aldosterone [23]. Interestingly, this effect is independent of blood pressure and mediated by the suppression of the expression of TGF, FGF, TIMP, and ROS production suggesting that the inhibition of aldosterone activity by angiotensin-(1–7) occurs locally in the kidney [23]. Angiotensin-(1–7) may inhibit angiotensin II-mediated effects on aldosterone not only by counterbalancing effects mediated by the activation of Mas receptor [23] but also by acting as natural-biased ligand for the $AT_1$ receptor, behaving as a natural competitive neutral antagonist for $AT_1$ in G protein-dependent signaling while simultaneously acting as an agonist for β-arrestin-related signaling [24].

In summary, aldosterone/mineralocorticoid receptor-dependent signaling pathways are under upstream regulation by at least two major axes of the RAAS: classical axis (ACE/Ang II) and nonclassical axis (ACE2/Ang-(1–7)). The relative ratio of these two axes determines aldosterone production and activity, and reciprocally aldosterone production might affect upstream mechanisms of RAAS. For the better understanding of the regulation of aldosterone/mineralocorticoid receptor-dependent pathways and optimal pharmacotherapy of diseases associated with aldosterone overactivation, one needs to take into account the regulatory

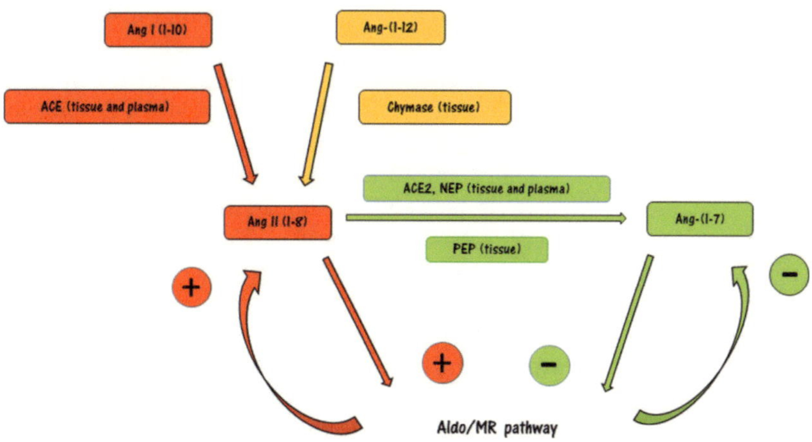


**Figure 2.**
*Scheme showing the reciprocal regulation of major angiotensins and aldosterone/mineralocorticoid pathway. Abbreviations: PEP, prolyl endopeptidase (see **Figure 1** for other abbreviations and colors coding).*

role of at least two major angiotensin pathways, the balance of which determines aldosterone/mineralocorticoid receptor-dependent pathways. Here, we review the complexity of local angiotensin pathways focusing on their role in various tissues in heart failure with particular emphasis on nonclassical pathways including protective ACE2/Ang-(1–7) axis and detrimental Ang-(1–12)/chymase/Ang II axis.

## 2. Classical (ACE/Ang II/$AT_1R$) and nonclassical (ACE2/Ang-(1–7)/MasR) axes of RAAS

The classical RAAS pathway involves renin secreted by the kidney to produce Ang I from angiotensinogen (derived from the liver) (**Figures 1** and **2**). Ang I is then converted mainly through ACE to Ang II which predominantly stimulates the $AT_1$ receptor, the major culprit receptor for Ang II-induced cardiovascular pathology. Indeed, overactivation of $AT_1R$ contributes to the pathophysiology of heart failure inducing cardiac fibrosis, inflammation, cell proliferation, coronary vasoconstriction, and cardiomyocyte hypertrophy, as well as apoptosis [25], cardiac remodeling [25, 26], vascular stiffness and atherosclerosis [27], endothelial dysfunction, oxidative stress, or insulin resistance [28]. Ang II may also stimulate $AT_2R$ that has a vasoprotective profile—anti-inflammatory, antifibrotic, and anti-apoptotic—involving the activation of bradykinin/NO/cGMP system [29]. $AT_2R$ is linked also to the regulation of vascular and cardiac growth responses [30]. Activation of $AT_2R$ after cardiac injury decreases sympathetic overstimulation and stimulates cardiac regeneration with increasing coronary vasodilation [31]. It was also shown that $AT_2R$ stimulation may indirectly increase ACE2 activity, Ang-(1–7), and MasR expression level [32]. Additionally, in physiological conditions, $AT_2R$ may downregulate [33] or directly inhibit $AT_1R$ [34–36]; however, physiological $AT_2R$ activation occurs mostly at embryonal stage (responsible for fetus development), while in adulthood $AT_2R$ expression is low [36, 37]. Nevertheless, it may still be detectable in different organs, including the heart in particular in pathological conditions. Both $AT_1R$ and $AT_2R$ are located on cell surfaces or nuclear membranes [38–40].

The second dominant RAAS pathway opposing the classical axis (ACE/Ang II/$AT_1R$) is the ACE2-dependent pathway, leading to the generation of Ang-(1–7) acting on Mas receptors. The major player in this system, ACE2, converts Ang I to Ang-(1–9), Ang II to Ang-(1–7), and Ang A to alamandine [41]. Ang-(1–7) is the main opposing signaling peptide to Ang II with a broad range of effects in different organs. The most significant activity of Ang-(1–7) includes vasodilation and anti-proliferative and anti-inflammatory effects that are mediated by Mas receptors [42]. Alamandine (the product of Ang A and Ang-(1–7)), despite its similarity in function to Ang-(1–7), acts on different receptors identified as Mas-related G protein-coupled receptor member D (MrgDR) [43]. Both of these vasoprotective angiotensins induce endothelial-dependent vasorelaxation and central nervous system-dependent cardiovascular effects [41], but their activity is not always identical [44, 45]. Importantly, the Mas receptor was found in cardiomyocytes and cardiac endothelial cells [46–48], as well as on cardiac fibroblasts [49]. MasR genetic deletion leads to impairment of cardiac function and endothelial dysfunction pointing to the important protective role of this receptor in cardiac and vascular physiology. Although there is equivocal evidence that Ang-(1–7) has vasoprotective, cardioprotective, and anti-inflammatory effects, still it is not clear if all of the effects of ACE2 pathway are mediated by Ang-(1–7) and by MasR. Ang-(1–7), alamandine, and bradykinin could act in concert as their concentrations increase simultaneously with decreased ACE/ACE2 ratio and Ang-(1–7)-mediated effects in some systems are inhibited by $B_2$ receptor antagonists [50]. Although evidence supporting the protective role of ACE2/Ang-(1–7) axis is convincing, it is still not clear if ACE2 is the only enzyme that plays a key role in Ang-(1–7) generation in various pathologies.

The major difference between ACE and ACE2 (which are quite similar in structure: 42% of amino acids are identical in the extracellular domain) is that ACE acts as dipeptidyl carboxypeptidase (removing a dipeptide from the C-terminus of substrate), while ACE2 acts as a mono-carboxypeptidase (removing a single amino acid) [2, 3]. Both enzymes are type I transmembrane proteins with an extracellular N-terminal domain containing the catalytic site and an intracellular C-terminal tail. ACE inhibitors do not act on ACE2 catalytic activity, the latter is affected by MLN 4760, a prototypic ACE2 inhibitor [51]. In the healthy heart, ACE2 is present in cardiomyocytes, fibroblasts, and coronary endothelial cells [52], while ACE is mainly found in endothelial cells [53]. ACE2 catalytic efficiency is 400-fold higher with Ang II as a substrate than with Ang I, suggesting a dominant role for ACE2 in Ang II metabolism as compared with Ang I metabolism. In this way, ACE2 counterbalances ACE activity mainly at the level of Ang II. In fact, ACE increases Ang II levels, and ACE2 decreases Ang II levels resulting in the activation of MasR instead of $AT_1R$. The relative significance of ACE2 converting Ang I to Ang-(1–9) and Ang A to alamandine seems to be of less importance, but further studies are needed.

The discovery of ACE2 in 2000 [3] and subsequent studies documenting opposite actions of ACE2/Ang-(1–7)/MasR axis as compared to ACE/Ang II/$AT_1R$ axis have revealed this pathway as a major protective arm of RAAS.

## 3. Other angiotensin pathways, enzymes, and receptors

In addition to ACE/Ang II/$AT_1$ and ACE2/Ang-(1–7)/MasR axes, the couple of other angiotensin axes has been proposed as important counterparts of RAAS including the protective axes of Ang III/aminopeptidase N(APN)/Ang IV/insulin-regulated aminopeptidase (IRAP)/$AT_4R$ and Ang II/aminopeptidase A(APA)/Ang III/$AT_2R$/NO/cGMP [54] (**Figure 1**). Additionally, the prorenin/renin/prorenin receptor was proposed to constitute an important vasopressor pathway in addition to the ACE/Ang II/$AT_1$ axis, with an emerging role for the prorenin receptor (PRR) [55] that may affect intracellular signaling pathways in an angiotensin-independent manner [56, 57]. On the other hand, the generation of Ang III stimulating directly $AT_2R$ and $AT_4R$ after conversion of Ang III to Ang IV represents a novel vasoprotective arm of angiotensin pathways regulating RAAS with vasodilator properties, as well as promoting endothelial cell proliferation [58, 59].

Additionally, intracellular Ang II in various tissues may be generated in a non-ACE-dependent way from Ang-(1–12) via chymase, particularly in pathological conditions [59, 60] (**Figure 1**). The detrimental effects of Ang-(1–12)/chymase/Ang II axis seem to play an important role, for example, in heart failure [61]. Ang-(1–12) when activated may lead to tissue remodeling and potentiated vascular as well as cardiac contractility [62, 63]. The independence of intracellular Ang II production from extracellular system was confirmed by studies showing that chronic administration of losartan and lisinopril did not influence cardiac Ang II content, despite antihypertensive effects of these treatments linked to circulating angiotensins [59].

Many other enzymes are also implicated in the generation of Ang II (besides ACE and chymase), including chymostatin-sensitive Ang II-generating enzyme

(CAGE), endopeptidase-2, meprin [64], cathepsins D and G, or tonin [65–67]. Various types of aminopeptidases (-A,-N,-M,-B) were suggested to take part in the generation of Ang III or Ang IV. Production of Ang-(1–9) may be mediated by carboxypeptidase A (CP-A) or cathepsin, while the generation of Ang-(1–7) can occur by activation of prolyl endopeptidase (PEP), neutral endopeptidase [68], neprilysin (NEP) [69–71], or thimet oligopeptidase (TOP) [72]. Prolyl endopeptidase has also an influence on tissue angiotensins which makes it an interesting target for pharmacotherapy [73].

The physiological and pathophysiological relevance of these multiple enzymes in the regulation of the angiotensin pathways influencing the RAAS network as well as the pathophysiological importance of prorenin/renin/prorenin receptor pathways (**Figure 1**) still needs to be delineated. Currently, among nonclassical pathways influencing angiotensin pathways, protective ACE2/Ang-(1–7)/MasR axis and detrimental Ang-(1–12)/chymase/Ang II axis are best characterized and seem to play a major role in heart failure. Both of them could influence the activity of aldosterone/mineralocorticoid receptor-dependent pathways (**Figure 2**).

## 4. Alterations of RAAS in heart failure

It is well known that overactivation of RAAS plays a crucial role in heart failure progression, while the inhibition of RAAS (by ACE-I, ARB, and MRA) represents a cornerstone for the current pharmacotherapy of HF [74]. It is clear that systemic RAAS and local angiotensin pathways in tissues act independently as alterations in systemic and tissue-derived angiotensins in HF progression do not coincide. Moreover, the range of concentrations of angiotensins in plasma and tissue differs, that is, cardiac Ang II concentration is about 100-fold higher than that of plasma [75]. This phenomenon may result from intrinsic cardiac Ang I production, which was estimated to represent about 90% of cardiac Ang I and about 75% cardiac Ang II [76], the rest being regulated by RAAS components taken to the tissue from the systemic circulation, for example, by plasma-derived renin [77]. Cardiac intrinsic angiotensin pathway activity gains particular importance in course of heart failure, activating additional mechanisms leading to increased Ang II production [78]. Cardiac intrinsic angiotensin pathways are upregulated in HF progression mainly through increased ACE/ACE2 ratio, leading to excessive Ang II production and through activation of intracellular chymase-dependent axis responsible for additional Ang II production [53, 79]. Both of these pathways lead to cardiac Ang II generation and $AT_1R$ stimulation.

Indeed, apart from ACE the second major cardiac intrinsic mechanism leading to excessive Ang II production in course of HF utilizes an intracellular source of Ang-(1–12) and chymase (present in different cell types, including mast cells, cardiac fibroblasts, and vascular endothelial cells [87, 88]). In HF, chymase-dependent conversion of Ang-(1–12) to Ang II [4, 62, 89–91] was proposed to play a role of an independent intracrine pathway accounting for trophic, contractile, and pro-arrhythmic effects of Ang II in the human heart as well as in resistance arteries [92]. Interestingly, it was shown that MR antagonists decrease Ang-(1–12) production and by this may additionally decrease the detrimental effects of Ang II [14]. The combined inhibition of chymase and ACE compared to ACE inhibition alone provided an added benefit in terms of left ventricular function and adverse cardiac remodeling [93, 94]. Chymase-specific inhibitor improved cardiac function in human myocardial infarction (MI) [95] and significantly attenuated cardiac diastolic dysfunction accompanied by fibrosis in an experimental dog model of tachycardiac-induced HF [96]. There is also evidence for local (intracellular) chymase activity that generates Ang II in the vascular wall [73, 95]. In relation to ACE, chymase is much more specific in Ang II production and does not break down bradykinin [87, 88, 97]. In contrast to ACE, chymase is not present in plasma and contributes only to tissue-based angiotensin pathways [87]. There is evidence for ACE inhibition-dependent chymase activation, which may explain a secondary increase in Ang II level in a large group of patients treated with ACE-I [93, 98].

In contrast to ACE and chymase, ACE2 has cardioprotective effects (influencing left ventricle remodeling and function) in HF [80]. In turn, loss of ACE2 leads to deterioration of cardiac function [81] and deleterious effects linked to increased Ang II production [49]. The ACE2 activity may be regulated by cardiac sheddases, which are located near ACE2 in the cellular membrane and their activation results in the secretion of a soluble form of tissue ACE2 into the circulation and decreases its activity in the heart. ADAM 17 (known as TACE) was proposed to act as a local sheddase [82, 83]. In humans, there are 21 sheddases described, among them 13 are proteolytically active [84], suggesting that besides ADAM 17 there may be other sheddases involved in ACE2 regulation. Shedding of ACE2 may be stimulated by Ang II acting through $AT_1R$, which induces phosphorylation and activation of ADAM 17. Circulating soluble form of ACE2 was recognized as one of the markers of worsening HF prognosis [85, 86] that, in our opinion, might reflect the increased shedding of ACE2 from the heart and dominance of ACE/Ang II/$AT_1$ axis in the heart.

In our recent study [99], in a unique murine model of HF that is characterized by a long-term development of end-stage HF [100], we demonstrated that changes in the profile of systemic versus tissue angiotensin pathways seem independent of each other. As shown in **Figure 3**, a significant increase in local Ang-(1–7) and alamandine content in the heart and aorta was observed at the early stage of HF and was followed by a decrease of Ang-(1–7) and alamandine in the heart and in the aorta at the late HF stage with simultaneous increase in Ang-(1–12). We concluded that HF progression in this murine model of HF was associated with a pronounced activation of the local ACE/Ang II pathway that was counterbalanced by a prominent ACE2/Ang-(1–7) activation with distinct pattern of changes in ACE/ACE2 balance in plasma. We tempted to speculate that the dominance of ACE2/Ang-(1–7) over ACE/Ang II in the adaptive phase of HF may contribute to the late onset of apparent cardiac dysfunction in this model and the balance between ACE/Ang II and ACE2/Ang-(1–7) in favor of the first axis determines the progression to the end stage of heart failure. Interestingly, the balance between ACE/Ang II and ACE2/Ang-(1–7) seems to correspond with aldosterone plasma concentration, low in the early phase and increased at the end stage of HF in this model (unpublished data).

Up to 45% of patients with reduced ejection fraction present elevated plasma angiotensin II levels despite ACE-I and MRA therapy [101, 102]. Moreover, for heart failure patients, with preserved ejection fraction and diastolic disturbance (which form up to 40% of HF patients), ACE-I are much less effective [103]. Lack of sufficient effectiveness of ACE-I and MRA therapy seems to support the notion of an ACE-independent local angiotensin pathway that may independently regulate Ang II production as well as $AT_1R$ stimulation and may represent an important contributing mechanism to heart failure progression. Clearly, the Ang II-generating mechanisms in HF are not well-controlled by current therapy, and this is also one of the reasons why additional treatment with MRA is frequently required and highly effective in HF patients.

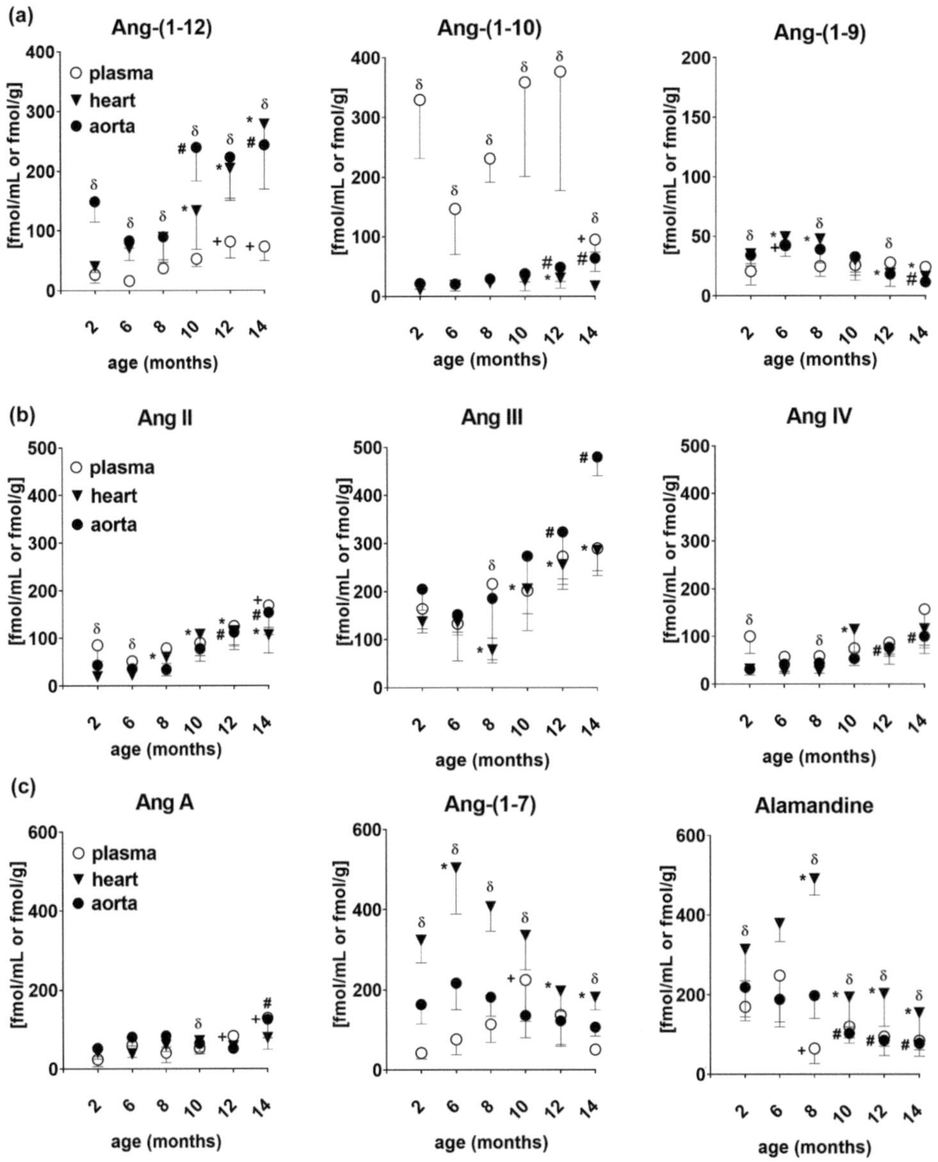


**Figure 3.**
*Angiotensin profile in plasma, the heart, and the aorta in Tgαq*44 mice. Concentration of Ang-(1–12), Ang-(1–10), and Ang-(1–9) (a), Ang II, Ang III and Ang IV (b), Ang A, Ang-(1–7), and alamandine (c) in plasma, aorta, and heart homogenates. *P < 0.05 for the heart tissue of a given group of Tgαq*44 mice vs. 2-month-old Tgαq*44 mice; #P < 0.05 for the aorta tissue of a given Tgαq*44 group vs. 2-month-old Tgαq*44 mice; +P < 0.05 for plasma of a given Tgαq*44 group vs. 2-month-old Tgαq*44 mice (one-way ANOVA with Tukey post hoc test or Kruskal-Wallis); δP < 0.05 hearts vs. plasma (t-test or Wilcoxon test). Reprinted with permission from [99].*

## 5. Quantification of angiotensin peptides and clinical needs

To better understand the regulation of angiotensin pathways and its impact on aldosterone/mineralocorticoid receptor-dependent pathways, the reliable quantification of endogenous angiotensin peptides is needed, in particular for angiotensins that are representatives of classical ACE/Ang II and nonclassical ACE2/Ang-(1–7) pathways. As the physiological levels of angiotensin peptides in biological samples are extremely low (fmol/mL in plasma or fmol/g tissue in organs), the analytical approaches require very sensitive methods among which enzyme-linked immunosorbent assay (ELISA), radioimmunoassay (RIA), and liquid chromatography combined with RIA (LC-RIA) or mass spectrometry detection (LC-MS) are used so far (**Table 1**).

| Origin | Angiotensin peptides (endogenous level in healthy subjects*) | Analytical approach | Ref. |
|---|---|---|---|
| *Plasma* | | | |
| **Mouse** | **Ang II** (24–215 fmol); **Ang-(1–7)** (ca. 142 fmol) | ELISA | [109, 110] |
| | **Ang I** (20–328 fmol); **Ang II** (15–48 fmol) | LC-RIA | [99, 111] |
| | **Alamandine** (40–263 fmol); **Ang I** (57–180 fmol)<br>**Ang II** (28–86 fmol); **Ang III** (50–176 fmol)<br>**Ang IV** (35–118 fmol); **Ang A** (10–50 fmol)<br>**Ang-(1–12)** (8–75 fmol); **Ang-(1–9)** (8–46 fmol)<br>**Ang-(1–7)** (23–72 fmol) | LC-MS | [99, 106] |
| **Rat** | **Ang II** (72–95 pmol) | ELISA | [112, 113] |
| | **Ang I** (40–137 fmol); **Ang II** (25–130 fmol) | RIA | [114, 115] |
| | **Ang I** (10–130 fmol); **Ang II** (5–30 fmol)<br>**Ang III** (4–8 fmol); **Ang IV** (2.5–7 fmol)<br>**Ang-(2–10)** (26–70 fmol); **Ang-(1–9)** (2–6 fmol)<br>**Ang-(3–10)** (5–30 fmol); **Ang-(1–7)** (1.4–15 fmol)<br>**Ang-(2–7)** (2.6–7 fmol); **Ang-(3–7)** (ca. 8 fmol)<br>**Ang-(4–8)** (ca. 8 fmol) | LC-RIA | [116–120] |
| **Human** | **Ang-(4–10)** (ca. 16 fmol); **Ang-(5–10)** (ca. 80 fmol)<br>**Ang-(6–10)** (ca. 12 nmol) | FLD-EIA | [121] |
| | **Ang II** (ca. 18 fmol) | LC-MS | [122] |
| | **Ang I** (ca. 20 fmol); **Ang II** (ca. 14 fmol)<br>**Ang III** (ca. 3.0 fmol); **Ang-(1–9)** (<0.4 fmol)<br>**Ang-(2–10)** (ca. 2.4 fmol); **Ang-(2–9)** (<2.1 fmol)<br>**Ang-(1–7)** (1.0–9.5 fmol); **Ang-(2–7)** (<1.1 fmol) | LC-RIA | [123, 124] |
| *Serum* | | | |
| **Rat** | **Ang II** (42–87 fmol); **Ang-(1–7)** (2220–6310 fmol) | CZE-PDA | [125] |
| *Urine* | | | |
| **Rat** | **Ang I** (ca. 0.5 pmol); **Ang II** (ca. 1.25 pmol)<br>**Ang-(1–7)** (ca. 0.5 pmol) | RIA | [115] |
| **Human** | **Ang-(1–7)** (ca. 0.11 pmol) | LC-RIA | [126] |
| *Kidney* | | | |
| **Mouse** | **Ang I** (60–184 fmol); **Ang II** (159–328 fmol) | LC-RIA | [111, 127] |
| **Rat** | **Ang I** (52–1050 fmol); **Ang II** (90–250 fmol)<br>**Ang III** (ca. 50 fmol); **Ang IV** (ca. 6 fmol)<br>**Ang-(1–9)** (ca. 64 fmol); **Ang-(2–10)** (ca. 300 fmol)<br>**Ang-(3–10)** (ca. 90 fmol); **Ang-(1–7)** (24–120 fmol)<br>**Ang-(2–7)** (ca. 50 fmol) | LC-RIA | [117, 118, 128] |
| *Adrenal gland* | | | |
| **Mouse** | **Ang I** (ca. 7 fmol); **Ang II** (ca. 300 fmol) | LC-RIA | [111] |
| **Rat** | **Ang I** (6–180 fmol); **Ang II** (545–2000 fmol)<br>**Ang III** (ca. 150 fmol); **Ang IV** (ca. 10 fmol)<br>**Ang-(1–9)** (<62 fmol); **Ang-(2–10)** (3–80 fmol)<br>**Ang-(3–10)** (ca. 3 fmol); **Ang-(1–7)** (30–180 fmol)<br>**Ang-(2–7)** (15–40 fmol); **Ang-(3–7)** (ca. 90 fmol) | LC-RIA | [117, 118, 128] |

| Origin | Angiotensin peptides (endogenous level in healthy subjects*) | Analytical approach | Ref. |
|---|---|---|---|
| *Lungs* | | | |
| **Mouse** | **Ang I** (ca. 5 fmol); **Ang II** (ca. 90 fmol) | LC-RIA | [111] |
| **Rat** | **Ang I** (2–3 fmol); **Ang II** (70–90 fmol)<br>**Ang-(1–9)** (ca. 4.6 fmol); **Ang-(1–7)** (<4.4 fmol) | LC-RIA | [117, 128] |
| *Liver* | | | |
| **Mouse** | **Ang I** (1.9–39 fmol); **Ang II** (42–204 fmol) | LC-RIA | [127] |
| *Heart* | | | |
| **Mouse** | **Ang I** (5.3–36 fmol); **Ang II** (49–201fmol) | LC-RIA | [111, 127] |
| | **Alamandine** (70–320 fmol); **Ang I** (5–50 fmol)<br>**Ang II** (10–100 fmol); **Ang III** (50–150 fmol)<br>**Ang IV** (15–35 fmol); **Ang A** (25–55 fmol)<br>**Ang-(1–12)** (20–280 fmol); **Ang-(1–9)** (35–50 fmol)<br>**Ang-(1–7)** (125–330 fmol) | LC-MS | [99, 106] |
| **Rat** | **Ang I** (5–25 fmol); **Ang II** (6–20 fmol);<br>**Ang III** (ca. 5 fmol); **Ang IV** (ca. 1 fmol);<br>**Ang-(1–9)** (<3.8 fmol)<br>**Ang-(2–10)** (ca. 2.5 fmol); **Ang-(3–10)** (ca. 2 fmol)<br>**Ang-(1–7)** (3.5–8 fmol); **Ang-(2–7)** (ca. 5 fmol) | LC-RIA | [117, 120, 128] |
| *Brain* | | | |
| **Mouse** | **Ang I** (ca. 2 fmol); **Ang II** (ca. 5 fmol) | LC-RIA | [111] |
| **Rat** | **Ang I** (<4 fmol); **Ang II** (8–16 fmol)<br>**Ang-(1–9)** (ca. 20 fmol); **Ang-(1–7)** (<13 fmol) | LC-RIA | [117, 128] |
| **Rat (medulla)** | **Ang I** (1.5–520 fmol); **Ang II** (3–900 fmol)<br>**Ang III** (ca. 3 fmol); **Ang IV** (ca. 90 fmol)<br>**Ang-(2–10)** (1.2–80 fmol); **Ang-(3–10)** (1.4–45 fmol)<br>**Ang-(1–7)** (5–720 fmol); **Ang-(2–7)** (ca. 7 fmol)<br>**Ang-(3–7)** (ca. 180 fmol) | LC-RIA | [116, 120] |
| *Aorta* | | | |
| **Mouse** | **Alamandine** (ca. 185 fmol); **Ang I** (ca. 16 fmol)<br>**Ang II** (ca. 15 fmol); **Ang III** (ca. 122 fmol)<br>**Ang IV** (ca. 30 fmol); **Ang A** (ca. 52 fmol)<br>**Ang-(1–12)** (ca. 57 fmol); **Ang-(1–9)** (ca. 25 fmol)<br>**Ang-(1–7)** (ca. 240 fmol) | LC-MS | [99] |
| **Rat** | **Ang I** (<10 fmol); **Ang II** (76–200 fmol)<br>**Ang-(1–9)** (<19 fmol); **Ang-(1–7)** (<20 fmol) | LC-RIA | [117, 128] |
| *Adipose* | | | |
| **Rat (BAT)** | **Ang I** (ca. 8 fmol); **Ang II** (42–60 fmol)<br>**Ang-(1–9)** (ca. 8 fmol); **Ang-(1–7)** (<8 fmol) | LC-RIA | [117, 128] |
| **Rat (WAT)** | **Ang II** (18–56 pmol); **Ang-(1–7)** (190–648 pmol) | CZE-PDA | [125] |

**The range of Ang peptides endogenous levels in healthy subjects was roughly estimated based on published data and expressed per milliliter (mL) of plasma, per mg of creatinine excreted per day for urine, and per g of tissue for organs; BAT, brown adipose tissue; WA, white adipose tissue; LC-RI, liquid chromatography combined with radioimmunoassay; LC-MS, liquid chromatography combined with mass spectrometry; RIA, radioimmunoassay; FLD-EIA, immunofluorescence assay; CZE-PDA, capillary zone electrophoresis with PDA detection.*

**Table 1.**
*The range of endogenous levels of angiotensin peptides in various biological matrices and the most commonly used analytical approaches for their quantification.*

The immunoassay-based methods have many drawbacks, among others, being the lack of specific antibodies as the antibodies used currently in ELISA kits for Ang II quantification cross-react with Ang III (36–100%), Ang IV

(33–100%), and Ang A (100%) which leads to the overestimation of the real concentration of Ang II in measured samples and does not allow to discern the role of individual angiotensin peptides. The limitations of immunoassay-based approaches are overcome by a highly specific, sensitive LC-MS technique. As LC-MS relies on the initial identification of studied peptides based on their molecular weight followed by detection of peptide fragmentation signatures, this approach is highly specific for individual angiotensins [105, 106]. Indeed, in a number of studies including our own [99, 106–108], LC-MS enabled a comprehensive analysis of various angiotensin peptides in in vivo, in vitro, and ex vivo studies (**Table 1**).

It seems that the pattern of Ang peptides measured in plasma could be of the clinical value and LC-MS could offer adequate analytical potential to foster development of angiotensin profiling in clinical field. After optimization, introduction of such analyses into the clinic may provide fundamental information in many current clinical challenges such as treatment of resistant hypertension or reversal of pathological cardiac remodeling. At the same time, angiotensin profiling could lead to a better understanding of upstream mechanisms of classical and nonclassical pathways of RAAS in the regulation of aldosterone/mineralocorticoid receptor-dependent pathways.

## 6. Conclusion

The diverse role of the aldosterone/mineralocorticoid receptor-dependent pathway in physiology and pathology needs to be analyzed in the context of the increasingly complex network of angiotensins. In fact a number of noncanonical mechanisms of angiotensin pathways represent possible novel upstream targets to inhibit aldosterone/mineralocorticoid receptor-dependent pathways, for example, the ACE2/Ang-(1–7) pathway and their novel regulatory elements such as sheddases (ADAM 17) or apelin (which increases ACE2 promotor activity) [129], as well as Ang-(1–12)/chymase/Ang II pathway. As expected, interventions blocking Ang-(1–12)/chymase/Ang II as well as enhancing ACE2/Ang-(1–7) diminished aldosterone production [124, 130]. It remains to be determined, however, which of the novel pharmacotherapies, shown to be effective in experimental heart failure including chymase inhibitors [131], recombinant human ACE2 [132–134], Ang-(1–7) [135], or combined angiotensin receptor antagonist and neprilysin inhibitor (ARNI) [104], are most effective in reducing the activity of aldosterone/mineralocorticoid receptor-dependent signaling. To exploit further these novel mechanisms pharmacotherapeutically, it is important to better understand the heterogeneity of local angiotensin pathways in various organs and their effects on aldosterone/mineralocorticoid receptor-dependent pathways.

Finally, we believe that the profiling of angiotensins in clinical facilities, at least for these two angiotensins (i.e., Ang II, Ang-(1–7)) with opposite actions on MR and aldosterone production, may prove to be a good tool to optimize the pharmacotherapy of RAAS including treatment with MRA.

## Acknowledgements

This publication is based upon work from the EU COST Action ADMIRE BM1301 in aldosterone and mineralocorticoid receptor (MR) physiology and pathophysiology (www.admirecosteu.com).

## Author details

Urszula Tyrankiewicz[1], Agnieszka Kij[1], Tasnim Mohaissen[1], Mariola Olkowicz[2], Ryszard T. Smolenski[3] and Stefan Chlopicki[1,4*]

1 Jagiellonian Centre for Experimental Therapeutics, Jagiellonian University, Krakow, Poland

2 Department of Chemistry, University of Waterloo, Waterloo, Ontario, Canada

3 Department of Biochemistry, Medical University of Gdansk, Gdansk, Poland

4 Chair of Pharmacology, Jagiellonian University Medical College, Krakow, Poland

*Address all correspondence to: stefan.chlopicki@jcet.eu

## References

[1] Patel S, Rauf A, Khan H, Abu-Izneid T. Renin-angiotensin-aldosterone (RAAS): The ubiquitous system for homeostasis and pathologies. Biomedicine & Pharmacotherapy. 2017;**94**:317-325

[2] Tipnis SR, Hooper NM, Hyde R, Karran E, Christie G, Turner AJ. A human homolog of angiotensin-converting enzyme. Cloning and functional expression as a captopril-insensitive carboxypeptidase. Journal of Biological Chemistry. 2000;**275**(43):33238-33243

[3] Donoghue M, Hsieh F, Baronas E, Godbout K, Gosselin M, Stagliano N, et al. A novel angiotensin-converting enzyme-related carboxypeptidase (ACE2) converts angiotensin I to angiotensin 1-9. Circulation Research. 2000;**87**(5):E1-E9

[4] Ahmad S, Varagic J, Groban L, Dell'Italia LJ, Nagata S, Kon ND, et al. Angiotensin-(1-12): A chymase-mediated cellular angiotensin II substrate. Current Hypertension Reports. 2014;**16**(5):429

[5] Holappa M, Vapaatalo H, Vaajanen A. Many faces of renin-angiotensin system—Focus on eye. Open Ophthalmology Journal. 2017;**11**:122-142

[6] Milliez P, Girerd X, Plouin PF, Blacher J, Safar ME, Mourad JJ. Evidence for an increased rate of cardiovascular events in patients with primary aldosteronism. Journal of the American College of Cardiology. 2005;**45**(8):1243-1248

[7] Andreozzi F, Laratta E, Sciacqua A, Perticone F, Sesti G. Angiotensin II impairs the insulin signaling pathway promoting production of nitric oxide by inducing phosphorylation of insulin receptor substrate-1 on Ser(312) and Ser(616) in human umbilical vein endothelial cells. Circulation Research. 2004;**94**(9):1211-1218

[8] Nakashima H, Suzuki H, Ohtsu H, Chao JY, Utsunomiya H, Frank GD, et al. Angiotensin II regulates vascular and endothelial dysfunction: Recent topics of angiotensin II type-1 receptor signaling in the vasculature. Current Vascular Pharmacology. 2006;**4**(1):67-78

[9] Kawai T, Forrester SJ, O'Brien S, Baggett A, Rizzo V, Eguchi S. AT1 receptor signaling pathways in the cardiovascular system. Pharmacological Research. 2017;**125**(Pt A):4-13

[10] Miyata K, Rahman M, Shokoji T, Nagai Y, Zhang GX, Sun GP, et al. Aldosterone stimulates reactive oxygen species production through activation of NADPH oxidase in rat mesangial cells. Journal of the American Society of Nephrology. 2005;**16**(10):2906-2912

[11] Munzel T, Gori T, Keaney JF Jr, Maack C, Daiber A. Pathophysiological role of oxidative stress in systolic and diastolic heart failure and its therapeutic implications. European Heart Journal. 2015;**36**(38):2555-2564

[12] Keidar S, Gamliel-Lazarovich A, Kaplan M, Pavlotzky E, Hamoud S, Hayek T, et al. Mineralocorticoid receptor blocker increases angiotensin-converting enzyme 2 activity in congestive heart failure patients. Circulation Research. 2005;**97**(9):946-953

[13] Kong EL, Zhang JM, An N, Tao Y, Yu WF, Wu FX. Spironolactone rescues renal dysfunction in obstructive jaundice rats by upregulating ACE2 expression. Journal of Cell Communication and Signaling. 2019;**13**(1):17-26

[14] Whaley-Connell A, Habibi J, Wei Y, Gutweiler A, Jellison J, Wiedmeyer CE, et al. Mineralocorticoid receptor antagonism attenuates glomerular filtration barrier remodeling in the transgenic Ren2 rat. American Journal of Physiology. Renal Physiology. 2009;**296**(5):F1013-F1022

[15] Kucharewicz I, Pawlak R, Matys T, Pawlak D, Buczko W. Antithrombotic effect of captopril and losartan is mediated by angiotensin-(1-7). Hypertension. 2002;**40**(5):774-779

[16] Kaiqiang J, Minakawa M, Fukui K, Suzuki Y, Fukuda I. Olmesartan improves left ventricular function in pressure-overload hypertrophied rat heart by blocking angiotensin II receptor with synergic effects of upregulation of angiotensin converting enzyme 2. Therapeutic Advances in Cardiovascular Disease. 2009;**3**(2):103-111

[17] Sukumaran V, Veeraveedu PT, Gurusamy N, Yamaguchi K, Lakshmanan AP, Ma ML, et al. Cardioprotective effects of telmisartan against heart failure in rats induced by experimental autoimmune myocarditis through the modulation of angiotensin-converting enzyme-2/angiotensin 1-7/Mas receptor axis. International Journal of Biological Sciences. 2011;**7**(8):1077-1092

[18] Wang XX, Ye Y, Gong H, Wu J, Yuan J, Wang SJ, et al. The effects of different angiotensin II type 1 receptor blockers on the regulation of the ACE-AngII-AT1 and ACE2-Ang(1-7)-Mas axes in pressure overload-induced cardiac remodeling in male mice. Journal of Molecular and Cellular Cardiology. 2016;**97**:180-190

[19] Zhong JC, Ye JY, Jin HY, Yu X, Yu HM, Zhu DL, et al. Telmisartan attenuates aortic hypertrophy in hypertensive rats by the modulation of ACE2 and profilin-1 expression. Regulatory Peptides. 2011;**166**(1-3):90-97

[20] Ishiyama Y, Gallagher PE, Averill DB, Tallant EA, Brosnihan KB, Ferrario CM. Upregulation of angiotensin-converting enzyme 2 after myocardial infarction by blockade of angiotensin II receptors. Hypertension. 2004;**43**(5):970-976

[21] Harada E, Yoshimura M, Yasue H, Nakagawa O, Nakagawa M, Harada M, et al. Aldosterone induces angiotensin-converting-enzyme gene expression in cultured neonatal rat cardiocytes. Circulation. 2001;**104**(2):137-139

[22] Itcho K, Oki K, Kobuke K, Ohno H, Yoneda M, Hattori N. Angiotensin 1-7 suppresses angiotensin II mediated aldosterone production via JAK/STAT signaling inhibition. The Journal of Steroid Biochemistry and Molecular Biology. 2019;**185**:137-141

[23] Chen Y, Zhao W, Liu C, Meng W, Zhao T, Bhattacharya SK, et al. Molecular and cellular effect of angiotensin 1-7 on hypertensive kidney disease. American Journal of Hypertension. 2019;**32**(5):460-467

[24] Galandrin S, Denis C, Boularan C, Marie J, M'Kadmi C, Pilette C, et al. Cardioprotective angiotensin-(1-7) peptide acts as a natural-biased ligand at the angiotensin II type 1 receptor. Hypertension. 2016;**68**(6):1365-1374

[25] Gavras H, Lever AF, Brown JJ, Macadam RF, Robertson JI. Acute renal failure, tubular necrosis, and myocardial infarction induced in the rabbit by intravenous angiotensin II. Lancet. 1971;**2**(7714):19-22

[26] Ikeda Y, Nakamura T, Takano H, Kimura H, Obata JE, Takeda S, et al. Angiotensin II-induced cardiomyocyte hypertrophy and cardiac fibrosis

in stroke-prone spontaneously hypertensive rats. The Journal of Laboratory and Clinical Medicine. 2000;**135**(4):353-359

[27] Daugherty A, Cassis L. Chronic angiotensin II infusion promotes atherogenesis in low density lipoprotein receptor −/− mice. Annals of the New York Academy of Sciences. 1999;**892**:108-118

[28] Karnik SS, Unal H, Kemp JR, Tirupula KC, Eguchi S, Vanderheyden PM, et al. International Union of Basic and Clinical Pharmacology. XCIX. Angiotensin receptors: Interpreters of pathophysiological angiotensinergic stimuli [corrected]. Pharmacological Reviews. 2015;**67**(4):754-819

[29] Kaschina E, Namsolleck P, Unger T. AT2 receptors in cardiovascular and renal diseases. Pharmacological Research. 2017;**125**(Pt A):39-47

[30] Singh KD, Karnik SS. Angiotensin receptors: Structure, function, signaling and clinical applications. Journal of Cell Signalling. 2016;**1**(2)

[31] Skorska A, von Haehling S, Ludwig M, Lux CA, Gaebel R, Kleiner G, et al. The CD4(+)AT2R(+) T cell subpopulation improves post-infarction remodelling and restores cardiac function. Journal of Cellular and Molecular Medicine. 2015;**19**(8):1975-1985

[32] Zhu LP, Carretero OA, Xu J, Harding P, Ramadurai N, Gu XS, et al. Activation of angiotensin II type 2 receptor suppresses TNF-alpha-induced ICAM-1 via NF-kappa B: Possible role of ACE2. American Journal of Physiology-Heart and Circulatory Physiology. 2015;**309**(5):H827-H834

[33] Tanaka M, Tsuchida S, Imai T, Fujii N, Miyazaki H, Ichiki T, et al. Vascular response to angiotensin II is exaggerated through an upregulation of AT1 receptor in AT2 knockout mice. Biochemical and Biophysical Research Communications. 1999;**258**(1):194-198

[34] Bedecs K, Elbaz N, Sutren M, Masson M, Susini C, Strosberg AD, et al. Angiotensin II type 2 receptors mediate inhibition of mitogen-activated protein kinase cascade and functional activation of SHP-1 tyrosine phosphatase. The Biochemical Journal. 1997;**325**(Pt 2): 449-454

[35] AbdAlla S, Lother H, Abdel-Tawab AM, Quitterer U. The angiotensin II AT2 receptor is an AT1 receptor antagonist. The Journal of Biological Chemistry. 2001;**276**(43):39721-39726

[36] de Gasparo M, Catt KJ, Inagami T, Wright JW, Unger T. International Union of Pharmacology. XXIII. The angiotensin II receptors. Pharmacological Reviews. 2000;**52**(3):415-472

[37] Jones ES, Vinh A, McCarthy CA, Gaspari TA, Widdop RE. AT2 receptors: Functional relevance in cardiovascular disease. Pharmacology & Therapeutics. 2008;**120**(3):292-316

[38] Cook JL, Mills SJ, Naquin R, Alam J, Re RN. Nuclear accumulation of the AT1 receptor in a rat vascular smooth muscle cell line: Effects upon signal transduction and cellular proliferation. Journal of Molecular and Cellular Cardiology. 2006;**40**(5):696-707

[39] Cook JL, Mills SJ, Naquin RT, Alam J, Re RN. Cleavage of the angiotensin II type 1 receptor and nuclear accumulation of the cytoplasmic carboxy-terminal fragment. American Journal of Physiology. Cell Physiology. 2007;**292**(4):C1313-C1322

[40] Cook JL, Re R, Alam J, Hart M, Zhang Z. Intracellular angiotensin

II fusion protein alters AT1 receptor fusion protein distribution and activates CREB. Journal of Molecular and Cellular Cardiology. 2004;**36**(1):75-90

[41] Villela DC, Passos-Silva DG, Santos RA. Alamandine: A new member of the angiotensin family. Current Opinion in Nephrology and Hypertension. 2014;**23**(2):130-134

[42] Keidar S, Kaplan M, Gamliel-Lazarovich A. ACE2 of the heart: From angiotensin I to angiotensin (1-7). Cardiovascular Research. 2007;**73**(3):463-469

[43] Santos RA, Simoes e Silva AC, Maric C, Silva DM, Machado RP, de Buhr I, et al. Angiotensin-(1-7) is an endogenous ligand for the G protein-coupled receptor Mas. Proceedings of the National Academy of Sciences of the United States of America. 2003;**100**(14):8258-8263

[44] Menon J, Soto-Pantoja DR, Callahan MF, Cline JM, Ferrario CM, Tallant EA, et al. Angiotensin-(1-7) inhibits growth of human lung adenocarcinoma xenografts in nude mice through a reduction in cyclooxygenase-2. Cancer Research. 2007;**67**(6):2809-2815

[45] Lautner RQ, Villela DC, Fraga-Silva RA, Silva N, Verano-Braga T, Costa-Fraga F, et al. Discovery and characterization of alamandine: A novel component of the renin-angiotensin system. Circulation Research. 2013;**112**(8):1104-1111

[46] Dias-Peixoto MF, Santos RA, Gomes ER, Alves MN, Almeida PW, Greco L, et al. Molecular mechanisms involved in the angiotensin-(1-7)/Mas signaling pathway in cardiomyocytes. Hypertension. 2008;**52**(3):542-548

[47] Zhong J, Basu R, Guo D, Chow FL, Byrns S, Schuster M, et al. Angiotensin-converting enzyme 2 suppresses pathological hypertrophy, myocardial fibrosis, and cardiac dysfunction. Circulation. 2010;**122**(7):717-728, 18 p following 728

[48] Sampaio WO, Souza dos Santos RA, Faria-Silva R, da Mata Machado LT, Schiffrin EL, Touyz RM. Angiotensin-(1-7) through receptor Mas mediates endothelial nitric oxide synthase activation via Akt-dependent pathways. Hypertension. 2007;**49**(1):185-192

[49] Patel VB, Zhong JC, Grant MB, Oudit GY. Role of the ACE2/angiotensin 1-7 axis of the renin-angiotensin system in heart failure. Circulation Research. 2016;**118**(8):1313-1326

[50] Kozlovski VI, Lomnicka M, Bartus M, Sternak M, Chlopicki S. Anti-thrombotic effects of nebivolol and carvedilol: Involvement of beta2 receptors and COX-2/PGI2 pathways. Pharmacological Reports. 2015;**67**(5):1041-1047

[51] Dales NA, Gould AE, Brown JA, Calderwood EF, Guan B, Minor CA, et al. Substrate-based design of the first class of angiotensin-converting enzyme-related carboxypeptidase (ACE2) inhibitors. Journal of the American Chemical Society. 2002;**124**(40):11852-11853

[52] Gallagher PE, Ferrario CM, Tallant EA. Regulation of ACE2 in cardiac myocytes and fibroblasts. American Journal of Physiology. Heart and Circulatory Physiology. 2008;**295**(6):H2373-H2379

[53] Weber KT, Sun Y. Recruitable ACE and tissue repair in the infarcted heart. Journal of the Renin-Angiotensin-Aldosterone System. 2000;**1**(4):295-303

[54] Li XC, Zhang JF, Zhuo JL. The vasoprotective axes of the

renin-angiotensin system: Physiological relevance and therapeutic implications in cardiovascular, hypertensive and kidney diseases. Pharmacological Research. 2017;**125**:21-38

[55] Saris JJ, 't Hoen PA, Garrelds IM, Dekkers DH, den Dunnen JT, Lamers JM, et al. Prorenin induces intracellular signaling in cardiomyocytes independently of angiotensin II. Hypertension. 2006;**48**(4):564-571

[56] Zhuo JL, Ferrao FM, Zheng Y, Li XC. New frontiers in the intrarenal renin-angiotensin system: A critical review of classical and new paradigms. Frontiers in Endocrinology (Lausanne). 2013;**4**:166

[57] Blair-West JR, Carey KD, Denton DA, Madden LJ, Weisinger RS, Shade RE. Possible contribution of brain angiotensin III to ingestive behaviors in baboons. American Journal of Physiology. Regulatory, Integrative and Comparative Physiology. 2001;**281**(5):R1633-R1636

[58] Zulli A, Burrell LM, Buxton BF, Hare DL. ACE2 and AT4R are present in diseased human blood vessels. European Journal of Histochemistry. 2008;**52**(1):39-44

[59] Ferrario CM, Ahmad S, Varagic J, Cheng CP, Groban L, Wang H, et al. Intracrine angiotensin II functions originate from noncanonical pathways in the human heart. American Journal of Physiology. Heart and Circulatory Physiology. 2016;**311**(2):H404-H414

[60] Isa K, Garcia-Espinosa MA, Arnold AC, Pirro NT, Tommasi EN, Ganten D, et al. Chronic immunoneutralization of brain angiotensin-(1-12) lowers blood pressure in transgenic (mRen2)27 hypertensive rats. American Journal of Physiology. Regulatory, Integrative and Comparative Physiology. 2009;**297**(1):R111-R115

[61] Urata H, Hoffmann S, Ganten D. Tissue angiotensin II system in the human heart. European Heart Journal. 1994;**15**(Suppl D):68-78

[62] Jessup JA, Trask AJ, Chappell MC, Nagata S, Kato J, Kitamura K, et al. Localization of the novel angiotensin peptide, angiotensin-(1-12), in heart and kidney of hypertensive and normotensive rats. American Journal of Physiology. Heart and Circulatory Physiology. 2008;**294**(6):H2614-H2618

[63] McDonald JE, Padmanabhan N, Petrie MC, Hillier C, Connell JM, McMurray JJ. Vasoconstrictor effect of the angiotensin-converting enzyme-resistant, chymase-specific substrate [pro(11)(D)-Ala(12)] angiotensin I in human dorsal hand veins: in vivo demonstration of non-ace production of angiotensin II in humans. Circulation. 2001;**104**(15):1805-1808

[64] Stephenson SL, Kenny AJ. The metabolism of neuropeptides. Hydrolysis of peptides by the phosphoramidon-insensitive rat kidney enzyme 'endopeptidase-2' and by rat microvillar membranes. Biochemical Journal. 1988;**255**(1):45-51

[65] Patil J, Stucki S, Nussberger J, Schaffner T, Gygax S, Bohlender J, et al. Angiotensinergic and noradrenergic neurons in the rat and human heart. Regulatory Peptides. 2011;**167**(1):31-41

[66] Uehara Y, Urata H, Ideishi M, Arakawa K, Saku K. Chymase inhibition suppresses high-cholesterol diet-induced lipid accumulation in the hamster aorta. Cardiovascular Research. 2002;**55**(4):870-876

[67] Borges JC, Silva JA Jr, Gomes MA, Lomez ES, Leite KM, Araujo RC, et al. Tonin in rat heart with experimental hypertrophy. American Journal of Physiology. Heart and Circulatory Physiology. 2003;**284**(6):H2263-H2268

[68] Welches WR, Brosnihan KB, Ferrario CM. A comparison of the properties and enzymatic-activities of 3 angiotensin processing enzymes—Angiotensin-converting enzyme, prolyl endopeptidase and neutral endopeptidase 24.11. Life Sciences. 1993;**52**(18):1461-1480

[69] Allred AJ, Diz DI, Ferrario CM, Chappell MC. Pathways for angiotensin-(1-7) metabolism in pulmonary and renal tissues. American Journal of Physiology-Renal Physiology. 2000;**279**(5):F841-F850

[70] Campbell DJ, Anastasopoulos F, Duncan AM, James GM, Kladis A, Briscoe TA. Effects of neutral endopeptidase inhibition and combined angiotensin converting enzyme and neutral endopeptidase inhibition on angiotensin and bradykinin peptides in rats. The Journal of Pharmacology and Experimental Therapeutics. 1998;**287**(2):567-577

[71] Chappell MC, Gomez MN, Pirro NT, Ferrario CM. Release of angiotensin-(1-7) from the rat hindlimb: Influence of angiotensin-converting enzyme inhibition. Hypertension. 2000;**35**(1 Pt 2):348-352

[72] Ferrario CM. Contribution of angiotensin-(1-7) to cardiovascular physiology and pathology. Current Hypertension Reports. 2003;**5**(2):129-134

[73] Jeong JK, Diano S. Prolyl carboxypeptidase and its inhibitors in metabolism. Trends in Endocrinology and Metabolism. 2013;**24**(2):61-67

[74] Ponikowski P, Voors AA, Anker SD, Bueno H, Cleland JG, Coats AJ, et al. R. Document, 2016 ESC Guidelines for the diagnosis and treatment of acute and chronic heart failure: The Task Force for the diagnosis and treatment of acute and chronic heart failure of the European Society of Cardiology (ESC). Developed with the special contribution of the Heart Failure Association (HFA) of the ESC. European Journal of Heart Failure. 2016;**18**(8):891-975

[75] Dell'Italia LJ, Meng QC, Balcells E, Wei CC, Palmer R, Hageman GR, et al. Compartmentalization of angiotensin II generation in the dog heart. Evidence for independent mechanisms in intravascular and interstitial spaces. Journal of Clinical Investigation. 1997;**100**(2):253-258

[76] de Lannoy LM, Danser AH, van Kats JP, Schoemaker RG, Saxena PR, Schalekamp MA. Renin-angiotensin system components in the interstitial fluid of the isolated perfused rat heart. Local production of angiotensin I. Hypertension. 1997;**29**(6):1240-1251

[77] Danser AHJ, Vankats JP, Admiraal PJJ, Derks FHM, Lamers JMJ, Verdouw PD, et al. Cardiac renin and angiotensins—Uptake from plasma versus in-situ synthesis. Hypertension. 1994;**24**(1):37-48

[78] Barlucchi L, Leri A, Dostal DE, Fiordaliso F, Tada H, Hintze TH, et al. Canine ventricular myocytes possess a renin-angiotensin system that is upregulated with heart failure. Circulation Research. 2001;**88**(3):298-304

[79] Ihara M, Urata H, Kinoshita A, Suzumiya J, Sasaguri M, Kikuchi M, et al. Increased chymase-dependent angiotensin II formation in human atherosclerotic aorta. Hypertension. 1999;**33**(6):1399-1405

[80] Dong B, Yu QT, Dai HY, Gao YY, Zhou ZL, Zhang L, et al. Angiotensin-converting enzyme-2 overexpression improves left ventricular remodeling and function in a rat model of diabetic cardiomyopathy. Journal of

the American College of Cardiology. 2012;**59**(8):739-747

[81] Kassiri Z, Zhong J, Guo D, Basu R, Wang X, Liu PP, et al. Loss of angiotensin-converting enzyme 2 accelerates maladaptive left ventricular remodeling in response to myocardial infarction. Circulation. Heart Failure. 2009;**2**(5):446-455

[82] Lambert DW, Yarski M, Warner FJ, Thornhill P, Parkin ET, Smith AI, et al. Tumor necrosis factor-alpha convertase (ADAM17) mediates regulated ectodomain shedding of the severe-acute respiratory syndrome-coronavirus (SARS-CoV) receptor, angiotensin-converting enzyme-2 (ACE2). The Journal of Biological Chemistry. 2005;**280**(34):30113-30119

[83] Patel VB, Clarke N, Wang Z, Fan D, Parajuli N, Basu R, et al. Angiotensin II induced proteolytic cleavage of myocardial ACE2 is mediated by TACE/ADAM-17: A positive feedback mechanism in the RAS. Journal of Molecular and Cellular Cardiology. 2014;**66**:167-176

[84] Edwards DR, Handsley MM, Pennington CJ. The ADAM metalloproteinases. Molecular Aspects of Medicine. 2008;**29**(5):258-289

[85] Putko BN, Wang Z, Lo J, Anderson T, Becher H, Dyck JR, et al. Circulating levels of tumor necrosis factor-alpha receptor 2 are increased in heart failure with preserved ejection fraction relative to heart failure with reduced ejection fraction: Evidence for a divergence in pathophysiology. PLoS One. 2014;**9**(6):e99495

[86] Uri K, Fagyas M, Kertesz A, Borbely A, Jenei C, Bene O, et al. Circulating ACE2 activity correlates with cardiovascular disease development. Journal of the Renin-Angiotensin-Aldosterone System. 2016;**17**(4)

[87] Urata H, Kinoshita A, Misono KS, Bumpus FM, Husain A. Identification of a highly specific chymase as the major angiotensin II-forming enzyme in the human heart. The Journal of Biological Chemistry. 1990;**265**(36):22348-22357

[88] Dell'Italia LJ, Collawn JF, Ferrario CM. Multifunctional role of chymase in acute and chronic tissue injury and remodeling. Circulation Research. 2018;**122**(2):319-336

[89] Ahmad S, Varagic J, VonCannon JL, Groban L, Collawn JF, Dell'Italia LJ, et al. Primacy of cardiac chymase over angiotensin converting enzyme as an angiotensin-(1-12) metabolizing enzyme. Biochemical and Biophysical Research Communications. 2016;**478**(2):559-564

[90] Patella V, de Crescenzo G, Lamparter-Schummert B, De Rosa G, Adt M, Marone G. Increased cardiac mast cell density and mediator release in patients with dilated cardiomyopathy. Inflammation Research. 1997;**46**(Suppl 1):S31-S32

[91] Ferrario CM, Ahmad S, Nagata S, Simington SW, Varagic J, Kon N, et al. An evolving story of angiotensin-II-forming pathways in rodents and humans. Clinical Science (London, England). 2014;**126**(7):461-469

[92] Petrie MC, Padmanabhan N, McDonald JE, Hillier C, Connell JMC, McMurray JJV. Angiotensin converting enzyme (ACE) and non-ACE dependent angiotensin II generation in resistance arteries from patients with heart failure and coronary heart disease. Journal of the American College of Cardiology. 2001;**37**(4):1056-1061

[93] Wei CC, Hase N, Inoue Y, Bradley EW, Yahiro E, Li M, et al. Mast cell chymase limits the cardiac efficacy of Ang I-converting enzyme

inhibitor therapy in rodents. The Journal of Clinical Investigation. 2010;**120**(4):1229-1239

[94] Reyes S, Varagic J, Ahmad S, VonCannon J, Kon ND, Wang H, et al. Novel cardiac intracrine mechanisms based on Ang-(1-12)/chymase axis require a revision of therapeutic approaches in human heart disease. Current Hypertension Reports. 2017;**19**(2):16

[95] Jin D, Takai S, Nonaka Y, Yamazaki S, Fujiwara M, Nakamura Y. A chymase inhibitory RNA aptamer improves cardiac function and survival after myocardial infarction. Molecular Therapy—Nucleic Acids. 2019;**14**:41-51

[96] Matsumoto T, Wada A, Tsutamoto T, Ohnishi M, Fujii M, Yamamoto T, et al. Chronic chymase inhibition prevented cardiac fibrosis and improved diastolic dysfunction in the progression of heart failure. Circulation. 2002;**106**(19):99-100

[97] Balcells E, Meng QC, Johnson WH Jr, Oparil S, Dell'Italia LJ. Angiotensin II formation from ACE and chymase in human and animal hearts: Methods and species considerations. The American Journal of Physiology. 1997;**273**(4 Pt 2): H1769-H1774

[98] Zablocki D, Sadoshima J. The one-two punch: Knocking out angiotensin II in the heart. The Journal of Clinical Investigation. 2010;**120**(4):1028-1031

[99] Tyrankiewicz U, Olkowicz M, Skorka T, Jablonska M, Orzylowska A, Bar A, et al. Activation pattern of ACE2/Ang-(1-7) and ACE/Ang II pathway in course of heart failure assessed by multiparametric MRI in vivo in Tgalphaq*44 mice. Journal of Applied Physiology. 1985, 2018;**124**(1):52-65

[100] Mackiewicz U, Czarnowska E, Brudek M, Pajak B, Duda M, Emanuel K, et al. Preserved cardiomyocyte function and altered desmin pattern in transgenic mouse model of dilated cardiomyopathy. Journal of Molecular and Cellular Cardiology. 2012;**52**(5):978-987

[101] Athyros VG, Mikhailidis DP, Kakafika AI, Tziomalos K, Karagiannis A. Angiotensin II reactivation and aldosterone escape phenomena in renin-angiotensin-aldosterone system blockade: Is oral renin inhibition the solution? Expert Opinion on Pharmacotherapy. 2007;**8**(5):529-535

[102] Juillerat L, Nussberger J, Menard J, Mooser V, Christen Y, Waeber B, et al. Determinants of angiotensin II generation during converting enzyme inhibition. Hypertension. 1990;**16**(5):564-572

[103] Fukuta H, Goto T, Wakami K, Ohte N. Effect of renin-angiotensin system inhibitors on mortality in heart failure with preserved ejection fraction: A meta-analysis of observational cohort and randomized controlled studies. Heart Failure Reviews. 2017;**22**(6):775-782

[104] Jhund PS, McMurray JJV. The neprilysin pathway in heart failure: A review and guide on the use of sacubitril/valsartan. Heart. 2016;**102**(17):1342-1347

[105] Cui L, Nithipatikom K, Campbell WB. Simultaneous analysis of angiotensin peptides by LC-MS and LC-MS/MS: Metabolism by bovine adrenal endothelial cells. Analytical Biochemistry. 2007;**369**(1):27-33

[106] Olkowicz M, Chlopicki S, Smolenski RT. A primer to angiotensin peptide isolation, stability, and analysis by nano-liquid chromatography with mass detection. Methods in Molecular Biology. 2017;**1614**:175-187

[107] Olkowicz M, Debski J, Jablonska P, Dadlez M, Smolenski RT. Application of a new procedure for liquid chromatography/mass spectrometry profiling of plasma amino acid-related metabolites and untargeted shotgun proteomics to identify mechanisms and biomarkers of calcific aortic stenosis. Journal of Chromatography. A. 2017;**1517**:66-78

[108] Olkowicz M, Radulska A, Suraj J, Kij A, Walczak M, Chlopicki S, et al. Development of a sensitive, accurate and robust liquid chromatography/mass spectrometric method for profiling of angiotensin peptides in plasma and its application for atherosclerotic mice. Journal of Chromatography. A. 2015;**1393**:37-46

[109] Chen J, Zhao Y, Chen S, Wang J, Xiao X, Ma X, et al. Neuronal over-expression of ACE2 protects brain from ischemia-induced damage. Neuropharmacology. 2014;**79**:550-558

[110] Tsukuda K, Mogi M, Iwanami J, Min LJ, Jing F, Ohshima K, et al. Influence of angiotensin II type 1 receptor-associated protein on prenatal development and adult hypertension after maternal dietary protein restriction during pregnancy. Journal of the American Society of Hypertension. 2012;**6**(5):324-330

[111] Campbell DJ, Alexiou T, Xiao HD, Fuchs S, McKinley MJ, Corvol P, et al. Effect of reduced angiotensin-converting enzyme gene expression and angiotensin-converting enzyme inhibition on angiotensin and bradykinin peptide levels in mice. Hypertension. 2004;**43**(4):854-859

[112] Waghe P, Sarath TS, Gupta P, Kandasamy K, Choudhury S, Kutty HS, et al. Arsenic causes aortic dysfunction and systemic hypertension in rats: Augmentation of angiotensin II signaling. Chemico-Biological Interactions. 2015;**237**:104-114

[113] Tufino C, Villanueva-Lopez C, Ibarra-Barajas M, Bracho-Valdes I, Bobadilla-Lugo RA. Experimental gestational diabetes mellitus induces blunted vasoconstriction and functional changes in the rat aorta. BioMed Research International. 2014;**2014**:329634

[114] Nishiyama A, Seth DM, Navar LG. Renal interstitial fluid angiotensin I and angiotensin II concentrations during local angiotensin-converting enzyme inhibition. Journal of the American Society of Nephrology. 2002;**13**(9):2207-2212

[115] Gilliam-Davis S, Payne VS, Kasper SO, Tommasi EN, Robbins ME, Diz DI. Long-term AT1 receptor blockade improves metabolic function and provides renoprotection in Fischer-344 rats. American Journal of Physiology. Heart and Circulatory Physiology. 2007;**293**(3):H1327-H1333

[116] Chappell MC, Brosnihan KB, Diz DI, Ferrario CM. Identification of angiotensin-(1-7) in rat brain. Evidence for differential processing of angiotensin peptides. Journal of Biological Chemistry. 1989;**264**(28):16518-16523

[117] Campbell DJ, Duncan AM, Kladis A, Harrap SB. Angiotensin peptides in spontaneously hypertensive and normotensive Donryu rats. Hypertension. 1995;**25**(5):928-934

[118] Senanayake PS, Smeby RR, Martins AS, Moriguchi A, Kumagai H, Ganten D, et al. Adrenal, kidney, and heart angiotensins in female murine Ren-2 transfected hypertensive rats. Peptides. 1998;**19**(10):1685-1694

[119] Ocaranza MP, Lavandero S, Jalil JE, Moya J, Pinto M, Novoa U, et al.

Angiotensin-(1-9) regulates cardiac hypertrophy in vivo and in vitro. Journal of Hypertension. 2010;**28**(5):1054-1064

[120] Senanayake PD, Moriguchi A, Kumagai H, Ganten D, Ferrario CM, Brosnihan KB. Increased expression of angiotensin peptides in the brain of transgenic hypertensive rats. Peptides. 1994;**15**(5):919-926

[121] Hildebrand D, Merkel P, Eggers LF, Schluter H. Proteolytic processing of angiotensin-I in human blood plasma. PLoS One. 2013;**8**(5):e64027

[122] Schulz A, Jankowski J, Zidek W, Jankowski V. Absolute quantification of endogenous angiotensin II levels in human plasma using ESI-LC-MS/MS. Clinical Proteomics. 2014;**11**(1):37

[123] Lawrence AC, Evin G, Kladis A, Campbell DJ. An alternative strategy for the radioimmunoassay of angiotensin peptides using amino-terminal-directed antisera: Measurement of eight angiotensin peptides in human plasma. Journal of Hypertension. 1990;**8**(8):715-724

[124] Nussberger J, Brunner DB, Nyfeler JA, Linder L, Brunner HR. Measurement of immunoreactive angiotensin-(1-7) heptapeptide in human blood. Clinical Chemistry. 2001;**47**(4):726-729

[125] Rubio-Ruiz ME, Del Valle-Mondragon L, Castrejon-Tellez V, Carreon-Torres E, Diaz-Diaz E, Guarner-Lans V. Angiotensin II and 1-7 during aging in metabolic syndrome rats. Expression of AT1, AT2 and Mas receptors in abdominal white adipose tissue. Peptides. 2014;**57**:101-108

[126] Ferrario CM, Martell N, Yunis C, Flack JM, Chappell MC, Brosnihan KB, et al. Characterization of angiotensin-(1-7) in the urine of normal and essential hypertensive subjects. American Journal of Hypertension. 1998;**11**(2):137-146

[127] Mazzolai L, Pedrazzini T, Nicoud F, Gabbiani G, Brunner HR, Nussberger J. Increased cardiac angiotensin II levels induce right and left ventricular hypertrophy in normotensive mice. Hypertension. 2000;**35**(4):985-991

[128] Campbell DJ, Kladis A, Duncan AM. Nephrectomy, converting enzyme inhibition, and angiotensin peptides. Hypertension. 1993;**22**(4):513-522

[129] Kuba K, Zhang L, Imai Y, Arab S, Chen M, Maekawa Y, et al. Impaired heart contractility in Apelin gene-deficient mice associated with aging and pressure overload. Circulation Research. 2007;**101**(4):e32-e42

[130] Shefer G, Marcus Y, Knoll E, Dolkart O, Foichtwanger S, Nevo N, et al. Angiotensin 1-7 is a negative modulator of aldosterone secretion in vitro and in vivo. Hypertension. 2016;**68**(2):378-384

[131] Kanefendt F, Thuss U, Becka M, Boxnick S, Berse M, Schultz A, et al. Pharmacokinetics, safety, and tolerability of the novel chymase inhibitor BAY 1142524 in healthy male volunteers. Clinical Pharmacology in Drug Development. 2018

[132] Basu R, Poglitsch M, Yogasundaram H, Thomas J, Rowe BH, Oudit GY. Roles of angiotensin peptides and recombinant human ACE2 in heart failure. Journal of the American College of Cardiology. 2017;**69**(7):805-819

[133] Patel VB, Lezutekong JN, Chen X, Oudit GY. Recombinant human ACE2 and the angiotensin 1-7 axis as potential new therapies for heart failure. The Canadian Journal of Cardiology. 2017;**33**(7):943-946

[134] Oudit GY, Penninger JM. Recombinant human angiotensin-converting enzyme 2 as a new renin-angiotensin system peptidase for heart failure therapy. Current Heart Failure Reports. 2011;**8**(3):176-183

[135] Luo D, Zhuang X, Luo C, Long M, Deng C, Liao X, et al. Continuous angiotensin-(1-7) infusion improves myocardial calcium transient and calcium transient alternans in ischemia-induced cardiac dysfunction rats. Biochemical and Biophysical Research Communications. 2015;**467**(4):645-650

Chapter 6

# Primary Aldosteronism: A Glimpse into the Most Common Endocrine Cause of Arterial Hypertension

*Gian Paolo Rossi and Teresa M. Seccia*

## Abstract

Compelling evidences showed that primary aldosteronism (PA) is a quite common disease. In spite of this, hypertensive patients are seldom screened for PA and, therefore, many patients are mislabelled as (low-renin) essential hypertension thereby remaining exposed to the nefarious consequences of long-term hyperaldosteronism. In this chapter we reviewed the clinical aspects of PA and the evidences supporting the need of implementing strategies aimed at diagnosing early PA patients. After reporting the prevalence rates of PA in different cohorts of hypertensive patients, we examined the reasons why PA is rarely searched for. The cardiovascular and renal damage associated with PA were also discussed, with particular emphasis to endothelial dysfunction, vascular remodeling, left ventricular changes, fibrosis, diastolic dysfunction, atrial fibrillation and chronic kidney disease. Studies supporting the concept that PA-associated organ damage can be prevented and even regressed with a timely diagnosis were also reviewed. A flowchart illustrating the proposal of a simplified diagnostic algorithm for screening and subtyping of PA, which allows circumventing the complexity of a diagnostic workup centred on confirmatory tests, is also proposed. Finally, the principles of treatment for PA are discussed.

**Keywords:** endocrine hypertension, primary aldosteronism, subtyping, diagnosis, adrenal vein sampling, outcome

## 1. Epidemiology

Primary aldosteronism (PA) is regarded by most practicing physicians as a 'needle in the haystack' [1], notwithstanding compelling evidences supporting the opposite view that is quite common. At the dawn of this millennium, based on small single-centre retrospective studies, the prevalence rate of PA was estimated to range from 1.4–32% (median 8.8%), i.e. so widely that no firm conclusions could be drawn on how common PA was, likely because of differences in the selection of the patient's cohorts and heterogeneous diagnostic criteria used in the various studies [2].

In 2006, the PA Prevalence in Hypertensives (PAPY) study, a prospective survey of consecutive newly diagnosed hypertensive patients referred to specialized hypertension centres, exploited for the first time use of a predefined protocol and standardized diagnostic criteria to diagnose PA [3]. This seminal study provided solid evidences that among referred hypertensive patients the prevalence of PA was high, i.e. 11.2% [3]. Moreover, by calling attention to the fact that the only subtype of PA that could be diagnosed with certainty is aldosterone-producing adenoma (APA), this study introduced the 'four-corners criteria' to diagnose PA due to APA, a concept thereafter adopted in the PASO criteria [4] and recently revised to take into consideration the availability, thanks to Gomez-Sanchez's laboratory, of a monoclonal antibody for human aldosterone synthase (CYP11B2) that allowed the immunohistochemical demonstration of aldosterone biosynthesis in adrenocortical nodule(s) of excised adrenals [5, 6].

It should be acknowledged, though, that estimates of the prevalence of PA are meaningless figures without specification of the cohort of hypertensive patients that are being considered. For example, in a general population survey in Japan, Ito et al. reported a prevalence of PA of 6.8% in prehypertensive subjects and 3.3% and 3.2%, respectively, in stage I and II hypertensive patients [7]. In the Bussolengo study, which involved hypertensive patients seen in general practice in Verona province in Italy, 34% were found to have an elevated aldosterone-to-renin ratio (ARR) suggesting PA [8]. Although the actual rate of those with confirmed PA remained uncertain, because no further tests could be undertaken, those findings suggested a high prevalence of PA among such unselected hypertensive patients. In line with this suggestion, in a similar study involving general practitioners in Torino (Italy), 5.9% of the patients were found to have PA [9]. Altogether these results led to the proposal that the screening for PA should be wider [10] than a screening only in selected categories of patients recommended by current guidelines [11].

Undoubtedly, screening should be exploited in patients with drug-resistant hypertension, which represent the cohort at the highest cardiovascular risk, not only because of the uncontrolled blood pressure (BP) values, but also because of the common concurrence of hypertension-mediated organ damage (HMOD) [9, 11–14]. In a single-centre study carefully carried out in Greece by Douma et al. in drug-resistant hypertension patients, who were studied after wash-out from interfering drugs, 20.6% were found to have a high ARR [15]. The rate fell to about 11% when the authors used the BP-lowering response to spironolactone to confirm their diagnosis. They considered this rate to be not as high as they expected [15]. However, yet unpublished data from the AVIS-2 study, the largest registry of patients submitted to adrenal vein sampling (AVS) for the subtyping of PA worldwide, indicated

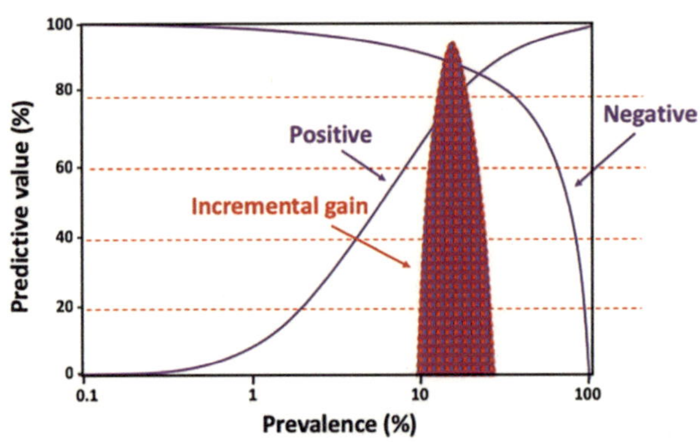


**Figure 1.**
*Prevalence of a disease affects positive and negative predictive values. Furthermore, the diagnostic gain of a test is maximized when the prevalence of the disease is between 10 and 30%. Since primary aldosteronism (PA) was found to involve 11.2% in the hypertensive patients referred to the specialized centres for hypertension, and to be even more prevalent in the 'resistant' hypertensives, implementation of the screening strategies for PA furnishes an unambiguous gain in these categories, besides being of crucial relevance for identifying the patients who can benefit of the targeted treatment.*

that between 20.1 and 49.5% of PA patients, depending on the criteria used to define this condition, have drug-resistant hypertension. Hence, resistant hypertension is a common presentation of PA. On the whole, these results showed that, at least among referred hypertensives who are carefully investigated, more than 11% have PA, with a rate that increases together with the stage of hypertension.

Hence, besides supporting the original contention of Conn [16], these findings showed that PA is by no means an exceptionally rare cause of human hypertension. Therefore, they have implications of paramount importance for the implementation of screening strategies in the hypertensive patients as the diagnostic gain of a diagnostic test is maximized when the prevalence of the disease that is sought for is between 10 and 30% (**Figure 1**).

## 2. Why PA is under-detected?

In spite of the fact that compelling evidences support the notion that PA is a common curable form of secondary hypertension, this condition remains markedly underdiagnosed for a number of reasons. The first is the misbelief that it is rare and therefore it is not worth of a search. The second entails the fact that hypokalaemia, which for decades has been considered the hallmark of PA, occurs only in less than half of the hypertensive patients, with APA and in less than 20% of those with bilateral adrenal hyperplasia (BAH, also known as idiopathic hyperaldosteronism, IHA) [3]. The third reason is a general phenomenon in medicine: the time lag occurring between publication of scientific data, their incorporation into practice guidelines and implementation of guidelines' recommendations in clinical practice. A survey of general practitioners in Italy and Germany documented that this is true also for PA: only 1 and 2%, respectively, in these countries were ever screened for PA by their general practitioners [17]. The fourth major reasons for the underscreening and consequent underdiagnosis of PA relate, in our view, to the fact that the diagnostic workup of patients for PA is perceived by practicing physicians as too complex to undertake and interpret. The recommended measure to prepare the hypertensive patients pharmacologically with a complete wash-out from drugs, which is totally unjustified, or better a switch to non-interfering drugs before undertaking the screening tests, is perceived as risky, even though evidence supporting the safety of a transient withdrawal of antihypertensive treatment exists [18, 19]. Uses of different assays to measure renin and aldosterone and of different units of measure are further factors undoubtedly confusing the interpretation of the screening test, which led us to develop an app that has been made freely available to address these difficulties [20] (https://siia.it/attivita-ricerca/iniziative/una-app-per-calcolare-l-arr/).

As a result of the under diagnosis, far too many PA patients are misdiagnosed as (low-renin) essential hypertension and remain exposed to the nefarious consequences of long-term exposure to hyperaldosteronism [21, 22], which are described in the next section.

## 3. Cardiovascular and renal damage associated with PA

Patients with PA have higher cardiovascular morbidity and mortality than age-, sex- and BP-matched patients with essential hypertension [9, 13, 14, 23, 24]. This is because aldosterone excess, in the presence of a normal-to-high salt intake, has deleterious effects on the cardiovascular system that aggravate those of high BP, as convincingly demonstrated in both experimental and clinical studies [25–28].

In 1991, Karl Weber's and Richardo Rocha's laboratories provided unambiguous evidences that uni-nephrectomized salt-fed rats infused with aldosterone developed prominent inflammation and fibrosis in the heart and kidneys. Moreover, they showed that these changes could be prevented by pretreatment with mineralocorticoid receptor antagonists, as spironolactone, even at sub-antihypertensive doses, suggesting that aldosterone can cause fibrosis independently of its pressor effects [25, 29]. Moreover, in animal models, aldosterone infusion was shown to cause endothelial dysfunction via reactive oxygen species (ROS) generation; increased expression of NADPH oxidase subunits p22phox, gp91phox and p47phox; formation of peroxynitrite; oxidation of the NOS cofactor BH4 (5,6,7,8-tetrahydrobiopterin); and decreased G6PD (glucose-6-phosphate dehydrogenase) [30, 31].

In 1996, at a time when PA was still regarded as a 'benign' form of arterial hypertension, we reported that PA patients developed more left ventricular (LV) hypertrophy (LVH) than age-, sex- and BP-matched essential hypertensive patients, [32] and that this was particularly evident in those who showed more florid PA phenotypes due to an APA [13]. These findings were thereafter extended to show that they are more prone to develop fibrosis, atrial fibrillation [33], vascular remodeling [34], endothelial dysfunction [35, 36], increased carotid intima-media thickness and femoral pulse wave velocity, more frequently than those with essential hypertension [13, 14, 32, 37].

Moreover, the occurrence of LVH, LV fibrosis, impaired diastolic function, atrial dilatation and electric remodeling in PA (rev in [38]) explains why these patients were found to have a 12-fold higher risk of developing atrial fibrillation, the most common arrhythmia worldwide, than essential hypertensive patients in a French retrospective study [39]. Accordingly, adrenalectomy was found to lower the risk of atrial fibrillation in PA patients in the long-term longitudinal phase of the PAPY study [33]. Collectively these evidences support the concept that aldosterone favors atrial fibrillation [38] and that PA patients are more susceptible to heart failure with onset of atrial fibrillation [13, 40] because of a 'stiffer' LV causing LV diastolic dysfunction and fibrosis, which lead to a greater dependency of the LV on the atrial kick for its filling.

PA patients also develop more renal damage with development of proteinuria and/or chronic kidney disease. In 1988, Danforth et al. first reported moderate to severe renal parenchymal damage in renal biopsies of patients with PA [41], a finding confirmed two decades later by Nishimura et al. [42] and, in 2006, by the PAPY study, which reported higher albumin excretion rate in PA patients than in matched essential hypertensives [14].

The important notion to be considered in this context is that most of the hypertension-mediated organ damage associated with PA can be prevented and even regressed, at least partially, with a timely diagnosis. For example, in a long-term observational study, long-term regression of LVH and a decrease incidence of AF were documented [43]. Moreover, in the longitudinal phase of the PAPY study, we found that incident AF was significantly decreased by adrenalectomy, but not by long-term medical treatment [33]. In line with such findings Hundemer et al. [40] reported that PA patients with persistently suppressed renin despite treatment with mineralocorticoid receptor antagonists had a higher risk of AF than essential hypertensives, or patients on treatment with mineralocorticoid receptor antagonists and increased renin (suggesting optimal mineralocorticoid receptor blockade), or adrenalectomized PA patients.

A long-term follow-up study by Sechi et al. [44] showed that in PA renal damage could be reversed by target treatment, a finding thereafter supported by Hundemer et al. [45], who showed that glomerular filtration rate declined more in PA patients treated with mineralocorticoid receptor antagonists than in essential hypertension patients and in PA cured with adrenalectomy. Rapid regression of microalbuminuria in PA suggests that urinary albumin excretion is, at least in part, due to functional rather than structural renal changes, i.e. glomerular hyperfiltration and decreased intrarenal vascular resistance. Elegant studies by Hall et al. in dogs exposed to hyperaldosteronism while renal perfusion pressure was maintained constant support this contention [46].

Thus, early screening and identification of PA patients who need surgery is needed to prevent/regress morbid events caused by hyperaldosteronism.

## 4. Screening of PA

The diagnosis of PA requires demonstration of an excessive aldosterone secretion autonomous of the renin-angiotensin system [11]. This implies concomitant measurement of plasma aldosterone and renin levels, $Na^+$ and $K^+$ in serum and 24-hour urine, followed by calculation of the aldosterone-to-renin ratio (ARR) [11]. Nowadays, the measurement of direct renin concentration has replaced plasma renin activity (PRA) in many laboratories because it is simpler, quicker and more accurate in the low range typically seen in PA [47]. However, the optimal cutoff value of the ARR is still a matter of debate and for optimal use they should be determined at each centre. Based on a prospective validation using a solid diagnosis of PA due to APA diagnosed as previously mentioned, we use 2.06 ng/dl/mUI/L (=20.6 ng/mUI) if renin is estimated by DRC or 26 ng/dl/ng/ml/h if renin was measured as PRA [47]. The aforementioned ARR-App can render the interpretation of results straightforward for practicing physicians and avoids the errors that might occur with unit conversion and calculations [20].

## 5. Confirmatory tests

Confirmatory tests are still used in most centres, even though there is clear-cut evidence that at the prevalence rate of PA seen in referral centres, i.e. between 11 and 30%, their negative predictive value largely exceeds their positive predictive value [48], and, therefore, these tests function as 'exclusion tests'. These tests stand on the unproven hypothesis that aldosterone secretion is unresponsive to maneuvers that perturbate renin. By such premise, they will identify only the subset of PA cases that are unresponsive to salt or volume suppression of aldosterone secretion, notably a minority of the cases of PA [6, 49].

Therefore, as discussed in depth elsewhere, this is a highly controversial issue [49]. Most studies supporting the use of these tests did not follow the STARD recommendations [50]: they attempted to validate the confirmatory tests not against a gold reference standard, as the diagnosis of APA, but against another confirmatory test, also based on the presumed autonomy of aldosterone secretion from the renin-angiotensin system [49]. Therefore, they were affected by a tautology bias. The only demonstration of CYP11B2-positive nodules at pathology, besides biochemical cure of PA after adrenalectomy, provides, in our view, a conclusive diagnosis of PA, which can be an APA or unilateral multinodular adrenocortical hyperplasia [5]. Given the availability of monoclonal antibodies for human CYP11B2, we recently amended the 'four corners' with the addition of immunohistochemical detection of CYP11B2 in the resected adrenal for the diagnosis of APA [3]. Likely considering the complexity and the intrinsic inaccuracy of the confirmatory tests, the last Endocrine Society guidelines for the first time foresaw the possibility of skipping these tests in patients with a florid PA phenotype and to proceed directly to subtyping (see later) [11].

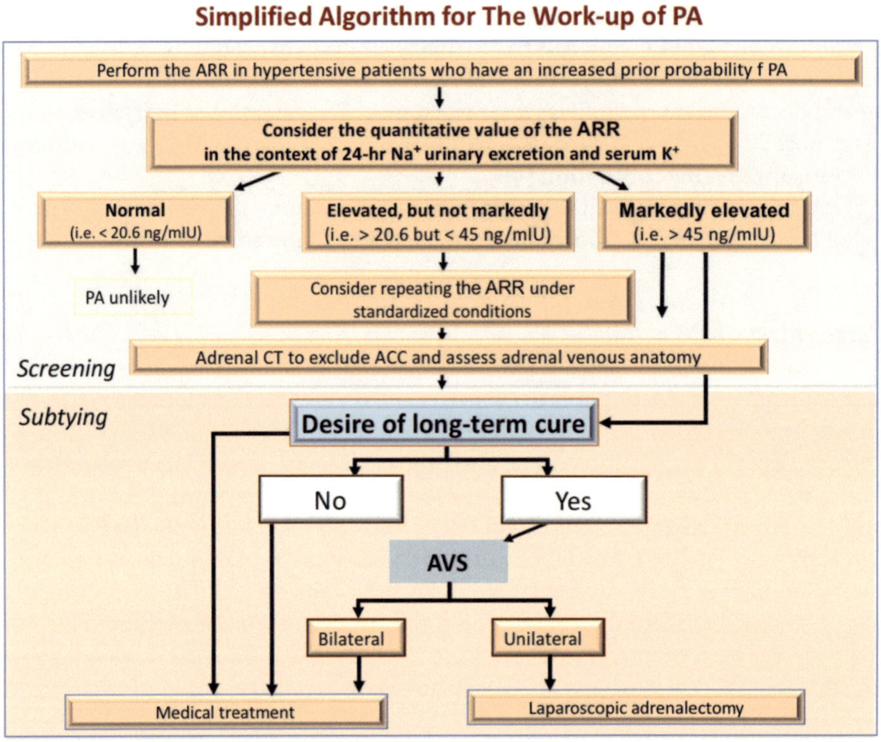


**Figure 2.**
*The flow-chart describes a simplified diagnostic algorithm for the work-up of primary aldosteronism (PA). The work up is schematically divided into screening, which is based on measurement of plasma aldosterone and renin and levels and calculation of the aldosterone-to-renin ratio (ARR), and subtyping that requires adrenal vein sampling (AVS). In the screening, given the important information conveyed by the quantitative value of the ARR, this test should not be regarded as positive or negative. Instead its actual value should be used to stratify the patients for probability of PA. The ARR value must be assessed in the context of 24-hr Na+ urinary excretion and serum K+. See text for explanation. Given the unreliable results of the so called "confirmatory tests", the authors do not recommend their use. A clear-cut advantage of this algorithm is its simplicity with ensuing cutting costs and, moreover, its being feasible in most centres. AVS is key for subtyping of primary aldosteronism (PA), which is indicated only in patients wishing to accomplish long-term cure. Adrenal imaging by CT should be performed preliminarily to AVS for two main reasons: to exclude malignant neoplasms (adrenocortical carcinoma, ACC) and to assess the anatomy of adrenal veins which can guide interventionists in performing AVS.*

In a recent large-size study comprising an exploratory and validation cohort, we investigated the accuracy of one such 'confirmatory' tests, the captopril challenge. This study provided unambiguous evidence that when a solid diagnosis of APA was used as reference index, the quantitative information conveyed by the ARR was accurate enough to avoid use of any confirmatory tests and to skip confirmatory tests [51]. In fact, neither the fall of plasma aldosterone concentration after captopril administration nor the fall of the ARR value furnished any diagnostic gain over baseline ARR values in these two very large cohorts of patients [51]. These results call for a simplification of the diagnostic algorithm as depicted in **Figure 2**. This strategy decreases the complexity, costs and time of the diagnostic workup for PA and therefore could extend the screening to most hypertensive patients, even in municipalities with low levels of access to specialized medical care.

## 6. Subtyping of PA

The most common forms of PA are unilateral causes of PA, mostly APA and rarely unilateral multinodular hyperplasia, and bilateral forms (BAH or IHA).

*DOI: http://dx.doi.org/10.5772/intechopen.87228*

As unilateral PA is best treated with unilateral laparoscopic adrenalectomy, while bilateral forms require lifelong mineralocorticoid receptor antagonists, the distinction between APA and IHA is crucial for choosing the appropriate treatment [11, 52].

There are at last 10 key reasons why AVS should be used to reliably discriminate between unilateral and bilateral PA, as reviewed in depth elsewhere [53]. AVS, albeit minimally invasive and safe [54], is technically difficult and expensive and potentially affected by several factors [55, 56]. For these reasons it should be performed only in properly selected patients and in centres with a skilled multidisciplinary team that has extensive expertise [11]. As a preliminary test for adrenalectomy, it should be reserved for patients seeking long-term cure of PA with surgery, who are reasonable candidates for general anesthesia and adrenalectomy. Importantly, AVS should be performed after correction of hypokalaemia, if present, and adjustment of antihypertensive medications to allow correct interpretation of the AVS results [11]. Patients with genetically confirmed familial forms of PA [57] usually have bilateral forms of PA and therefore should not be submitted to this test unless they have a CT detectable node.

## 7. Treatment of PA

The Endocrine Society guidelines [11] state that a lateralized aldosterone secretion should be demonstrated before undertaking surgery in patients who are candidates for general anesthesia and wish to achieve long-term cure. Laparoscopic adrenalectomy is currently the best treatment that it can be performed during a short hospital stay at a very low operative risk [58].

Overall, surgery cured PA in 33–72% of patients and resulted in marked improvements in 40–50% of patients [54]. This wide variation of results is explained by the fact that at some centres adrenalectomy is performed on the basis of imaging alone that can be misleading in a substantial proportion of patients [54]. When performed after demonstration of lateralized aldosterone, excess adrenalectomy cured or determined a marked improvement of hypertension in ~82% of the patients, while practically all were biochemically cured from the hyperaldosteronism [54]. Even when antihypertensive treatment cannot be withdrawn after adrenalectomy, the number and/or the doses of antihypertensive drugs could be markedly decreased, and/or resistant hypertension was resolved at long term [54]. Adrenalectomy can also lead to a considerable improvement in several indexes of quality of life.

The outcome for blood pressure was found to be predicted by the duration of hypertension and vascular remodeling, both of which are associated with delayed diagnosis (28). Overall available evidence supports the concept that the sooner the diagnosis is made and adrenalectomy performed, the better the outcome [54]. Failure to achieve cure of PA can be the result of concurrent essential hypertension or an inaccurate diagnosis (AVS not performed or results incorrectly interpreted). In fact, both the PASO study [4] and the larger AVIS-2 study (manuscript submitted) showed a huge variability in AVS success even at major referral centres. Due to the high prevalence of both PA and primary (essential) hypertension, up to one third of patients with PA would be expected to have concurrent primary hypertension. Adrenalectomy can cure only PA, but not hypertension, in these patients.

For patients who are not candidates for surgery or do not show lateralized aldosterone excess, a treatment based on mineralocorticoid receptor antagonists, such as spironolactone, canrenone, potassium canrenoate and eplerenone (which is more selective but also more expensive, weaker and shorter acting than the other antagonists and is not generally available), is a reasonable alternative to adrenalectomy.

Spironolactone was found to regress LVH even at doses (37 mg daily) that did not completely normalize BP in both PA and low-renin hypertension, supporting a role of aldosterone in LVH development [59]. The occurrence of gynaecomastia and impotence, the more annoying side effects of the mineralocorticoid receptor antagonists, is dose-dependent, which suggests the use of reduced doses in combination, if necessary, with other agents, such as long-acting calcium channel blockers, angiotensin-converting enzyme inhibitors or angiotensin receptor blockers. Amiloride and triamterene have been also proposed in addition to the first-line treatment with mineralocorticoid receptor antagonists if BP control is not optimal [60], but these drugs are not available as single agent in some counties, and, moreover, the combined therapy needs monitoring of serum potassium and creatinine. Angiotensin-converting enzyme inhibitors and angiotensin receptor blockers can be particularly useful, as they effectively control the counter-regulatory stimulation of the renin-angiotensin system triggered by the diuretic action of the mineralocorticoid receptor antagonists. Aldosterone synthase inhibitors are also being developed and tested in phase III trials as an effective strategy to control hyperaldosteronism [61, 62].

## 8. Future developments

Mutations in the selectivity filter of potassium channels of the KCNJ5 type and other genes involved in the regulation of cytosolic calcium in adrenocortical cells [57, 63] play an important role in upregulating aldosterone secretion. Few germline mutations associated with bilateral adrenal hyperplasia and severe PA have been identified, thus allowing identification of further forms of familial hyperaldosteronism (6). These discoveries have triggered enormous investigative efforts, whose results, which are difficult to anticipate at this time, might lead to change our understanding and our diagnostic and therapeutic approach to PA. For the time being, following a few simple rules and a streamlined approach (**Figure 2**), physicians can successfully and cost-effectively identify and treat many patients with the so-called 'essential' hypertension whose high blood pressure is instead caused by hyperaldosteronism. In these patients the clue to PA is a low plasma renin, which responds little nothing to stimulatory maneuvers. Identification of PA is particularly beneficial when hypertension is severe and/or resistant to treatment, because specific treatment can bring blood pressure under control despite withdrawal or a prominent reduction in the number and dosage of antihypertensive medications.

## Acknowledgements

This publication is based upon the work from the EU COST Action ADMIRE BM1301 in Aldosterone and Mineralocorticoid Receptor Physiology and Pathophysiology www.admirecosteu.com. The authors' work herein reviewed was supported by research grants from FORICA (the Foundation for advanced Research in Hypertension and Cardiovascular diseases), the Società Italiana dell'Ipertensione Arteriosa and grants from the Ministry of University and Scientific Research (MIUR) and The University of Padova.

## Conflict of interest

Both authors have read and approved the manuscript. There is no conflict of interest and financial disclosure.

## Author details

Gian Paolo Rossi* and Teresa M. Seccia
Hypertension Unit, Department of Medicine-DIMED, University of Padova, Padova, Italy

*Address all correspondence to: gianpaolo.rossi@unipd.it

## References

[1] Rossi GP. Primary aldosteronism: A needle in a haystack or a yellow cab on fifth avenue? Current Hypertension Reports. 2004;**6**(1):1-4

[2] Rossi GP, Seccia TM, Pessina AC. Primary aldosteronism - part I: Prevalence, screening, and selection of cases for adrenal vein sampling. Journal of Nephrology. 2008;**21**(4):447-454

[3] Rossi GP, Bernini G, Caliumi C, Desideri G, Fabris B, Ferri C, et al. A prospective study of the prevalence of primary aldosteronism in 1,125 hypertensive patients. Journal of the American College of Cardiology. 2006;**48**(11):2293-2300

[4] Williams TA, Lenders JWM, Mulatero P, Burrello J, Rottenkolber M, Adolf C, et al. Investigators PASO (PASO). Outcomes after adrenalectomy for unilateral primary aldosteronism: An international consensus on outcome measures and analysis of remission rates in an international cohort. The Lancet Diabetes and Endocrinology. 2017;**5**(9):689-699

[5] Gioco F, Seccia TM, Gomez-Sanchez EP, Rossi GP, Gomez-Sanchez CE. Adrenal histopathology in primary aldosteronism: Is it time for a change? Hypertension. 2015;**66**(4):724-730

[6] Seccia TM, Caroccia B, Gomez-Sanchez EP, Gomez-Sanchez CE, Rossi GP. The biology of Normal zona glomerulosa and aldosterone-producing adenoma: Pathological implications. Endocrine Reviews. 2018;**39**(6):1029-1056

[7] Ito Y, Takeda R, Karashima S, Yamamoto Y, Yoneda T, Takeda Y. Prevalence of primary aldosteronism among prehypertensive and stage 1 hypertensive subjects. Hypertension Research. 2010;**34**(1):98-102

[8] Olivieri O, Ciacciarelli A, Signorelli D, Pizzolo F, Guarini P, Pavan C, et al. Aldosterone to renin ratio in a primary care setting: The Bussolengo study. The Journal of Clinical Endocrinology and Metabolism. 2004;**89**(9):4221-4226

[9] Monticone S, Burrello J, Tizzani D, Bertello C, Viola A, Buffolo F, et al. Prevalence and clinical manifestations of primary Aldosteronism encountered in primary care practice. Journal of the American College of Cardiology. 2017;**69**(14):1811-1820

[10] Maiolino G, Calò LA, Rossi GP. The time has come for systematic screening for primary Aldosteronism in all hypertensives. Journal of the American College of Cardiology. 2017;**69**(14):1821-1823

[11] Funder JW, Carey RM, Mantero F, Murad MH, Reincke M, Shibata H, et al. The management of primary aldosteronism: Case detection, diagnosis, and treatment: An endocrine society clinical practice guideline. The Journal of Clinical Endocrinology and Metabolism. 2016;**101**(5):1889-1916

[12] Brown JM, Underwood PC, Ferri C, Hopkins PN, Williams GH, Adler GK, et al. Aldosterone dysregulation with aging predicts renal vascular function and cardiovascular risk. Hypertension. 2014;**63**(6):1205-1211

[13] Rossi GP, Sacchetto A, Pavan E, Palatini P, Graniero GR, Canali C, et al. Remodeling of the left ventricle in primary aldosteronism due to Conn's adenoma. Circulation. 1997;**95**(6):1471-1478

[14] Rossi GP, Bernini G, Desideri G, Fabris B, Ferri C, Giacchetti G, et al. Renal damage in primary aldosteronism: Results of the PAPY Study. Hypertension. 2006;**48**(2):232-238

[15] Douma S, Petidis K, Doumas M, Papaefthimiou P, Triantafyllou A, Kartali N, et al. Prevalence of primary hyperaldosteronism in resistant hypertension: A retrospective observational study. Lancet. 2008;**371**(9628):1921-1926

[16] Conn JW. Presidential address. I. Painting background. II. Primary aldosteronism, a new clinical syndrome. The Journal of Laboratory and Clinical Medicine. 1955;**45**(1):3-17

[17] Mulatero P, Monticone S, Burrello J, Veglio F, Williams TA, Funder J. Guidelines for primary aldosteronism: Uptake by primary care physicians. Journal of Hypertension. 2016;**34**(11):2253-2257

[18] Mulatero P, Rabbia F, Milan A, Paglieri C, Morello F, Chiandussi L, et al. Drug effects on aldosterone/plasma renin activity ratio in primary aldosteronism. Hypertension. 2002;**40**(6):897-902

[19] Stowasser M, Ahmed AH, Pimenta E, Taylor PJ, Gordon RD. Factors affecting the aldosterone/renin ratio. Hormone and Metabolic Research. 2012;**44**(3):170-176

[20] Rossi GP, Bisogni V. A useful tool to improve the case detection rate of primary aldosteronism: The aldosterone -renin ratio (ARR)-app. Journal of Hypertension. 2016;**34**(5):1019-1021

[21] Rossi GP, Gioco F, Fassina A, Gomez-Sanchez CE. Normoaldosteronemic aldosterone-producing adenoma: Immunochemical characterization and diagnostic implications. Journal of Hypertension. 2015;**33**(12):2546-2549

[22] Baudrand R, Guarda FJ, Fardella C, Hundemer G, Brown J, Williams G, et al. Continuum of renin-independent Aldosteronism in Normotension. Hypertension. 2017;**69**(5):950-956

[23] Rossi GP, Cesari M, Cuspidi C, Maiolino G, Cicala MV, Bisogni V, et al. Long-term control of arterial hypertension and regression of left ventricular hypertrophy with treatment of primary aldosteronism. Hypertension. 2013;**62**(1):62-69

[24] Gaddam KK, Pimenta E, Husain S, Calhoun DA. Aldosterone and cardiovascular disease. Current Problems in Cardiology. 2009;**34**(2):51-84

[25] Weber KT, Brilla CG. Pathological hypertrophy and cardiac interstitium. Fibrosis and renin-angiotensin-aldosterone system. Circulation. 1991;**83**(6):1849-1865

[26] Young M, Funder JW. Eplerenone, but not steroid withdrawal, reverses cardiac fibrosis in deoxycorticosterone/salt-treated rats. Endocrinology. 2004;**145**(7):3153-3157

[27] Wang Q, Clement S, Gabbiani G, Horisberger J-D, Burnier M, Rossier BC, et al. Chronic hyperaldosteronism in a transgenic mouse model fails to induce cardiac remodeling and fibrosis under a normal-salt diet. American Journal of Physiology. Renal Physiology. 2004;**286**(6):F1178-F1184

[28] Rickard AJ, Funder JW, Fuller PJ, Young MJ. The role of the glucocorticoid receptor in mineralocorticoid/salt-mediated cardiac fibrosis. Endocrinology. 2006;**147**(12):5901-5906

[29] Rocha R, Rudolph AE, Frierdich GE, Nachowiak DA, Kekec BK, Blomme EA, et al. Aldosterone induces a vascular inflammatory phenotype in the rat heart. American Journal of Physiology. Heart and Circulatory Physiology. 2002;**283**(5):H1802-H1810

[30] Brown NJ. Aldosterone and end-organ damage. Current Opinion in Nephrology and Hypertension. 2005;**14**(3):235-241

[31] Leopold JA, Dam A, Maron BA, Scribner AW, Liao R, Handy DE, et al. Aldosterone impairs vascular reactivity by decreasing glucose-6-phosphate dehydrogenase activity. Nature Medicine. 2007;**13**(2):189-197

[32] Rossi GP, Sacchetto A, Visentin P, Canali C, Graniero GR, Palatini P, et al. Changes in left ventricular anatomy and function in hypertension and primary aldosteronism. Hypertension. 1996;**27**(5):1039-1045

[33] Rossi GP, Maiolino G, Flego A, Belfiore A, Bernini G, Fabris B, et al. Adrenalectomy lowers incident atrial fibrillation in primary aldosteronism patients at long term. Hypertension. 2018;**71**(4):585-591

[34] Rossi GP, Bolognesi M, Rizzoni D, Seccia TM, Piva A, Porteri E, et al. Vascular remodeling and duration of hypertension predict outcome of adrenalectomy in primary aldosteronism patients. Hypertension. 2008;**51**(5):1366-1371

[35] Swedberg K, Zannad F, McMurray JJV, Krum H, Van Veldhuisen DJ, Shi H, et al. Eplerenone and atrial fibrillation in mild systolic heart failure: Results from the EMPHASIS-HF (Eplerenone in mild patients hospitalization and SurvIval Study in heart failure) study. Journal of the American College of Cardiology. 2012;**59**(18):1598-1603

[36] Farquharson CA, Struthers AD. Aldosterone induces acute endothelial dysfunction in vivo in humans: Evidence for an aldosterone-induced vasculopathy. Clinical Science (London, England). 2002;**103**(4):425-431

[37] Rossi GP, Di BV, Ganzaroli C, Sacchetto A, Cesari M, Bertini A, et al. Excess aldosterone is associated with alterations of myocardial texture in primary aldosteronism. Hypertension. 2002;**40**(1):23-27

[38] Seccia TM, Caroccia B, Adler GK, Maiolino G, Cesari M, Rossi GP. Arterial hypertension, atrial fibrillation, and hyperaldosteronism: The triple trouble. Hypertension. 2017;**69**(4):545-550

[39] Milliez P, Girerd X, Plouin PF, Blacher J, Safar ME, Mourad JJ. Evidence for an increased rate of cardiovascular events in patients with primary aldosteronism. Journal of the American College of Cardiology. 2005;**45**(8):1243-1248

[40] Hundemer GL, Curhan GC, Yozamp N, Wang MVA. Incidence of atrial fibrillation and mineralocorticoid receptor activity in patients with medically and surgically treated primary Aldosteronism. JAMA Cardiology. 2018;**3**(8):768-774

[41] Danforth D, Orlando M, Javadpour N. Renal changes in primary aldosteronism. The Journal of Urology. 1977;**117**(2):140-144

[42] Nishimura M, Uzu T, Fujii T, Kuroda S, Nakamura S, Inenaga T, et al. Cardiovascular complications in patients with primary aldosteronism. American Journal of Kidney Diseases. 1999;**33**(2):261-266

[43] Rossi GP, Cesari M, Cuspidi C, Maiolino G, Cicala MV, Bisogni V, et al. Response to effectiveness of adrenalectomy and aldosterone antagonists for long-term treatment of primary aldosteronism. Hypertension. 2013;**62**(4):4-5

[44] Sechi LA, Novello M, Lapenna R, Baroselli S, Nadalini E, Colussi GL, et al. Long-term renal outcomes in patients with primary aldosteronism. Journal of the American Medical Association. 2006;**295**(22):2638-2645

[45] Hundemer GL, Curhan GC, Yozamp N, Wang M, Vaidya A. Renal outcomes in medically and surgically treated primary Aldosteronism. Hypertension. 2018;**72**(3):658-666

[46] Hall JE, Granger JP, MJS J, Premen AJ. Role of renal hemodynamics and arterial pressure in aldosterone "escape". Hypertension. 1984;**6**(2 Pt 2): I183-I192

[47] Rossi GP, Ceolotto G, Rossitto G, Seccia TM, Maiolino G, Berton C, et al. Prospective validation of an automated chemiluminescence-based assay of renin and aldosterone for the work-up of arterial hypertension. Clinical Chemistry and Laboratory Medicine. 2016;**54**(9):1441-1450

[48] Rossi GP, Belfiore A, Bernini G, Desideri G, Fabris B, Ferri C, et al. Comparison of the captopril and the saline infusion test for excluding aldosterone-producing adenoma. Hypertension. 2007;**50**(2):424-431

[49] Rossi GP, Seccia TM, Pessina AC. A diagnostic algorithm—The holy grail of primary aldosteronism. Nature Reviews Endocrinology. 2011;7(12):697-699

[50] Bossuyt PM, Reitsma JB, Bruns DE, Gatsonis CA, Glasziou PP, Irwig LM, et al. For reporting of diagnostic accuracy S. the STARD statement for reporting studies of diagnostic accuracy: Explanation and elaboration. Clinical Chemistry. 2003;**49**(1):7-18

[51] Maiolino G, Rossitto G, Bisogni V, Cesari M, Seccia TM, Plebani M, et al. Quantitative value of aldosterone-renin ratio for detection of aldosterone-producing adenoma: The aldosterone-renin ratio for primary aldosteronism (AQUARR) study. Journal of the American Heart Association. 2017;**6**(5):e005574

[52] Rossi GP, Auchus RJ, Brown M, Lenders JWM, Naruse M, Plouin PF, et al. An expert consensus statement on use of adrenal vein sampling for the subtyping of primary aldosteronism. Hypertension. 2014;**63**(1):151-160

[53] Rossi GP, Mulatero P, Satoh F. 10 good reasons why adrenal vein sampling is the preferred method for referring primary aldosteronism patients for adrenalectomy. Journal of Hypertension. 2019;**37**(3):603-611

[54] Rossi GP, Barisa M, Allolio B, Auchus RJ, Amar L, Cohen D, et al. The adrenal vein sampling international Study (AVIS) for identifying the major subtypes of primary aldosteronism. The Journal of Clinical Endocrinology and Metabolism. 2012;**97**(5):1606-1614

[55] Seccia TM, Miotto D, Battistel M, Motta R, Barisa M, Maniero C, et al. A stress reaction affects assessment of selectivity of adrenal venous sampling and of lateralization of aldosterone excess in primary aldosteronism. European Journal of Endocrinology. 2012;**166**(5):869-875

[56] Miotto D, De Toni R, Pitter G, Seccia TM, Motta R, Vincenzi M, et al. Impact of accessory hepatic veins on adrenal vein sampling for identification of surgically curable primary aldosteronism. Hypertension. 2009;**54**(4):885-889

[57] Lenzini L, Prisco S, Caroccia B, Rossi GP. Saga of familial hyperaldosteronism. Hypertension. 2018;**71**(6):1010-1014

[58] Iacobone M, Citton M, Viel G, Rossi GP, Nitti D. Approach to the surgical management of primary aldosteronism. Gland Surgery. 2015;**4**(1):69-81

[59] Ori Y, Chagnac A, Korzets A, Zingerman B, Herman-Edelstein M, Bergman M, et al. Regression of left ventricular hypertrophy in patients with primary aldosteronism/low-renin hypertension on low-dose spironolactone. Nephrology, Dialysis, Transplantation. 2013;**28**(7):1787-1793

[60] Quinkler M, Stewart PM. Treatment of primary aldosteronism. Best Practice & Research: Clinical Endocrinology & Metabolism. 2010;**24**(6):923-932

[61] Amar L, Azizi M, Menard J, Peyrard S, Plouin P-F. Sequential comparison of aldosterone synthase inhibition and mineralocorticoid blockade in patients with primary aldosteronism. Journal of Hypertension. 2013;**31**(3):624-629

[62] Tamargo J, Solini A, Ruilope LM. Comparison of agents that affect aldosterone action. Seminars in Nephrology. 2014;**34**(3):285-306

[63] Lenzini L, Rossi GP. The molecular basis of primary aldosteronism: From chimeric gene to channelopathy. Current Opinion in Pharmacology. 2015;**21**:35-42

Chapter 7

# Potential Benefit of Mineralocorticoid Receptor Antagonists in Kidney Diseases

*Jonatan Barrera-Chimal, Lionel Lattenist and Frederic Jaisser*

## Abstract

Since the last two decades, a major paradigm shift occurred in our understanding of the physiological and pathophysiological roles of the mineralocorticoid receptor (MR). Expression of the MR in cells/tissues not involved in sodium/potassium balance and extracellular volume homeostasis, i.e., the primary role of the aldosterone/MR complex, paved the way to the discovery of unsuspected implications of MR in a variety of cellular processes and pathological consequences. It also opens the possibility for quick translation to the bedside using available MR antagonists (MRAs) such as spironolactone, canrenone, or eplerenone or using the more recently developed various nonsteroidal MRAs that are not yet marketed. Landmark clinical trials like RALES, EPHESUS, or EMPHASIS well established that MRAs provide great benefits in patients with heart failure and spironolactone or eplerenone have been recommended in these patients. The deep understanding provided by preclinical studies in various domains stimulated the possibility to extend the use of MRAs to new fields, including renal diseases even if MRAs are currently contraindicated or used with great caution in patients with renal function impairment due to the higher risk of hyperkalemia associated with MRA therapy in this at-risk population. The present review presents preclinical data supporting potential indications in renal diseases.

**Keywords:** aldosterone, renal, hypertension

## 1. Pathophysiological basis: MR activation in the kidney—where and what are the consequences?

### 1.1 MR expression in the kidney

Besides the well-known expression of MR in the so-called aldosterone-sensitive distal nephron (ASDN) encompassing DCT1-2, CNT, and CDD, MR is also expressed in a variety of other cell types within the kidney [1–5]. In basal condition, MR is expressed in the vasculature in both endothelium [6] and smooth muscle cells [1]. MR expression has also been reported in the mesangium [7], podocytes [8], fibroblasts [9], and immune cells (macrophages, dendritic cells, T lymphocytes) [10–13]. In **Figure 1**, we summarize the effects reported for MR antagonists in different target cells within the kidney that represent potential

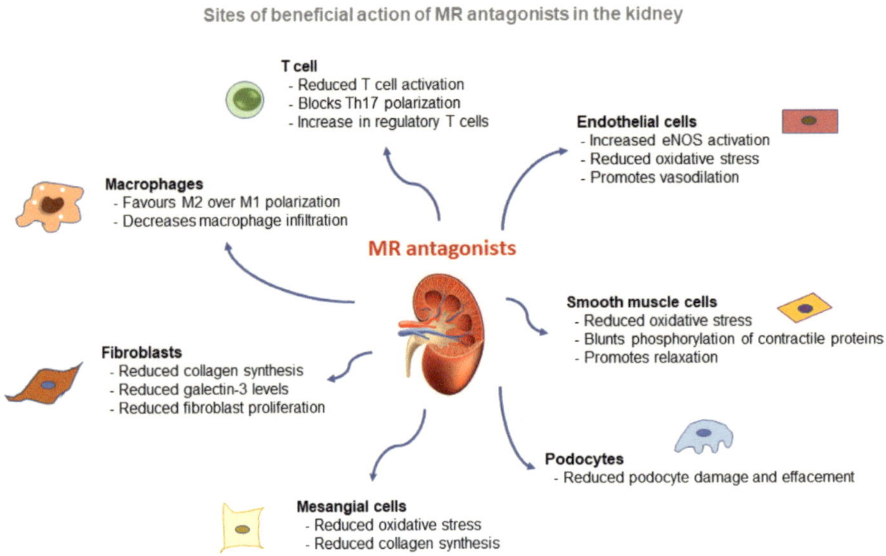


**Figure 1.**
*MR antagonists display beneficial effects against kidney diseases by acting in several cell types and by different mechanisms.*

beneficial mechanisms acting against kidney disease progression, and that will be detailed below. It is important to mention that MR expression might be upregulated in some pathological conditions such as diabetes [14], heavy proteinuria [15], vascular aging [16], and hypertension [17], leading to potential increased MR signaling. The specific physiological role of MR in the cells where its expression has been reported remains to be elucidated; however, it was recently proposed that MR in endothelial, smooth muscle, and inflammatory cells may be an evolutionary mechanism to prevent hemorrhage by promoting vasoconstriction and thrombosis and to promote wound healing by the activation of inflammation and vascular remodeling [18].

## 1.2 MR activation: what is the ligand?

The classical ligand of the MR is aldosterone, but glucocorticoids can bind with similar affinity with that of MR. Of note ligand-receptor dissociation is faster for glucocorticoid than aldosterone, resulting in higher transactivation potency for aldosterone as compared to glucocorticoids, especially at low concentration. However, a selectivity mechanism allows aldosterone to preferentially activate the MR in the presence of glucocorticoids, despite much higher local concentration of glucocorticoids than aldosterone. The 11β-hydroxysteroid dehydrogenase type 2 (11β-HSD2) converts corticosterone/cortisol to compounds with low affinity for the MR [19]. The cellular aldosterone/glucocorticoid selectivity therefore depends on the expression level/activity of the HSD2. In the kidney, cells from the ASDN and endothelium express HSD2, while this is debated for the smooth muscle cells [20]. In podocytes, mesangial cells, and immune cells, for example, HSD2 is not expressed, therefore supporting the fact that glucocorticoids may be the main ligands of MR in these cells. It should be stressed, however, that there may be species differences as well as induction of HSD2 expression in some pathological conditions, allowing aldosterone to activate MR. This has not been carefully analyzed yet [1].

### 1.3 Major pathophysiological mechanisms involved in MR and kidney diseases

#### *1.3.1 MR and renal hemodynamic alterations*

Experimental evidence in rodent models of acute kidney injury (AKI) supports the concept that MR contributes to vascular tone regulation [1]. The benefit of MRA in renal ischemia-reperfusion injury is associated with improved renal hemodynamics and decreased renal vascular resistance [21, 22]. We recently showed that MR expressed in mouse smooth muscle cells contributes to renal injury induced by ischemia (through a mechanism involving oxidative stress and Rac1 activation) [23], as well as in acute CsA nephrotoxicity (due to increased vascular L-type calcium channel activity thereby resulting in decreased renal artery vasoconstriction and overall improvement in renal hemodynamics) [24]. Of note, the endothelial MR was not directly involved since endothelial MR gene inactivation had no effect in ischemia-reperfusion or CsA-induced renal injuries [23, 24]. Whether MR expressed in the renal vasculature contributes to renal injury in other settings like diabetes or chronic kidney diseases remains to be explored.

#### *1.3.2 MR and oxidative stress*

Multiple in vitro and in vivo studies have shown the significance of oxidative stress induced by aldosterone/MR and its detrimental consequences on kidney injury. In vivo, the DOCA-salt causes oxidative DNA damage [25], and aldosterone infusion produces an MR-dependent increase in NADPH oxidase activity and ROS generation in the kidney [26, 27]. MR expressed in the smooth muscle cell may have a major role as we recently demonstrated in ischemia-reperfusion injury using smooth muscle MR KO mice [23]. In vascular cells, aldosterone increased ROS which in turn modifies the cysteinyl thiols in the eNOS-activating region of endothelin-1 B receptor to decrease endothelin-1-stimulated eNOS activity, impairing the vasodilatory pathway. These effects have repercussions on renal hemodynamics and function in kidney ischemia/reperfusion injury in both rat and mouse [21–23]. In rat mesangial cells, aldosterone directly stimulates superoxide anion generation, which is accompanied by an increase in NADPH oxidase activity and translocation of p47phox and p67phox to the cell membrane [28]. Moreover, recent studies have shown that aldosterone induces mesangial cell apoptosis and that the administration of an antioxidant or MR antagonist attenuates the proapoptotic effects of aldosterone [29]. The increase in NADPH oxidase Nox2 plasma levels and urinary isoprostanes is also observed in patients with primary aldosteronism as compared to essential hypertensive patients [30]. Interestingly, adrenalectomy is associated with a reduction in both parameters [30]. Moreover, therapeutic MR antagonism reduced oxidative stress in diabetic [31] or kidney transplant patients [32].

#### *1.3.3 MR and inflammation*

A role for MR signaling in inflammation has been suggested since early studies showing that the treatment of rats with aldosterone and salt causes perivascular leukocyte infiltration and increased expression of inflammatory markers [1]. More recently, macrophages, dendritic cells, and T lymphocytes have been identified as MR-expressing cells [1, 11, 33]. The use of genetically modified mouse model deficient of MR in myeloid cells revealed that myeloid MR contributes to renal injury in a glomerulonephritis mouse model [8]. Moreover, our recent work showed that myeloid MR participates to CKD progression induced by AKI [34].

The deletion of MR in myeloid cells favored M2 polarization of renal macrophages leading to improved tissue repair and prevention of renal scaring, decreased function, and interstitial fibrosis. Interestingly MRA administration using the nonsteroidal MRA finerenone has similar effects, blunting CKD development after ischemia-reperfusion injury in rodents [22, 34] and in the large white pig [34]. The role of myeloid MR in the progression of CKD in other models of kidney disease has to be further studied. The role of MR expressed in T cell has not been explored in kidney disease. However, T-cell MR knockout mice prevented cardiac hypertrophy, fibrosis, and dysfunction compared with littermate control mice after abdominal aortic constriction suggesting that MR in T cells may also play a pro-inflammatory role [13]. In dendritic cells, MR stimulation with aldosterone induces the secretion of IL-6 and TGF-β, two pro-inflammatory cytokines able to polarize the adaptive immune response toward a Th17 phenotype [35]. MR antagonism with spironolactone reduced heart and kidney damage in a hypertension rat model due to blockade of Th17 polarization and the induction of regulatory T cells [36]. Pharmacological MR blockade improves the chronic inflammatory state associated with CV disease [1, 33]. Altogether, these data suggest that aldosterone/MR modulates innate and adaptive immunity, which may have a critical role in end-organ damage.

#### *1.3.4 MR and fibrosis*

Fibrosis and extracellular matrix remodeling is a well-documented effect of MR activation in various tissues, including the kidney [1]. Aldosterone induces pro-fibrotic cytokine production and accumulation of collagen and other extracellular matrix components [9, 37, 38]. Aldosterone administration is associated with an increase in renal TGF-β, collagen, and connective tissue growth factor expression and medullary and cortical fibrosis [39]. Aldosterone also influences the production of plasminogen activator inhibitor-1 leading to glomerulosclerosis [40]. MR activation in renal fibroblasts results in rapid activation of growth factor receptors and induction of PI3K/MAPK signaling, which stimulates proliferation and therefore contributes to fibrosis expansion [41]. Several molecular MR targets may be involved in the pro-fibrotic response of Aldo/MR signaling. We recently deeply explored the role of neutrophil gelatinase-associated lipocalin (NGAL) that we identified as a novel aldosterone/MR target [42]. NGAL induction by the MR might be a mechanism for MR-induced fibrosis since mice deficient in NGAL are protected from aldosterone-induced kidney fibrosis (Jaisser, unpublished data). Galectin-3 also mediates the pro-fibrotic effects of aldosterone-MR, and galectin-3 KO mice are protected against aldosterone-induced kidney fibrosis [43]. Taken together increased MR activation which may promote kidney fibrosis by inducing fibroblast proliferation and the production of several pro-fibrotic molecules.

## 2. Preclinical data supporting the benefit of MR antagonists (MRA) in kidney diseases

### 2.1 Benefit of MRA on acute kidney injury (AKI) induced by ischemia/reperfusion (IR)

A reduction of renal blood flow is occurring in several clinical settings, and this is a major cause of AKI. A number of studies in rodents and in the Large White Pig preclinical model have shown that MR antagonism with steroidal and nonsteroidal MRAs prevents and treats AKI induced by IR. In an early study, it was shown that spironolactone is a useful strategy to prevent the acute kidney dysfunction and tubular injury induced by bilateral renal IR injury in the rat [44]. The sustained reduction in renal blood flow observed after 24 hours in the IR-untreated rats was prevented in the spironolactone-treated groups. This was reproduced using nonsteroidal MRAs in both rats and mice [21–23] leading to the discovery of a novel underlying mechanism related to the limitation of oxidative stress and impaired endothelin-B receptor signaling [21, 22]. Importantly MRA also have curative effects when administered within the first 3 hours post ischemia-reperfusion [21, 45, 46]. The benefit of MR antagonists in ischemic AKI was translated into the Large White Pig preclinical model in which MR antagonism with soludactone (potassium canrenoate, a soluble MRA used in clinics) prevented the effects of AKI including kidney dysfunction and structural injuries [23].

### 2.2 AKI to CKD transition

In recent years, special focus has been given to the chronic consequences of an AKI episode. Several clinical and experimental studies have shown that AKI is linked with increased risk for CKD development.

In the rat, CKD progression induced by a single event of ischemic AKI (characterized by proteinuria, kidney dysfunction, and severe structural injury including interstitial fibrosis, glomerulosclerosis, tubule dilation, and podocyte injury) is prevented by spironolactone [45] and finerenone [22, 47]. MR antagonism also prevents CKD induced by a mild ischemic period even when administered 3 hours after the ischemia episode [48]. The underlying mechanisms rely on the limitation of inflammatory events and the promotion of repair mechanisms held by M2-type macrophages and interleukin-4 receptor signaling [34]. Importantly, these benefits are also observed in the Large White Pig model: short-term soludactone administration before/after the ischemic event indeed prevents CKD progression at 3 months, with a reduction in fibrosis and proteinuria and improved renal function [34]. The data indicate that MRA treatment is an encouraging therapeutic option to prevent the AKI to CKD transition which identifies the MR expressed in inflammatory cells as a specific target in this setting.

### 2.3 MR antagonism in kidney fibrosis and CKD progression

Kidney fibrosis is a common endpoint of CKD from different origins. Accumulating evidences indicate that aldosterone and/or MR signaling plays a key role in CKD development in a number of animal models including nephron reduction [49, 50], hypertensive models [51, 52], unilateral ureteral obstruction [53, 54], and mineralocorticoid/salt models [55]. MR antagonism not only prevents glomerulosclerosis in the remnant kidney model but also induces regression of glomerulosclerosis as evidenced by Aldigier et al. on kidney biopsy 4 weeks after spironolactone treatment initiation in rats already presenting CKD [56]. Eplerenone also limited proteinuria in this model [50]. Renal injury observed in the Dahl-sensitive rat upon salt loading is greatly limited by eplerenone [57, 58] and the nonsteroidal MRA CS-3150 [59]. This may be related to a direct effect on podocyte, as underlined by Shibata et al., involving activation of Rac1 and possible increased Rac1-mediated transactivation of the podocyte MR [60].

### 2.4 Benefit of MR blockade in diabetic nephropathy

The beneficial effects of MRA in different models of type I and type II diabetic nephropathy or kidney injury related to metabolic disorders have been reported. Spironolactone administration for 3 weeks reduced renal collagen deposition in

STZ-induced diabetic rats [61]. This was thereafter reported for other MRAs such as eplerenone [62]. MRAs are also efficient in limiting progression of diabetic nephropathy in models of type 2 diabetes. Eplerenone reduced albuminuria, glomerular hypertrophy, and mesangial expansion in the db/db mouse model [62]. The novel nonsteroidal MRA AZ9977 has similar effects [63]. In the Otsuka Long-Evans Tokushima Fatty (OLETF) rats or Zucker obese rats, similar benefits have been reported after MRA treatment [64, 65].

### 2.5 Calcineurin inhibitor toxicity and kidney transplantation

Some studies showed a benefit of MR blockade in acute and chronic CsA nephrotoxicity, including effects on preventing structural and functional alterations [66–68]. The underlying mechanisms leading to this protection rely on hemodynamic effects (blunting the sustained vasoconstriction induced by CNI) [24, 68] or renal extracellular matrix remodeling [67]. The effect of MRA in experimental kidney transplantation has been tested in a model of chronic allograft dysfunction in the Dark-Agouti to Wistar-Furth rat with a reduced vasculopathy and glomerular macrophage influx and a trend to reduced proteinuria and glomerulosclerosis [69].

### 2.6 Glomerulonephritis and MR blockade

Although few studies have addressed this issue, it has been reported that spironolactone and the nonsteroidal MRA BR-4628 are beneficial in mouse models of glomerulonephritis [70–72]. The myeloid MR seems to play a key role in the kidney since genetic deletion of MR in myeloid cells, but not in podocyte, blunted glomerulonephritis development [8].

## 3. Conclusion

Preclinical evidences clearly support the concept of a benefit of MR antagonism to treat or delay kidney diseases from different origins including ischemic kidney disease, diabetic and hypertensive nephropathy, glomerulonephritis, and calcineurin inhibitor toxicity in the context of kidney transplant. The underlying mechanisms rely on improving local hemodynamics and reducing extracellular matrix remodeling and local inflammation (**Figure 1**). Whether this translates in clinics is already largely supported by several clinical trials, but definitive answers should be provided by well-designed, large clinical trials based on hard renal outcomes like limitation of CKD progression and/or cardiovascular outcomes. A recent study showed that in patients with heart failure with preserved ejection fraction, spironolactone treatment decreased the relative risk for cardiovascular death, heart failure hospitalization, or aborted cardiac arrest, despite an increase in the hyperkalemia risk [73]. Novel therapeutics limiting the risk of hyperkalemia upon MRA use is also warranted in these at-risk populations.

## Acknowledgements

This publication is based upon the work from the EU COST Action ADMIRE BM1301 in Aldosterone and Mineralocorticoid Receptor Physiology and Pathophysiology (www.admirecosteu.com). The authors' work was supported by grants from the Institut National de la Santé et de la Recherche Médicale, the Centre de Recherche Industrielle et Technique, the Agence Nationale de la

Recherche (ANR-16-CE14-0021-01), the French Medical Research Foundation (DEQ20160334885), and the National Autonomous University of Mexico—DGAPA—PAPIIT (IA200117 and IN202919 to JBC) and a public grant Fight-HF overseen by the French National Research Agency (ANR) as part of the "Investissements d'Avenir" program (reference: ANR-15-RHU-0004).

## Author details

Jonatan Barrera-Chimal[1], Lionel Lattenist[2] and Frederic Jaisser[2,3]*

1 Laboratorio de Fisiología Cardiovascular y Trasplante Renal, Unidad de Medicina Traslacional, Instituto de Investigaciones Biomédicas, Instituto Nacional de Cardiología Ignacio Chávez, Universidad Nacional Autónoma de México, Mexico City, Mexico

2 Clinical Investigation Centre, Lorraine University, Vandoeuvre-lès-Nancy, France

3 Centre de Recherche des Cordeliers, Sorbonne University, Paris Descartes University, Paris, France

*Address all correspondence to: frederic.jaisser@inserm.fr

## References

[1] Jaisser F, Farman N. Emerging roles of the mineralocorticoid receptor in pathology: Toward new paradigms in clinical pharmacology. Pharmacological Reviews. 2016;**68**(1):49-75

[2] Kolkhof P, Barfacker L. 30 years of the mineralocorticoid receptor: Mineralocorticoid receptor antagonists: 60 years of research and development. The Journal of Endocrinology. 2017;**234**(1):T125-T140

[3] Pitt B, Zannad F, Remme WJ, et al. The effect of spironolactone on morbidity and mortality in patients with severe heart failure. Randomized aldactone evaluation study investigators. The New England Journal of Medicine. 1999;**341**(10):709-717

[4] Pitt B, Remme W, Zannad F, et al. Eplerenone, a selective aldosterone blocker, in patients with left ventricular dysfunction after myocardial infarction. The New England Journal of Medicine. 2003;**348**(14):1309-1321

[5] Zannad F, McMurray JJ, Krum H, et al. Eplerenone in patients with systolic heart failure and mild symptoms. The New England Journal of Medicine. 2011;**364**(1):11-21

[6] Caprio M, Newfell BG, la Sala A, et al. Functional mineralocorticoid receptors in human vascular endothelial cells regulate intercellular adhesion molecule-1 expression and promote leukocyte adhesion. Circulation Research. 2008;**102**(11):1359-1367

[7] Nishiyama A, Yao L, Fan Y, et al. Involvement of aldosterone and mineralocorticoid receptors in rat mesangial cell proliferation and deformability. Hypertension. 2005;**45**(4):710-716

[8] Huang LL, Nikolic-Paterson DJ, Han Y, et al. Myeloid mineralocorticoid receptor activation contributes to progressive kidney disease. Journal of the American Society of Nephrology. 2014;**25**(10):2231-2240

[9] Nagai Y, Miyata K, Sun GP, et al. Aldosterone stimulates collagen gene expression and synthesis via activation of ERK1/2 in rat renal fibroblasts. Hypertension. 2005;**46**(4):1039-1045

[10] Belden Z, Deiuliis JA, Dobre M, Rajagopalan S. The role of the mineralocorticoid receptor in inflammation: Focus on kidney and vasculature. American Journal of Nephrology. 2017;**46**(4):298-314

[11] Bene NC, Alcaide P, Wortis HH, Jaffe IZ. Mineralocorticoid receptors in immune cells: Emerging role in cardiovascular disease. Steroids. 2014;**91**:38-45

[12] Rickard AJ, Morgan J, Tesch G, Funder JW, Fuller PJ, Young MJ. Deletion of mineralocorticoid receptors from macrophages protects against deoxycorticosterone/salt-induced cardiac fibrosis and increased blood pressure. Hypertension. 2009;**54**(3):537-543

[13] Sun XN, Li C, Liu Y, et al. T-cell mineralocorticoid receptor controls blood pressure by regulating interferon-gamma. Circulation Research. 2017;**120**(10):1584-1597

[14] Taira M, Toba H, Murakami M, et al. Spironolactone exhibits direct renoprotective effects and inhibits renal renin-angiotensin-aldosterone system in diabetic rats. European Journal of Pharmacology. 2008;**589**(1-3):264-271

[15] Quinkler M, Zehnder D, Eardley KS, et al. Increased expression of mineralocorticoid effector mechanisms in kidney biopsies of patients with

heavy proteinuria. Circulation. 2005;**112**(10):1435-1443

[16] Krug AW, Allenhofer L, Monticone R, et al. Elevated mineralocorticoid receptor activity in aged rat vascular smooth muscle cells promotes a proinflammatory phenotype via extracellular signal-regulated kinase 1/2 mitogen-activated protein kinase and epidermal growth factor receptor-dependent pathways. Hypertension. 2010;**55**(6):1476-1483

[17] DeLano FA, Schmid-Schonbein GW. Enhancement of glucocorticoid and mineralocorticoid receptor density in the microcirculation of the spontaneously hypertensive rat. Microcirculation. 2004;**11**(1):69-78

[18] Biwer LA, Wallingford MC, Jaffe IZ. Vascular mineralocorticoid receptor: Evolutionary mediator of wound healing turned harmful by our modern lifestyle. American Journal of Hypertension. 2019;**32**(2):123-134

[19] Farman N, Rafestin-Oblin ME. Multiple aspects of mineralocorticoid selectivity. American Journal of Physiology. Renal Physiology. 2001;**280**(2):F181-F192

[20] Odermatt A, Kratschmar DV. Tissue-specific modulation of mineralocorticoid receptor function by 11beta-hydroxysteroid dehydrogenases: An overview. Molecular and Cellular Endocrinology. 2012;**350**(2):168-186

[21] Barrera-Chimal J, Prince S, Fadel F, et al. Sulfenic acid modification of endothelin B receptor is responsible for the benefit of a nonsteroidal mineralocorticoid receptor antagonist in renal ischemia. Journal of the American Society of Nephrology. 2016;**27**(2):398-404

[22] Lattenist L, Lechner SM, Messaoudi S, et al. Nonsteroidal mineralocorticoid receptor antagonist finerenone protects against acute kidney injury-mediated chronic kidney disease: Role of oxidative stress. Hypertension. 2017;**69**(5):870-878

[23] Barrera-Chimal J, Andre-Gregoire G, Nguyen Dinh Cat A, et al. Benefit of mineralocorticoid receptor antagonism in AKI: Role of vascular smooth muscle Rac 1. Journal of the American Society of Nephrology. 2017;**28**(4):1216-1226

[24] Amador CA, Bertocchio JP, Andre-Gregoire G, et al. Deletion of mineralocorticoid receptors in smooth muscle cells blunts renal vascular resistance following acute cyclosporine administration. Kidney International. 2016;**89**(2):354-362

[25] Schupp N, Kolkhof P, Queisser N, et al. Mineralocorticoid receptor-mediated DNA damage in kidneys of DOCA-salt hypertensive rats. The FASEB Journal. 2011;**25**(3):968-978

[26] Shibata S, Nagase M, Yoshida S, Kawachi H, Fujita T. Podocyte as the target for aldosterone: Roles of oxidative stress and Sgk 1. Hypertension. 2007;**49**(2):355-364

[27] Nishiyama A, Yao L, Nagai Y, et al. Possible contributions of reactive oxygen species and mitogen-activated protein kinase to renal injury in aldosterone/salt-induced hypertensive rats. Hypertension. 2004;**43**(4):841-848

[28] Miyata K, Rahman M, Shokoji T, et al. Aldosterone stimulates reactive oxygen species production through activation of NADPH oxidase in rat mesangial cells. Journal of the American Society of Nephrology. 2005;**16**(10):2906-2912

[29] Mathew JT, Patni H, Chaudhary AN, et al. Aldosterone induces mesangial cell apoptosis both *in vivo* and *in vitro*. American Journal of Physiology. Renal Physiology. 2008;**295**(1):F73-F81

[30] Petramala L, Pignatelli P, Carnevale R, et al. Oxidative stress in patients affected by primary aldosteronism. Journal of Hypertension. 2014;**32**(10):2022-2029. discussion 2029

[31] Takebayashi K, Matsumoto S, Aso Y, Inukai T. Aldosterone blockade attenuates urinary monocyte chemoattractant protein-1 and oxidative stress in patients with type 2 diabetes complicated by diabetic nephropathy. The Journal of Clinical Endocrinology and Metabolism. 2006;**91**(6):2214-2217

[32] Ojeda-Cervantes M, Barrera-Chimal J, Alberu J, Perez-Villalva R, Morales-Buenrostro LE, Bobadilla NA. Mineralocorticoid receptor blockade reduced oxidative stress in renal transplant recipients: A double-blind, randomized pilot study. American Journal of Nephrology. 2013;**37**(5):481-490

[33] Girerd S, Frimat L, Ducloux D, et al. EPURE transplant (eplerenone in patients undergoing renal transplant) study: Study protocol for a randomized controlled trial. Trials. 2018;**19**(1):595

[34] Barrera-Chimal J, Rocha L, Amador-Martinez I, et al. Delayed spironolactone administration prevents the transition from acute kidney injury to chronic kidney disease through improving renal inflammation. Nephrology, Dialysis, Transplantation. 2018;**33**(12):2080-2091

[35] Herrada AA, Contreras FJ, Marini NP, et al. Aldosterone promotes autoimmune damage by enhancing Th17-mediated immunity. Journal of Immunology. 2010;**184**(1):191-202

[36] Amador CA, Barrientos V, Pena J, et al. Spironolactone decreases DOCA-salt-induced organ damage by blocking the activation of T helper 17 and the downregulation of regulatory T lymphocytes. Hypertension. 2014;**63**(4):797-803

[37] Martin-Fernandez B, Rubio-Navarro A, Cortegano I, et al. Aldosterone induces renal fibrosis and inflammatory M1-macrophage subtype via mineralocorticoid receptor in rats. PLoS One. 2016;**11**(1):e0145946

[38] Chen D, Chen Z, Park C, et al. Aldosterone stimulates fibronectin synthesis in renal fibroblasts through mineralocorticoid receptor-dependent and independent mechanisms. Gene. 2013;**531**(1):23-30

[39] Sun Y, Zhang J, Zhang JQ, Ramires FJ. Local angiotensin II and transforming growth factor-beta 1 in renal fibrosis of rats. Hypertension. 2000;**35**(5):1078-1084

[40] Brown NJ, Nakamura S, Ma L, et al. Aldosterone modulates plasminogen activator inhibitor-1 and glomerulosclerosis *in vivo*. Kidney International. 2000;**58**(3):1219-1227

[41] Huang LL, Nikolic-Paterson DJ, Ma FY, Tesch GH. Aldosterone induces kidney fibroblast proliferation via activation of growth factor receptors and PI3K/MAPK signalling. Nephron. Experimental Nephrology. 2012;**120**(4):e115-e122

[42] Latouche C, El Moghrabi S, Messaoudi S, et al. Neutrophil gelatinase-associated lipocalin is a novel mineralocorticoid target in the cardiovascular system. Hypertension. 2012;**59**(5):966-972

[43] Calvier L, Martinez-Martinez E, Miana M, et al. The impact of galectin-3 inhibition on aldosterone-induced cardiac and renal injuries. JACC: Heart Failure. 2015;**3**(1):59-67

[44] Mejia-Vilet JM, Ramirez V, Cruz C, Uribe N, Gamba G, Bobadilla NA. Renal ischemia-reperfusion injury is prevented by the mineralocorticoid receptor blocker spironolactone.

American Journal of Physiology. Renal Physiology. 2007;**293**(1):F78-F86

[45] Barrera-Chimal J, Perez-Villalva R, Rodriguez-Romo R, et al. Spironolactone prevents chronic kidney disease caused by ischemic acute kidney injury. Kidney International. 2013;**83**(1):93-103

[46] Sanchez-Pozos K, Barrera-Chimal J, Garzon-Muvdi J, et al. Recovery from ischemic acute kidney injury by spironolactone administration. Nephrology, Dialysis, Transplantation. 2012;**27**(8):3160-3169

[47] Barrera-Chimal J, Estrela GR, Lechner SM, et al. The myeloid mineralocorticoid receptor controls inflammatory and fibrotic responses after renal injury via macrophage interleukin-4 receptor signaling. Kidney International. 2018;**93**(6):1344-1355

[48] Barrera-Chimal J, Perez-Villalva R, Ortega JA, et al. Mild ischemic injury leads to long-term alterations in the kidney: Amelioration by spironolactone administration. International Journal of Biological Sciences. 2015;**11**(8):892-900

[49] Greene EL, Kren S, Hostetter TH. Role of aldosterone in the remnant kidney model in the rat. The Journal of Clinical Investigation. 1996;**98**(4):1063-1068

[50] Fujihara CK, Kowala MC, Breyer MD, et al. A novel aldosterone antagonist limits renal injury in 5/6 nephrectomy. Scientific Reports. 2017;7(1):7899

[51] Rocha R, Chander PN, Zuckerman A, Stier CT Jr. Role of aldosterone in renal vascular injury in stroke-prone hypertensive rats. Hypertension. 1999;**33**(1 Pt 2):232-237

[52] Zhou X, Ono H, Ono Y, Frohlich ED. Aldosterone antagonism ameliorates proteinuria and nephrosclerosis independent of glomerular dynamics in L-NAME/SHR model. American Journal of Nephrology. 2004;**24**(2):242-249

[53] Trachtman H, Weiser AC, Valderrama E, Morgado M, Palmer LS. Prevention of renal fibrosis by spironolactone in mice with complete unilateral ureteral obstruction. The Journal of Urology. 2004;**172**(4 Pt 2): 1590-1594

[54] Chen H, Sun F, Zhong X, Shao Y, Yoshimura A, Liu Y. Eplerenone-mediated aldosterone blockade prevents renal fibrosis by reducing renal inflammation, interstitial cell proliferation and oxidative stress. Kidney & Blood Pressure Research. 2013;**37**(6):557-566

[55] Lother A, Furst D, Bergemann S, et al. Deoxycorticosterone acetate/salt-induced cardiac but not renal injury is mediated by endothelial mineralocorticoid receptors independently from blood pressure. Hypertension. 2016;**67**(1):130-138

[56] Aldigier JC, Kanjanbuch T, Ma LJ, Brown NJ, Fogo AB. Regression of existing glomerulosclerosis by inhibition of aldosterone. Journal of the American Society of Nephrology. 2005;**16**(11):3306-3314

[57] Miura R, Nakamura K, Miura D, et al. Anti-inflammatory effect of spironolactone on human peripheral blood mononuclear cells. Journal of Pharmacological Sciences. 2006;**101**(3):256-259

[58] Kobayashi N, Hara K, Tojo A, et al. Eplerenone shows renoprotective effect by reducing LOX-1-mediated adhesion molecule, PKCepsilon-MAPK-p90RSK, and Rho-kinase pathway. Hypertension. 2005;**45**(4):538-544

[59] Arai K, Tsuruoka H, Homma T. CS-3150, a novel non-steroidal mineralocorticoid receptor antagonist,

prevents hypertension and cardiorenal injury in Dahl salt-sensitive hypertensive rats. European Journal of Pharmacology. 2015;**769**:266-273

[60] Shibata S, Nagase M, Yoshida S, et al. Modification of mineralocorticoid receptor function by Rac 1 GTPase: Implication in proteinuric kidney disease. Nature Medicine. 2008;**14**(12):1370-1376

[61] Fujisawa G, Okada K, Muto S, et al. Spironolactone prevents early renal injury in streptozotocin-induced diabetic rats. Kidney International. 2004;**66**(4):1493-1502

[62] Guo C, Martinez-Vasquez D, Mendez GP, et al. Mineralocorticoid receptor antagonist reduces renal injury in rodent models of types 1 and 2 diabetes mellitus. Endocrinology. 2006;**147**(11):5363-5373

[63] Bamberg K, Johansson U, Edman K, et al. Preclinical pharmacology of AZD 9977: A novel mineralocorticoid receptor modulator separating organ protection from effects on electrolyte excretion. PLoS One. 2018;**13**(2):e0193380

[64] Han SY, Kim CH, Kim HS, et al. Spironolactone prevents diabetic nephropathy through an anti-inflammatory mechanism in type 2 diabetic rats. Journal of the American Society of Nephrology. 2006;**17**(5):1362-1372

[65] Lachaux M, Barrera-Chimal J, Nicol L, et al. Short- and long-term administration of the non-steroidal mineralocorticoid receptor antagonist finerenone opposes metabolic syndrome-related cardio-renal dysfunction. Diabetes, Obesity & Metabolism. 2018;**20**(10):2399-2407

[66] Nielsen FT, Jensen BL, Marcussen N, Skott O, Bie P. Inhibition of mineralocorticoid receptors with eplerenone alleviates short-term cyclosporin A nephrotoxicity in conscious rats. Nephrology, Dialysis, Transplantation. 2008;**23**(9):2777-2783

[67] Feria I, Pichardo I, Juarez P, et al. Therapeutic benefit of spironolactone in experimental chronic cyclosporine A nephrotoxicity. Kidney International. 2003;**63**(1):43-52

[68] Perez-Rojas JM, Derive S, Blanco JA, et al. Renocortical mRNA expression of vasoactive factors during spironolactone protective effect in chronic cyclosporine nephrotoxicity. American Journal of Physiology. Renal Physiology. 2005;**289**(5):F1020-F1030

[69] Waanders F, Rienstra H, Boer MW, et al. Spironolactone ameliorates transplant vasculopathy in renal chronic transplant dysfunction in rats. American Journal of Physiology. Renal Physiology. 2009;**296**(5):F1072-F1079

[70] Ma FY, Han Y, Nikolic-Paterson DJ, Kolkhof P, Tesch GH. Suppression of rapidly progressive mouse glomerulonephritis with the non-steroidal mineralocorticoid receptor antagonist BR-4628. PLoS One. 2015;**10**(12):e0145666

[71] Gullulu M, Akdag I, Kahvecioglu S, Filiz G, Savci V. Aldosterone blockage in proliferative glomerulonephritis prevents not only fibrosis, but proliferation as well. Renal Failure. 2006;**28**(6):509-514

[72] Asai M, Monkawa T, Marumo T, et al. Spironolactone in combination with cilazapril ameliorates proteinuria and renal interstitial fibrosis in rats with anti-Thy-1 irreversible nephritis. Hypertension Research. 2004;**27**(12):971-978

[73] Beldhuis IE, Myhre PL, Claggett B, et al. Efficacy and safety of spironolactone in patients with HFpEF and chronic kidney disease. JACC: Heart Failure. 2019;**7**(1):25-32

Chapter 8

# Mineralocorticoid Receptor in Novel Target Tissues: A Closer Look at the Adipocyte

*Andrea Armani, Vincenzo Marzolla, Alessandra Feraco, Stefania Gorini, Caterina Mammi, Marco Infante and Massimiliano Caprio*

## Abstract

In addition to the well-documented role in the kidney, the mineralocorticoid receptor (MR) has been recently identified in different "non-classical" target tissues, such as the brain, the heart, vasculature, macrophages/monocytes, and adipose tissue. In this context, the MR is involved in adipocyte fundamental processes such as differentiation, autophagy, and adipokine secretion. Excessive activation of the MR contributes to metabolic derangements occurring in mice with obesity and metabolic syndrome. Interestingly, MR pharmacological blockade in murine models of obesity has led to protection from weight gain and adipocyte dysfunctions. Unfortunately, there is still a lack of knowledge on the metabolic effects of MR antagonists, and larger clinical studies are deemed necessary to clarify the metabolic role of MR blockade in humans. This review discusses the role of MR in adipose tissue, focusing on regulation by MR of key cellular processes occurring in the adipocyte. The molecular pathways affected by MR activation or blockade in adipose tissue have been investigated only in part. Hence, more studies are necessary to get more insights in the role of aldosterone/MR in this "non-classical" target tissue and to better understand its potential implications in obesity and metabolic syndrome.

**Keywords:** adipose tissue, autophagy, browning, insulin resistance, obesity

## 1. Introduction

Mineralocorticoid receptor (MR) activity in the distal nephron plays a well-known role in salt homeostasis and blood pressure regulation [1]. Importantly, studies performed since the late 1980s by different laboratories have revealed the presence of MR also in non renal tissues (i.e., heart, brain, adipose tissue (AT)) [2–4]. The discovery of expression of MR in adipocytes, cardiomyocytes, and vascular cells has promoted further research to investigate MR function in the pathophysiology of obesity [5–7], cardiovascular disease [8–10], and metabolic syndrome [11]. Both aldosterone and glucocorticoids are able to activate MR [12]. Expression of the enzyme 11b-hydroxysteroid dehydrogenase type 2 (11b-HSD2) favors MR activation by aldosterone in epithelial tissues, whereas in non-epithelial tissues (AT, cardiomyocyte), scarce expression of 11b-HSD2 suggests that MR is activated mainly by glucocorticoids [12].

However, it is still controversial whether increased circulating levels of aldosterone observed in obesity, metabolic syndrome, and primary aldosteronism (PA) can activate MR in non-epithelial tissues [13] and, in particular, in the adipocyte where this transcription factor regulates differentiation and modulates oxidative stress and adipokine expression [6, 14, 15]. Notably, preclinical studies in murine models of obesity suggest that MR blockade counteracts fat mass expansion and improves insulin sensitivity, indicating that pharmacological antagonism of MR may represent a valid approach to fight obesity [5, 6], even though human studies have not yet confirmed such anti-obesogenic effects for MR antagonists.

Although a deeper comprehension of MR function in the adipose cell, at a molecular level, requires further research, it appears clear right now that adipocyte-specific MR represents a topic of future research on AT dysfunctions and obesity.

This review examines the state of the art of research on adipocyte MR, describes AT function, and analyzes the contribution of altered function of MR in the pathophysiology of obesity and metabolic syndrome.

## 2. Adipose organ function

*Adipose tissue is composed of two distinct types of fat: white adipose tissue (WAT) and brown adipose tissue (BAT) with distinct morphology and function. Both types of fat affect whole-body metabolism.*

The adipose organ represents a multi-depot organ consisting of subcutaneous and visceral fat depots with a marked cellular heterogeneity, containing adipocytes, preadipocytes, endothelial cells, fibroblasts, and immune cells [16, 17]. The adipocyte is the most relevant cell type in the AT and mammals display at least two distinct types of adipocytes, characterized by diverse morphology and physiological function. White adipocytes are unilocular spherical cells with a peripheral flattened nucleus and a single large cytoplasmic lipid droplet. White adipocytes are cells specialized for storing energy in the form of triglycerides and display endocrine properties, being able to synthesize and release secretory proteins called "adipokines" involved in regulation of whole-body energy metabolism [16, 17]. On the other hand, brown adipocytes display a round central nucleus and a high number of cytoplasmic lipid droplets and mitochondria. Mitochondria in brown adipocytes are characterized by the expression of uncoupling protein 1 (UCP1) which is the hallmark of the brown adipocyte. UCP1 is a unique protein which allows uncoupling of oxidative phosphorylation from ATP synthesis, leading to dissipation of chemical energy as heat (non-shivering thermogenesis) [18]. WAT has storage and secretory function and contains mainly white adipocytes. In the brown adipose tissue (BAT), with thermogenic function, the prevalent type of adipocyte is the brown adipocyte. BAT function is regulated by the sympathetic nervous system, and its thermogenic activity maintains body temperature in the presence of cold exposure or during postnatal period [19]. Up until a few years ago, BAT function was considered relevant only in hibernating mammals and newborn humans, whereas adult humans were thought to lack BAT [20]. Notably, studies published in 2007 and 2009 performed using fluorodeoxyglucose positron-emission tomography (FDG PET) [21, 22] have revealed the presence of functional BAT also in healthy adult humans, detected as regions of increased tracer uptake [22, 23]. Human BAT has been detected in the supraclavicular and cervical regions, as well as in mediastinal, paravertebral, paraaortic, and suprarenal regions [21]. Cold exposure results in BAT activation both in mice and humans [24, 25] with parallel increase in energy expenditure and reduced fat mass, thus suggesting that BAT activity enhancement may be considered a valid approach to fight obesity also in humans [26].

## 3. Adipose tissue dysfunctions in obesity

*Dysfunctional adipose tissue is characterized by enlarged size of the adipocyte, altered expression of adipokines, pro-inflammatory polarization of resident macrophages, and defective thermogenic capacity.*

Altered metabolic regulation of AT leads to excessive WAT expansion through two possible mechanisms: increased cell number (hyperplasia) and/or increased cell size (hypertrophy) [27]. Deregulated enlargement of adipocyte size promotes macrophage recruitment within WAT, through production of chemokines such as MCP-1 and IL-8. Macrophage recruitment is also associated with changes in macrophage polarization toward a pro-inflammatory phenotype (M1), which contributes to insulin sensitivity alteration [28]. Increased content of immune cells such as $CD8^+$ T cells and IFN-$\gamma^+$T-helper type 1 cells, in the AT of obese subjects, may contribute to the low-grade chronic inflammation associated with obesity [29]. In the obese state, altered expansion of WAT is also accompanied by increased secretion of pro-inflammatory adipokines, such as leptin, TNF-α, and IL-6, paralleled by a reduced secretion of anti-inflammatory and insulin-sensitizing adipokines, thus promoting obesity-related complications. As discussed above, preclinical and human studies suggest that enhanced activity of brown adipocytes by stimulating thermogenic function can protect against obesity and associated alterations in glucose metabolism and lipid profile [24, 30]. Importantly, reduced amounts of BAT have been observed in overweight and obese subjects, indicating that impairment in brown adipocyte activity may favor AT dysfunctions [22]. Indeed, a recent study has shown that a specific single-nucleotide T to C variant in the FTO locus promotes obesity development through inactivation of genes involved in brown adipogenesis, further confirming the importance of the brown fat in counteracting AT metabolic alterations [31].

In the adipocyte, MR has a central role in signaling pathways regulating physiology and pathophysiology of AT. Research on MR function in AT has been summarized and discussed in the paragraphs below.

## 4. MR in adipogenesis

*MR plays a key role in regulating adipogenesis. Overactivation of MR promotes adipose tissue dysfunction. On the other hand, MR antagonism counteracts white adipocyte differentiation and promotes brown adipogenesis.*

The role of MR has been studied in adipocyte cultures and in murine models of obesity. MR activity has been shown to promote expression of adipocyte markers and stimulate differentiation of 3T3-L1 adipose cell cultures (**Figure 1**) [14], whereas MR antagonism counteracts adipogenesis in 3T3-L1 cells as well as in primary human adipocytes [32, 33]. In accordance with these data, primary adipocyte cultures obtained from mice knockout for MR have shown impaired adipogenesis [34], as well as knockdown of MR in cultures of human preadipocytes represses differentiation [32]. Altogether, these data show that MR impaired function represses white adipocyte differentiation. Notably, in vivo studies show increased expression of MR in adipose tissue of obese mice and humans, suggesting enhanced activity of this receptor in the obese state which may contribute to adipocyte dysfunctions [11]. Pharmacological MR antagonism in obese mice counteracts weight gain and excessive expansion of fat mass [5, 6] and, at a molecular level, prevents altered expression of adiponectin, PPAR-γ, and leptin [15] confirming that MR activity modulates expression of adipocyte marker genes and regulates AT function. Recent data by Feraco et al. have shown that adipocyte-specific MR-KO mice do not show

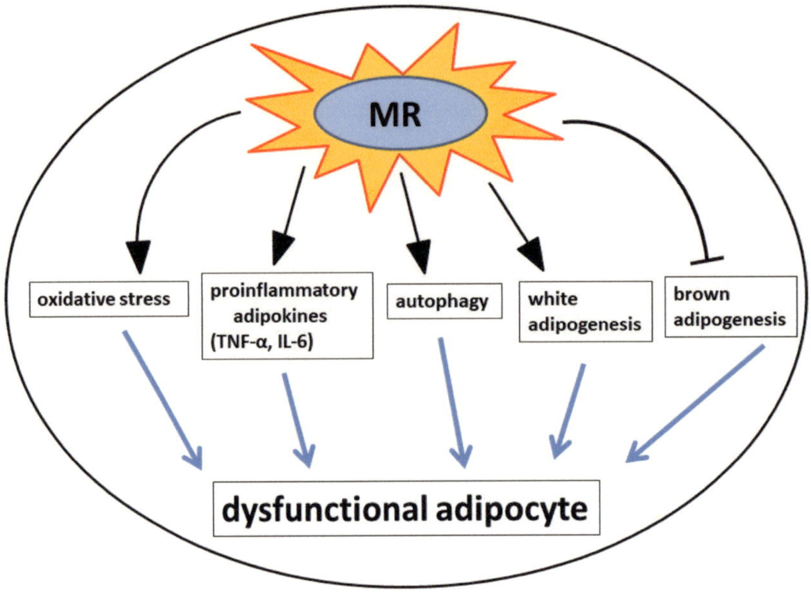


**Figure 1.**
*Involvement of MR in the pathophysiology of adipose tissue. MR overactivation results in detrimental effects on adipocyte metabolism. Upregulated activity of adipocyte MR promotes expression of enzymes involved in reactive oxygen species (ROS) production and pro-inflammatory adipokines such as TNF-α and IL-6. In the adipocyte, increased function of MR stimulates the autophagic flux which, in turn, promotes white adipocyte differentiation. Altogether, these effects lead to alterations of adipose tissue metabolism. MR activation also represses brown adipogenesis, reducing thermogenic capacity and favoring adipose tissue dysfunctions.*

changes in AT function or glucose tolerance, under both normal diet and high-fat diet (HFD), indicating a negligible role of MR in AT [35]. Nevertheless, these transgenic mice express a Cre-recombinase protein (adipoq-Cre) which removes MR only in mature adipose cells. This may indicate that MR activity is not required in mature adipose cells, suggesting that MR modulation may be crucial in regulating early stages of white adipogenesis.

Studies by Lombes and collaborators have shown that MR is expressed in brown adipocytes [36] where MR activation represses expression of UCP1 (**Figure 1**), which confers thermogenic function to BAT [37]. In accordance with these data, more recent studies by Caprio and colleagues revealed that MR blockade promotes brown adipogenesis in cultures of mouse primary preadipocytes derived from inguinal AT increasing expression of brown adipocyte markers such as PRDM16, CIDEA, and PPAR-γ coactivator 1α (PGC1-α) [5]. Moreover, mice upon pharmacological MR blockade showed upregulated expression of these markers in BAT, with a parallel increase in BAT activity, confirming the impact of MR function on brown adipocyte function also in vivo [5].

## 5. MR involvement in "browning" of adipose tissue

*Appearance of brown-like (brite) adipocytes in murine WAT takes place upon cold exposure. In mice, treatment with MR antagonist has been shown to promote browning and protect against fat mass expansion.*

White and brown adipocytes display distinct embryonic origin. White adipocytes are derived from myogenic factor 5 (myf5)-negative progenitors, whereas classical brown adipocytes (and skeletal muscle cells) are derived from myf5-positive precursors [38]. In addition, studies by Spiegelman and collaborators have identified a third type of adipocyte, termed "beige" (or "brite"), localized in murine WAT depots [39]. These "brown-like" adipocytes display classical brown adipocyte morphological and biochemical features (several cytoplasmic lipid droplets and high number of mitochondria), even if they are derived from myf5-negative precursors [26]. Importantly, β-adrenergic stimulation results in increased levels in UCP1 and uncoupled respiration rate in beige adipocytes, leading to the acquisition of brown fat features by WAT [39], a process known as "browning," and several preclinical studies have shown that browning protects mice against glucose and AT dysfunctions. Transgenic mice with fat tissue-specific overexpression of PRDM16, a transcriptional regulator involved in brown adipocyte development, displayed brite adipocyte formation in inguinal WAT. These mice also showed increased energy expenditure and improved glucose tolerance with high-fat feeding and parallel reduction in weight gain and fat mass [40]. Accordingly, another study showed that transgenic mice lacking PRDM16 in AT display defective browning, obesity, and insulin resistance, strongly indicating that brite adipocyte function, at least in mice, affects AT metabolism and whole-body energy expenditure [41]. Treatment of mice fed with HFD with the MR antagonists spironolactone (spiro) or drospirenone resulted in browning of white fat depots, reduced weight gain, and decreased fat mass expansion, as well as improved glucose tolerance [5]. In this study, transcriptional induction of a thermogenic gene program by MR antagonism was observed both in mice and in primary cultures of mouse adipocytes treated with spiro and drospirenone, indicating that MR blockade-mediated browning is cell autonomous.

However, further studies are required to better understand the molecular mechanisms regulated by MR which affect the thermogenic gene program of brite adipocytes.

The negative causal link between MR signaling and browning of WAT has been confirmed by Pisani et al. with Task1 −/− mice lacking the TWIK-related acid-sensitive K+ channel. These mice displayed increased WAT mass and impaired browning, as well as reduced BAT activity upon adrenergic stimulation. In brown adipocytes from Task1 −/− mice, MR antagonist treatment was able to rescue defective expression of UCP1, suggesting that the absence of Task1 activity can result in enhancement of MR function and subsequent downregulated expression of thermogenic genes [42].

## 6. Regulation of autophagy by MR in adipose cells

*The process of autophagy has been shown to regulate white and brown adipogenesis. Modulation of MR activity regulates the autophagic flux which, in turn, affects white and brown adipocyte differentiation.*

In the eukaryotic cells, autophagy regulates organelle and protein turnover maintaining cellular homeostasis and function [43]. Increased autophagic flux has been observed during adipocyte differentiation [44, 45]. Recent research has identified genes involved in autophagy regulation (atg). In particular, the role of atg5 and atg7 has been analyzed both in transgenic mice and in adipocyte cultures [45, 46]. Impaired adipose differentiation, i.e., altered morphology and decreased lipid droplet accumulation, has been observed in autophagy-related 5 (atg5)−/− mouse embryonic fibroblasts (MEFs), and, accordingly, newborn mice lacking atg5 display reduced fat mass [45]. Likewise, both 3T3-L1 preadipocytes lacking atg7 and atg7−/− MEFs display impaired adipogenesis, showing that also atg7 affects adipocyte maturation [46, 47]. Interestingly, Singh et al. have analyzed the metabolic profile of atg7-knockout mice showing that these mice have reduced WAT amount, paralleled by increased interscapular BAT. Moreover, browning of WAT has been also detected in atg7-KO mice. Indeed, WAT of atg7-KO mice displayed higher levels of UCP1 and PGC-1α, a master regulator of mitochondrial biogenesis, and higher levels of mitochondrial enzymes. Therefore, this study suggests that impaired autophagy leads to the formation of brite adipocytes in WAT. Recent data from Caprio and collaborators have shown that MR regulates the autophagic flux in murine adipocytes (**Figure 1**) [5]. Both in 3T3-L1 cells and primary murine adipocytes, aldosterone treatment increases autophagy, whereas MR blockade reduces the autophagic flux. In mice fed with HFD, pharmacological antagonism of MR leads to reduced AT autophagic flux inducing, in turn, browning of WAT. These data confirm the effects of impaired autophagy on browning of WAT observed in atg7-KO mice [46]. Evidence of a causal link between impairment in autophagy and induction of browning has been also demonstrated by treating murine adipocytes with either spiro or bafilomycin (autophagy inhibitor) or everolimus (autophagy activator) [5]. Both spiro and bafilomycin reduce autophagic flux with a concomitant increase in UCP1 levels, which indicates brown conversion of the adipose cell. Cotreatment with everolimus prevented UCP1 increase induced by spiro, indicating that decrease of autophagy is required for brown adipose conversion, whereas autophagy activation inhibits such process [5].

## 7. Metabolic effects of MR antagonism on adipose tissue metabolism

*Overactivity of adipocyte MR contributes to the development of adipose tissue dysfunctions. Pharmacological blockade of MR counteracts adipocyte oxidative stress and adipocyte hypertrophy, improving insulin sensitivity and stimulating BAT activity.*

Preclinical evidence suggests that increased expression of MR plays a role in AT dysfunctions. Increased levels of MR transcript have been detected in AT of obese humans and mice [11]. Data by Jaisser and collaborators has shown that adipocyte-specific MR overactivity leads to obesity and metabolic syndrome features in mice overexpressing MR in adipocytes (adipo-MROE mice) [11]. In particular, upregulated expression of MR in mouse adipocytes leads to increase in body weight and visceral AT hypertriglyceridemia, hypercholesterolemia, and impaired insulin response. Interestingly, in adipo-MROE mice, adipocyte area was increased and positively correlated with the MR expression in visceral AT. Hypertrophy of the adipocyte is a well-known feature of dysfunctional AT associated with local and systemic inflammation and impaired insulin sensitivity [48]. Accordingly, increased activity of MR promoted adipocyte hypertrophy associated with negative effects on glucose metabolism of adipo-MROE mice [11]. A recent study by Feraco et al. has investigated the effects of adipocyte-specific MR ablation on mouse AT and glucose metabolism. Mice lacking adipocyte MR (adipo-MRKO mice) do not show changes in fat mass, glucose, and lipid profile, suggesting that MR removal, at least in the mature adipocyte, does not alter AT function [35]. As discussed above, in adipo-MRKO mice the enzyme adipoq-Cre removes MR in mature adipocytes but does not alter MR function in preadipocytes, indicating that removal of MR in the early stages of adipogenesis may indeed affect AT and explain the metabolic effects of pharmacological blockade of MR observed in mice [5]. Accordingly with this hypothesis, treatment of preadipocyte cultures with MR antagonist represses differentiation [33].

Pharmacological antagonism of MR in obese mice protects against weight gain, fat mass expansion, and local inflammation [5, 6]. In the AT MR blockade counteracts adipocyte size enlargement, reduces the expression of pro-inflammatory adipokines (**Figure 1**), and promotes adiponectin production. In addition, MR antagonism reduces the expression of enzymes involved in reactive oxygen species

(ROS) production and, in parallel, increases the expression of ROS-eliminating enzymes, leading to decreased oxidative stress [6]. Increased oxidative stress has been detected in AT of murine models of obesity (mice fed with HFD or ob/ob mice), and mitochondrial dysfunction associated with obesity can contribute to production of ROS leading to carbonylation and impaired function of proteins such as IRS, contributing to AT dysfunction and insulin resistance [49]. In accordance with this, pharmacological blockade of MR reduces oxidative stress and improves insulin resistance in obese mice [6]. As mentioned above, treatment of mice fed with HFD with MR antagonists counteracts fat mass expansion and promotes also browning of WAT associated with improved glucose homeostasis. Therefore, preclinical studies with MR antagonists suggest that MR blockade counteracts AT dysfunctions dampening inflammation and oxidative stress and favoring brite adipocyte formation, at least in mice.

An increase in circulating levels of aldosterone is frequently observed in obese subjects, and recent data by Huby et al. suggest that leptin can contribute to the elevation of aldosterone [50]. This study reveals that the adipokine leptin can increase adrenal expression of the aldosterone synthase and plasma aldosterone levels, supporting the presence of a cross talk between AT and adrenal gland. In fact, increased secretion of leptin from the AT of obese subjects can lead to upregulated production of aldosterone which, in turn, may activate MR function in the adipocyte, further promoting leptin expression, fat expansion, and oxidative stress. Thus, in obesity, adipocyte MR might be overactivated by high plasma levels of aldosterone which further reinforces the dysregulated function of AT. There are very few studies that have investigated the role of adipocyte MR in humans. Karashima et al. have reported that treatment with MR antagonists for 12 months in subjects with primary aldosteronism (PA) led to reduction in blood pressure and visceral fat mass without changes in subcutaneous AT HOMA-IR, or in lipid profile [51]. To date, there are no other studies describing any effect of MR antagonism on human WAT. On the other hand, a recent study has shown that treatment with spiro in healthy adult subjects increases BAT volume and activity [52], indicating that MR blockade results in BAT function enhancement also in humans. These data suggest that the increase in thermogenic activity of BAT by MR antagonist-based therapies may represent a valuable approach to treat obesity.

## 8. Conclusion

A number of studies have shown that MR regulates AT physiology and can also contribute to the pathophysiology of obesity. In the adipocyte, MR has been shown to modulate transcript levels of adipogenic transcription factors, adipokines, and enzymes involved in ROS production (**Figure 1**) and scavenging. Notably, in murine models of obesity, treatment with MR antagonist is capable of counteracting excessive expansion, increased inflammation, and oxidative stress of AT. Moreover, in adipocyte cultures and obese mice, MR blockade can reduce the autophagic flux and promotes brown adipogenesis, upregulating BAT activity and inducing browning of WAT, a process that exerts favorable effects against glucose intolerance and AT dysfunction. Recent data have also shown that treatment with MR antagonist is able to enhance BAT activity in humans, further supporting the potential of MR antagonists as novel pharmacological agents in programs of metabolic rehabilitation for subjects with obesity and metabolic syndrome. However, the molecular mechanisms downstream MR, which mediate the mentioned effects on adipocyte function, are poorly known. Indeed, deeper understanding of the molecular pathways modulated by MR is necessary to design efficient therapies against AT dysfunctions and obesity.

## Acknowledgements

This publication is based upon work from the EU COST Action ADMIRE BM1301 in aldosterone and mineralocorticoid receptor (MR) physiology and pathophysiology (www.admirecosteu.com).

## Funding

This work was supported by grants of the Italian Ministry of Health (Ricerca Corrente), by grants from the Italian Ministry of Health "Bando 2011–2012 Progetti Collaborazione Ricercatori Italiani all'Estero" (Project Grant PE-2011-02347070 to M C), "Bando Giovani Ricercatori 2013" (Project Grant GR-2013-02357959 to AF), and by a grant of MIUR (Progetti di Ricerca di interesse Nazionale 2015 project code 2015ZTT5KB to M C, work package leader).

## Author details

Andrea Armani[1], Vincenzo Marzolla[1], Alessandra Feraco[1], Stefania Gorini[1], Caterina Mammi[1], Marco Infante[2] and Massimiliano Caprio[1,2,3*]

1 Laboratory of Cardiovascular Endocrinology, IRCCS San Raffaele Pisana, Rome, Italy

2 Unit of Endocrinology and Metabolic Diseases, Department of Systems Medicine, CTO A. Alesini Hospital, ASL Roma 2, University of Rome Tor Vergata, Rome, Italy

3 Department of Human Sciences and Promotion of the Quality of Life, San Raffaele Roma Open University, Rome, Italy

*Address all correspondence to: massimiliano.caprio@sanraffaele.it

## References

[1] Funder JW. Mineralocorticoid receptors: Distribution and activation. Heart Failure Reviews. 2005;**10**:15-22. DOI: 10.1007/s10741-005-2344-2

[2] Pearce PT, Funder JW. Steroid binding to cardiac type I receptors: In vivo studies. Journal of Hypertension. Supplement. 1988;**6**:S131-S133

[3] Rondinone CM, Rodbard D, Baker ME. Aldosterone stimulated differentiation of mouse 3T3-L1 cells into adipocytes. Endocrinology. 1993;**132**:2421-2426. DOI: 10.1210/endo.132.6.8504747

[4] Van Eekelen JA, Jiang W, de Kloet ER. Distribution of the mineralocorticoid and the glucocorticoid receptor mRNAs in the rat hippocampus. Journal of Neuroscience Research. 1988;**21**:88-94. DOI: 10.1002/jnr.490210113

[5] Armani A, Cinti F, Marzolla V. Mineralocorticoid receptor antagonism induces browning of white adipose tissue through impairment of autophagy and prevents adipocyte dysfunction in high-fat-diet-fed mice. The FASEB Journal. 2014;**28**:3745-3757. DOI: 10.1096/fj.13-245415

[6] Hirata A, Maeda N, Hiuge A. Blockade of mineralocorticoid receptor reverses adipocyte dysfunction and insulin resistance in obese mice. Cardiovascular Research. 2009;**84**:164-172. DOI: 10.1093/cvr/cvp191

[7] Wada T, Kenmochi H, Miyashita Y. Spironolactone improves glucose and lipid metabolism by ameliorating hepatic steatosis and inflammation and suppressing enhanced gluconeogenesis induced by high-fat and high-fructose diet. Endocrinology. 2010;**151**:2040-2049. DOI: 10.1210/en.2009-0869

[8] Gueret A, Harouki N, Favre J. Vascular smooth muscle mineralocorticoid receptor contributes to coronary and left ventricular dysfunction after myocardial infarction. Hypertension. 2016;**67**:717-723. DOI: 10.1161/HYPERTENSIONAHA.115.06709

[9] Marzolla V, Armani A, Mammi C. Essential role of ICAM-1 in aldosterone-induced atherosclerosis. International Journal of Cardiology. 2017;**232**:233-242. DOI: 10.1016/j.ijcard.2017.01.013

[10] McGraw AP, Bagley J, Chen WS. Aldosterone increases early atherosclerosis and promotes plaque inflammation through a placental growth factor-dependent mechanism. Journal of the American Heart Association. 2013;**2**(1):e000018. DOI: 10.1161/JAHA.112.000018

[11] Urbanet R, Nguyen Dinh Cat A, Feraco A. Adipocyte mineralocorticoid receptor activation leads to metabolic syndrome and induction of prostaglandin D2 synthase. Hypertension. 2015;**66**:149-157. DOI: 10.1161/HYPERTENSIONAHA.114.04981

[12] Armani A, Marzolla V, Fabbri A. Cellular mechanisms of MR regulation of adipose tissue physiology and pathophysiology. Journal of Molecular Endocrinology. 2015;**55**:R1-R10. DOI: 10.1530/JME-15-0122

[13] Funder JW. Aldosterone and mineralocorticoid receptors: Orphan questions. Kidney International. 2000;**57**:1358-1363. DOI: 10.1046/j.1523-1755.2000.00975.x

[14] Caprio M, Fève B, Claës A. Pivotal role of the mineralocorticoid receptor in corticosteroid-induced adipogenesis. The FASEB Journal.

2007;**21**:2185-2194. DOI: 10.1096/fj.06-7970com

[15] Guo C, Ricchiuti V, Lian BQ. Mineralocorticoid receptor blockade reverses obesity-related changes in expression of adiponectin, peroxisome proliferator-activated receptor-gamma, and proinflammatory adipokines. Circulation. 2008;**117**: 2253-2261. DOI: 10.1161/CIRCULATIONAHA.107.748640

[16] Cinti S. The adipose organ at a glance. Disease Models & Mechanisms. 2012;**5**:588-594. DOI: 10.1242/dmm.009662

[17] Coelho M, Oliveira T, Fernandes R. Biochemistry of adipose tissue: An endocrine organ. Archives of Medical Science. 2013;**9**:191-200. DOI: 10.5114/aoms.2013.33181

[18] Seale P, Kajimura S, Spiegelman BM. Transcriptional control of brown adipocyte development and physiological function of mice and men. Genes & Development. 2009;**23**:788-797. DOI: 10.1101/gad.1779209

[19] Cannon B, Nedergaard J. Brown adipose tissue: Function and physiological significance. Physiological Reviews. 2004;**84**:277-359. DOI: 10.1152/physrev.00015.2003

[20] Lean ME. Brown adipose tissue in humans. The Proceedings of the Nutrition Society. 1989;**48**:243-256

[21] Nedergaard J, Bengtsson T, Cannon B. Unexpected evidence for active brown adipose tissue in adult humans. American Journal of Physiology. Endocrinology and Metabolism. 2007;**293**:E444-E452. DOI: 10.1152/ajpendo.00691.2006

[22] Cypess AM, Lehman S, Williams G. Identification and importance of brown adipose tissue in adult humans. The New England Journal of Medicine. 2009;**360**:1509-1517. DOI: 10.1056/NEJMoa0810780

[23] Virtanen KA, Lidell ME, Orava J. Functional brown adipose tissue in healthy adults. The New England Journal of Medicine. 2009;**360**: 1518-1525. DOI: 10.1056/NEJMoa0808949

[24] Yoneshiro T, Aita S, Matsushita M. Recruited brown adipose tissue as an antiobesity agent in humans. The Journal of Clinical Investigation. 2013;**123**:3404-3408. DOI: 10.1172/JCI67803

[25] Ravussin Y, Xiao C, Gavrilova O. Effect of intermittent cold exposure on brown fat activation, obesity, and energy homeostasis in mice. PLoS One. 2014;**9**(1):e85876. DOI: 10.1371/journal.pone.0085876

[26] Harms M, Seale P. Brown and beige fat: Development, function and therapeutic potential. Nature Medicine. 2013;**19**:1252-1263. DOI: 10.1038/nm.3361

[27] Jo J, Gavrilova O, Pack S. Hypertrophy and/or hyperplasia: Dynamics of adipose tissue growth. PLoS Computational Biology. 2009;**5**(3):e1000324. DOI: 10.1371/journal.pcbi.1000324

[28] Nakamura K, Fuster JJ, Walsh K. Adipokines: A link between obesity and cardiovascular disease. Journal of Cardiology. 2014;**63**:250-259. DOI: 10.1016/j.jjcc.2013.11.006

[29] Reilly SM, Saltiel AR. Adapting to obesity with adipose tissue inflammation. Nature Reviews. Endocrinology. 2017;**13**:633-643. DOI: 10.1038/nrendo.2017.90

[30] Matsushita M, Yoneshiro T, Aita S. Impact of brown adipose tissue on body fatness and glucose metabolism in healthy humans. International

Journal of Obesity. 2014;**38**:812-817. DOI: 10.1038/ijo.2013.206

[31] Claussnitzer M, Dankel SN, Kim KH. FTO obesity variant circuitry and adipocyte browning in humans. The New England Journal of Medicine. 2015;**373**:895-907. DOI: 10.1056/NEJMoa1502214

[32] Armani A, Marzolla V, Rosano G. Mineralocorticoid vs glucocorticoid receptors: Solo players or team mates in the control of adipogenesis? International Journal of Obesity. 2014;**38**:1580-1581. DOI: 10.1038/ijo.2014.68

[33] Caprio M, Antelmi A, Chetrite G. Antiadipogenic effects of the mineralocorticoid receptor antagonist drospirenone: Potential implications for the treatment of metabolic syndrome. Endocrinology. 2011;**152**:113-125. DOI: 10.1210/en.2010-0674

[34] Hoppmann J, Perwitz N, Meier B. The balance between gluco- and mineralo-corticoid action critically determines inflammatory adipocyte responses. The Journal of Endocrinology. 2010;**204**:153-164. DOI: 10.1677/JOE-09-0292

[35] Feraco A, Armani A, Urbanet R. Minor role of mature adipocyte mineralocorticoid receptor in high fat induced obesity. The Journal of Endocrinology. 2018. DOI: 10.1530/JOE-18-0314. pii: JOE-18-0314. (In print)

[36] Zennaro MC, Le Menuet D, Viengchareun S. Hibernoma development in transgenic mice identifies brown adipose tissue as a novel target of aldosterone action. The Journal of Clinical Investigation. 1998;**101**:1254-1260. DOI: 10.1172/JCI1915

[37] Viengchareun S, Penfornis P, Zennaro MC. Mineralocorticoid and glucocorticoid receptors inhibit UCP expression and function in brown adipocytes. American Journal of Physiology. Endocrinology and Metabolism. 2001;**280**:E640-E649. DOI: 10.1152/ajpendo.2001.280.4.E640

[38] Kajimura S, Seale P, Spiegelman BM. Transcriptional control of brown fat development. Cell Metabolism. 2010;**11**:257-262. DOI: 10.1016/j.cmet.2010.03.005

[39] Wu J, Boström P, Sparks LM. Beige adipocytes are a distinct type of thermogenic fat cell in mouse and human. Cell. 2012;**150**:366-376. DOI: 10.1016/j.cell.2012.05.016

[40] Seale P, Conroe HM, Estall J. Prdm16 determines the thermogenic program of subcutaneous white adipose tissue in mice. The Journal of Clinical Investigation. 2011;**121**:96-105. DOI: 10.1172/JCI44271

[41] Cohen P, Levy JD, Zhang Y. Ablation of PRDM16 and beige adipose causes metabolic dysfunction and a subcutaneous to visceral fat switch. Cell. 2014;**156**:304-316. DOI: 10.1016/j.cell.2013.12.021

[42] Pisani DF, Beranger GE, Corinus A. The K+ channel TASK1 modulates beta-adrenergic response in brown adipose tissue through the mineralocorticoid receptor pathway. The FASEB Journal. 2016;**30**:909-922. DOI: 10.1096/fj.15-277475

[43] Mizushima N, Levine B. Autophagy in mammalian development and differentiation. Nature Cell Biology. 2010;**12**:823-830. DOI: 10.1038/ncb0910-823

[44] Novikoff AB, Novikoff PM, Rosen OM. Organelle relationships in cultured 3T3-L1 preadipocytes. The Journal of Cell Biology. 1980;**87**:180-196

[45] Baerga R, Zhang Y, Chen PH. Targeted deletion of autophagy-related 5 (atg5) impairs adipogenesis in a cellular model and in mice. Autophagy. 2009;**5**:1118-1130

[46] Singh R, Xiang Y, Wang Y. Autophagy regulates adipose mass and differentiation in mice. The Journal of Clinical Investigation. 2009;**119**:3329-3339. DOI: 10.1172/JCI39228

[47] Zhang Y, Goldman S, Baerga R. Adipose-specific deletion of autophagy-related gene 7 (atg7) in mice reveals a role in adipogenesis. Proceedings of the National Academy of Sciences of the United States of America. 2009;**106**:19860-19865. DOI: 10.1073/pnas.0906048106

[48] Klöting N, Fasshauer M, Dietrich A. Insulin-sensitive obesity. American Journal of Physiology. Endocrinology and Metabolism. 2010;**299**:E506-E515. DOI: 10.1152/ajpendo.00586.2009

[49] Le LS, Simard G, Martinez MC. Oxidative stress and metabolic pathologies: From an adipocentric point of view. Oxidative Medicine and Cellular Longevity. 2014;**2014**:908539. DOI: 10.1155/2014/908539

[50] Huby AC, Antonova G, Groenendyk J. Adipocyte-derived hormone leptin is a direct regulator of aldosterone secretion, which promotes endothelial dysfunction and cardiac fibrosis. Circulation. 2015;**132**:2134-2145. DOI: 10.1161/CIRCULATIONAHA.115.018226

[51] Karashima S, Yoneda T, Kometani M. Comparison of eplerenone and spironolactone for the treatment of primary aldosteronism. Hypertension Research. 2016;**39**:133-137. DOI: 10.1038/hr.2015.129

[52] Thuzar M, Law WP, Dimeski G. Mineralocorticoid antagonism enhances brown adipose tissue function in humans: A randomized placebo-controlled cross-over study. Diabetes, Obesity & Metabolism. 2019;**21**: 509-516. DOI: 10.1111/dom.13539

Chapter 9

# Investigating the Role of Mineralocorticoid Receptor Signaling in Cancer Biology in the Genomic Era

*Ozlen Konu and Seniye Targen*


## Abstract

In the last decades, advances that take place in the next-generation sequencing and bioinformatics research have helped reveal tissue- and cancer-specific gene expression patterns and mutation landscapes. Indeed, such data are now easily accessible via online genome browsers and different types and levels of public data compendia. Appropriate use of these tools eventually can lead to better patient stratification for diagnosis, prognosis, and therapy of cancers. Mineralocorticoid receptor (MR), encoded by NR3C2 gene, has long been implicated in the development and progression of multiple cancers. Nevertheless, MR has remained relatively understudied at the genomic and transcriptomic levels. In this review, we present the current, literature-based state of knowledge on the role of MR primarily in epithelial cancers. At the same time, we summarize the gene expression, mutation, and copy number variation data on MR obtained from The Cancer Genome Atlas (TCGA). We also show that MR expression could be a promising prognostic marker in different cancers using online tools for survival data analysis. Accordingly, this review strongly demonstrates the emerging potential of studying MR using available tools from the genomics/transcriptomics field for improving cancer diagnosis and prognostication.


**Keywords:** mineralocorticoid receptor, aldosterone, epithelial cancers, genomics, transcriptomics, prognosis, The Cancer Genome Atlas, www.cbioportal.org

## 1. Introduction

MR/NR3C2 belongs to the steroid receptor family and it adopts important roles in human physiology and pathology. Although MR has long been studied in renal and cardiovascular contexts, identification of MR in multiple epithelial cancers and presence of cross talk between steroid receptors in cancer-related processes make MR a promising candidate for cancer diagnosis and prognosis. Nevertheless, a focused yet comprehensive literature review about MR's expression in cancers and established role in cancer-associated hallmarks is lacking. Our literature search reveals that MR is expressed in cancerous as well as adjacent and/or normal tissue although the expression of MR can become deregulated during cancer development. Moreover, we provide an account of changes in ligand-dependent or -independent

MR signaling in association with cell proliferation, apoptosis, and senescence of cancer cells. We also identify future directions that can help target novel aspects of MR signaling for mechanistic studies as well as cancer therapeutics. In addition, we point out an emergent need for analyzing the range of genomic alterations and variability in MR expression and its potential association with prognosis across epithelial solid tumors using the existing genomic and transcriptomic resources. We exemplify the extent of variability in MR expression within and among patients based on the patient data found in The Cancer Genome Atlas (TCGA) [1]. Moreover, we demonstrate the profound potential of MR expression as a biomarker for cancer prognostication, i.e., estimation of the likelihood of developing future risks for cancer over a time period using TCGA datasets [2].

## 2. A concise literature review on MR in cancer biology

Herein an overview of the scientific literature on MR is provided using examples mainly from cancers of epithelial origin including the lung, colon, liver, kidney, pancreas, prostate, breast, and adrenal gland, revealing the understudied aspects of MR in the context of cancer biology.

### 2.1 Lung cancer

The presence of MR protein in lung cancer tissues has opened new avenues for MR research. Suzuki et al. [3] demonstrated by immunohistochemistry (IHC) that primary lung cancer tissues expressed MR protein along with HSD11B2 enzyme, required for MR receptor specificity through conversion of cortisol to cortisone. However, MR and HSD11B2 proteins, although present and significantly correlated with each other in lung adenocarcinomas, were non-existent in squamous cell, small cell, or large-cell carcinomas [3]. Next, Jeong and colleagues [4] studied gene expression signatures of all 48 nuclear receptors (NRs) including MR in non-small-cell lung cancers (NSCLCs) and corresponding normal lung tissues and found that short heterodimer partner (SHP) and progesterone receptor (PGR) predicted survival in patients with early-stage lung tumors. In the same study, the prognostic role of NRs was also investigated in corresponding normal tissues; and higher expressions of MR and nerve growth factor-induced gene B3, NGFIB3, were identified as predictors of good prognosis for survival and disease recurrence [4]. Furthermore, increasing aldosterone levels in the presence of VEGF inhibitors also proved to be a better indicator of prognosis in NSCLC patients [5]. However, future epidemiological as well as mechanistic studies are needed to address the cross talk between antiangiogenic drugs and MR signaling in lung cancer.

### 2.2 Colorectal cancer

In colon cancer, an observed decrease in the expression of MR in cancerous tissue in comparison to the adjacent normal mucosa has attributed MR a tumor suppressive role [6]. Tiberio et al. [7] further investigated how MR expression correlated with patient survival in colorectal carcinomas. In this study, the expressions of MR and tumor microvessel density marker protein CD34 were evaluated in tumor and normal colorectal mucosa by IHC, and an inverse correlation of expression was detected between them in colorectal cancers. Kaplan–Meier survival analysis has led to a conclusion that MR could be a tumor suppressor whose decreased expression is correlating well with poor patient survival based on a relatively small number of patients [7]. Recently, spironolactone, an MR antagonist, has also arisen as a tumor suppressor in colon carcinoma yet independent of MR and through RXRγ receptor signaling [8]. Moreover, recent studies showed that HSD11B2 inhibition, and hence potential dysregulation of MR signaling, could modify gut microbiota, known to be an important factor in colon carcinogenesis [9]. A better understanding of MR cross talk with other nuclear receptors and interaction with gut microbiota from patients treated with MR antagonists is needed in the future.

### 2.3 Breast cancer

MR expression in normal and diseased breast tissues was initially identified in the 1990s [10, 11]. MR and HSD11B2 proteins were shown to co-localize predominantly in the duct epithelia and to exhibit higher expressions in invasive ductal carcinoma than invasive lobular carcinoma [11]. More recently a study by Conde et al. [12] found that MR expression was peculiar to the cytoplasm of benign and cancerous breast lesions, whereas GR/NR3C1 expression was nuclear in benign breast lesions but showed cytoplasmic as well as nuclear distribution in cancer tissues. These findings might suggest a potential deregulation of GR signaling in malignant tissues, while the effects of MR on tumor development could be less ligand-dependent and/or ligand-insensitive in breast cancer. However, this remains to be assessed.

Induction of growth of lobulo-alveolar structures in mouse mammary gland by MR ligand aldosterone also pointed to the importance of MR signaling in breast biology [13–15]. Furthermore, the presence of progesterone, a potential MR ligand, in the breast tissue highlighted the significance of MR in breast cancers [16]. In addition, in vitro culturing of breast cancer cell lines provided further opportunities for understanding the impact of MR signaling in tumor growth. For example, in the breast cancer cell line PMC42 with detectable MR and HSD11B2 expression levels, aldosterone, alone, did not have an effect on cell proliferation yet when given together with the anti-mineralocorticoid spironolactone resulted in a significant decrease in cell numbers [17]. In another study, aldosterone and cortisol exerted progesterone-like effects such as induction of focal adhesion and reduced cell growth in the progesterone receptor-transfected MDA-MB-231 breast cancer cell line [18]. Recently, genomic and non-genomic actions of aldosterone through G-coupled estrogen receptor (GPER) and MR signaling pathways were demonstrated [19]. Rapid aldosterone exposure activated EGFR and ERK1/2 transduction pathway through MR and GPER in the HER2+ breast cancer cell line SkBr3 and breast tumor-derived endothelial cells [19]. Furthermore, direct interactions among GPER and MR as well as GPER and EGFR were shown, while a long-term exposure to aldosterone increased cell growth which could be inhibited by the silencing of MR expression [19]. These findings indicated possible contributions of GPER activity in the MR-dependent aldosterone signaling and EGFR activation in the regulation of cancer cell growth. However, the relationship between aldosterone and other modulators of GPER, e.g., estrogen, remains to be investigated in breast cancer. MR receptors can exhibit affinity to aldosterone and cortisol as well as other potential ligands likely to be found in the milieu of breast cancer, and thus studying MR, GR, GPER, and/or other receptor crosstalk could be important for better evaluating mammary gland physiology and pathology.

### 2.4 Liver cancer

As in the lung and colon cancers, MR expression was shown to be downregulated in a large cohort of liver cancer patient tissues [20]. Furthermore, in the same study, overexpression of MR suppressed cancer progression by inhibition of proliferation and induction of cell cycle arrest eventually leading to apoptosis. Aldosterone's effect on tumor growth was also tested, and its antiproliferative and apoptotic effects were reversed by spironolactone. All of these significantly implicated an evidence for decreased MR signaling in liver cancer pathogenesis [20]. Additionally, this study showed that MR suppressed the Warburg effect [20] by which cancer cells gain growth advantage over normal cells [21] leading to novel insights about MR signaling through cancer research.

Apart from cancer, fibrosis is another significant pathology of the liver. Fibrosis, the leading factor of liver carcinogenesis, occurs due to the accumulation of fibrogenic cells and extracellular matrix (ECM) proteins in excess [22, 23]. ECM is central to sustain cellular homeostasis and integrity, and deregulation of ECM is considered as a hallmark of cancer [24]. The role of aldosterone on ECM synthesis and potentially on liver fibrosis was previously shown in rats, although independent of MR itself [25]. On the other hand, spironolactone was shown to act as a potent provocateur of liver regeneration following partial hepatectomy [26]. As a result, these studies demonstrate the current need for better understanding the role of ligand-dependent and ligand-independent signaling of MR in different facets of liver pathologies including fibrosis, regeneration, and carcinoma.

### 2.5 Renal cancer

MR and aldosterone signaling have been extensively studied in kidney physiology and pathology for decades [27, 28] and to some degree, in renal carcinomas. Initially, the protein expressions of MR and HSD11B2 were characterized in a large cohort of renal cell neoplasms of different cellular origins using IHC. In this study, co-expression HSD11B2 and MR was shown in normal distal nephron, in chromophobe renal cell carcinoma (chRCC) and oncocytoma of distal nephron origin [29]. In renal cell carcinoma, aldosterone led to upregulation of KRAS oncogene (KRAS4A splice variant) resulting in increased survival and cell proliferation [30]. Yet another study revealed that aldosterone exerted its migratory/metastatic actions through G-protein-coupled estrogen receptor (GPER) in a murine renal cortical adenocarcinoma cell line and also in mice in vivo [31]. These findings implicated important oncogenic pathways and their crosstalk with MR and aldosterone signaling in renal cancers.

Hypertension is a well-established risk factor in kidney cancers potentially due to the genotoxic nature of aldosterone [32, 33]. Indeed, supraphysiological levels of aldosterone treatment induced DNA breaks and chromosomal aberrations in epithelial porcine kidney cells, whereas MR blockade by antagonists prevented formation of such aberrations [34]. Genotoxic effects of aldosterone were investigated further in the DOCA-salt-treated rat model used for inducing MR-dependent hypertension. DOCA-salt treatment caused inflammation, oxidative stress, DNA damage, and increased kidney cell proliferation [35]. Another study highlighted aldosterone-dependent induction of oxidative stress and DNA damage as well as activation of MR-dependent NFKB signaling pathway in kidney tubule cells [36]. Queisser et al. [37] further addressed the downstream signaling pathways triggered by aldosterone-induced oxidative stress both in vitro (porcine kidney cells with proximal tubular properties) and in vivo (rat kidneys). In these models, aldosterone treatment resulted in MR-dependent activation of ERK1/2 and its target, STAT3; and hence aldosterone exposure led to higher proliferation rates while diminishing apoptosis [37]. Accordingly, the role of aldosterone-induced MR signaling in deregulation of DNA damage response needs to be studied also in other epithelial cancers in more detail.

Senescence, evasion of which is another hallmark of cancer [38], was studied in the context of aldosterone signaling in different renal models. For example, p16$^{INK4a}$, a cyclin-dependent kinase inhibitor and a cellular senescence marker [39, 40], was induced in the kidneys and hearts of DOCA-salt-treated rats [41]. These effects could be reversed by antihypertensives and spironolactone, suggesting a potential role of MR signaling in the regulation of the senescent phenotype [41]. In another study, senescence was investigated in aldosterone-infused rats and cultured human proximal tubular cells. In both models, aldosterone-induced senescence-like characteristics were marked by senescence-associated beta-galactosidase staining, p21/Cdkn1a and p53 overexpression, and SIRT1 under-expression. MR blockade either using eplerenone (in vivo) or through gene silencing (in vitro) sufficiently reversed the aldosterone-induced senescence-like characteristics [42]. In line with this study, Kitada et al. [43] also showed the presence of aldosterone-induced senescence, characterized by increased p21 expression and beta-galactosidase staining, in human proximal tubular cells. Furthermore, a prolonged exposure to aldosterone triggered p21-mediated cytokine release, e.g., TNF alpha, which in turn led to apoptosis [43]. All of these have implicated MR signaling through interaction with aldosterone in the induction of senescence, an inherent autoregulatory mechanism of proliferating cells with established tumor suppressive activity. The role of MR/aldosterone-induced senescence in epithelial cancers however needs to be further studied since this can provide an effective route for therapeutic invention.

### 2.6 Pancreas cancer

Recently, MR has been ascribed a tumor suppressive role also in pancreatic ductal adenocarcinoma (PDAC) [44]. In PDAC patients, dysregulated expression of macrophage migration inhibitory factor (MIF) was associated with disease aggressiveness, and MIF-driven upregulation of miR-301b was shown to suppress MR expression [44]. In turn, MR expression resulted in the inhibition of epithelial to mesenchymal transition (EMT) and increased chemotherapeutic drug (gemcitabine) sensitivity. Consistently, survival data analysis further associated downregulation of MR expression with poor survival in PDAC patients [44]. However, PDAC remains one of the cancers receiving less attention in the MR field; future studies can address the role of genomic and non-genomic effects of MR signaling in PDAC.

### 2.7 Prostate cancer

Detection of 11 beta-hydroxysteroid dehydrogenase enzyme [45] and a functional MR in the androgen-dependent prostate cancer cell line LNCaP cells dates back to the early 1990s [46]. More recently, Dovio et al. [47] assessed GR and MR expression together with HSD11B-1 and HSD11B-2 enzyme activity upon inflammatory stimulus (IL1B stimulation) or basal conditions in the androgen-dependent and androgen-independent prostate cancer cell lines. Diverse expression patterns of MR, GR, and HSD11B enzyme activities were detected among cell lines, while downstream effects of IL1B exposure were inhibited by cortisol or dexamethasone in a cell line-dependent manner [47].

Another lead for the role of mineralocorticoids in prostate cancer has come from abiraterone acetate (AA), an androgen synthesis inhibitor, used for metastatic castration-resistant prostate cancer (mCRPC), which results in secondary mineralocorticoid excess [48]. Androgen-induced conformational changes in androgen receptor (AR) could be inhibited in the presence of mineralocorticoids (corticosterone or deoxycorticosterone). However, administration of corticosterone alone resulted in repression of AR transcriptional activity and cellular growth at concentrations present in the serum of AA-administered patients [49]. Pia et al. [50] focusing on identifying ways of eliminating adrenocorticotropic hormone (ACTH)-dependent AA-induced mineralocorticoid excess showed that a low effective dose of glucocorticoid together with MR antagonist and salt deprivation could be an ideal treatment. Indeed, the use of prednisone, a synthetic glucocorticoid, could overcome the effects of secondary mineralocorticoid excess in mCRPC patients treated with abiraterone [51]. Effect of eplerenone-abiraterone co-administration on secondary mineralocorticoid excess syndrome and progression-free survival (PFS) was evaluated and compared to prednisone-abiraterone co-administered in patients. No significant difference was obtained by means of mineralocorticoid excess syndrome characteristics and PFS between these two experimental groups; and this has raised AA-eplerenone as an alternative therapy for overcoming prednisone-induced side effects [52]. Enzalutamide is another antiandrogen drug used for treating metastatic prostate cancer patients; however, resistance gained against enzalutamide therapy remains a challenge. GR signaling induces antiandrogen resistance by hijacking AR function [53, 54]; hence, the therapeutic effects of enzalutamide-corticosteroid co-administration were addressed in prostate cancer cells [55]. Dexamethasone decreased the therapeutic effects of enzalutamide as well as increasing resistance. However, prednisolone and aldosterone diminished resistance to enzalutamide. Consistently, silencing of MR resulted in enhanced resistance to enzalutamide and AR activity [55]. Moreover, the effects of diverse antihypertensive medication on prostate cancer survival following radical prostatectomy were tested in the Finnish population, and overall, the antihypertensive treatment was associated with increased death risk [56]. These findings clearly establish the importance of AR and MR cross talk and complex ligand interactions in prostate cancer, which could be further studied in other cancers and cancer subtypes where AR signaling can play a role.

### 2.8 Adrenocortical cancer

Adrenal incidentalomas include adrenocortical adenomas, adrenocortical carcinomas, and pheochromocytoma [57, 58]. Aldosterone-producing adenomas (APA, i.e., benign tumors of the adrenal glands) account for 35% of the diseases of the primary aldosteronism spectrum [59, 60]. Somatic mutations occurring in KCNJ5, CACNA1D, ATP1A1, ATP2B3, and CTNNB1 genes give rise to sporadic APA [61]. In addition to the abovementioned mutations, regulatory RNAs such as miRNAs have also been shown to be important in modulating aldosterone levels and tumorigenesis [62–64]. On the other hand, adrenocortical cancers (ACC), some of which are hormone-producing, occur relatively rarely, and patients with ACC exhibit poor prognosis with a median survival of 5.5 years [65]. In the adrenocortical cell line H295R, aldosterone in vitro is shown to upregulate T-type calcium channel expression and currents, an effect reversed by spironolactone [66]. H295R cells have also been shown to express components of aldosterone signaling pathway including ENaC subunits, NEDD4L, SGK1, MR, and HSD11B2 [66, 67]. Although several factors, such as age, resection margin and proliferation scores, uterine steroid profiles, CpG island hypermethylation status, as well as levels of selected biomarkers, have been tested for their contribution in ACC prognosis, the importance of MR expression status is yet to be evaluated in ACC patients [65, 68, 69]. Future studies should investigate the role of activation/inactivation of MR-aldosterone signaling in diagnosis/prognosis of ACC for which significant amounts of genomic and transcriptomic data have recently become available (please see the next section for details).

## 3. Cancer genome and transcriptome analyses for MR using online tools

The advent of whole-genome sequencing and development and availability of genome browsers, such as UCSC genome browser [70, 71] and Ensembl [72, 73], in the early 2000s have enabled researchers to identify genes/genomic intervals that are important in human physiology and pathology. This is mainly done by association of genome fragments with informative tracks that range from expression values to the presence of copy number and single nucleotide variations (CNVs and SNVs, respectively). Cataloging and annotation of the human genome with regard to genomic and transcriptomic variation have also revolutionized cancer research [74, 75]. The NIH-driven giant effort named The Cancer Genome Atlas (TCGA) has published its first results in 2008 on the genomic and transcriptomic landscape of gliomas [76]. Over the years, TCGA has expanded to house thousands of cancer genomes/transcriptomes/proteomes from tens of different cancers allowing researchers from all over the world to have unlimited access to cancer-related datasets [1]. Many different web-based tools nowadays use TCGA and Catalog of Somatic Mutations in Cancer (COSMIC) [77] as primary resources and build on them to extract data from user-provided queries and/or to perform gene-specific or genome-wide secondary analyses, such as cbioportal.org [78, 79]. These webservers make use of a wide range of information and incorporate quantitative and statistical analyses and visualization tools and help users with little or no programming experience perform cancer bioinformatics analyses.

The expression of MR along with those of other nuclear receptors has been studied in a recent TCGA PanCancer transcriptomics study of bladder, breast, colon, head and neck, liver, and prostate cancers; and MR expression is shown to be downregulated in all [80]. To demonstrate the potential of TCGA in revealing the importance of MR in cancer research, we have used www.cbioportal.org webserver [78, 79] to visualize the next-generation RNA sequencing data from different cancers of TCGA provisional datasets for MR and showed that MR mRNA is expressed differentially across many tumor types (**Figure 1**). Among these, chromophobe renal cell carcinoma (chRCC) has the highest expression of MR followed by thyroid carcinoma (THCA), pheochromocytoma and paragangliomas (PCPG), and adrenocortical carcinoma (ACC), while carcinomas of the bladder, breast, cervix, esophagus, head, and neck exhibit high variability (**Figure 1**). It is also apparent that genomic alterations (gains and shallow deletions) are common in many of these TCGA dataset patients (**Figure 1**). Future analyses can focus on how these alterations are associated with MR expression in different cancers, especially in chRCC and ACC.

Overall, the observed rate of somatic mutations of MR has been shown to be significantly lower with respect to the expected rate suggesting MR does not tolerate well mutations with functional constraints [81]. On the other hand, functional mutations of MR have been identified in different contexts including renal pseudohypoaldosteronism as well as hypertension [81, 82]. In addition, relatively different residues in the DNA-binding domain of MR seem to be affected between type I pseudohypoaldosteronism and cancers [83]. Herein we have compiled the MR mutation landscape for cancers found in TCGA provisional datasets (cbioportal.org) showing the number (95 missense, 19 truncating totaling 0.9% somatic mutation frequency) as well as the distribution of mutations across the MR protein sequence (984 amino acids long) and the DNA-binding domain zinc finger, C4 type

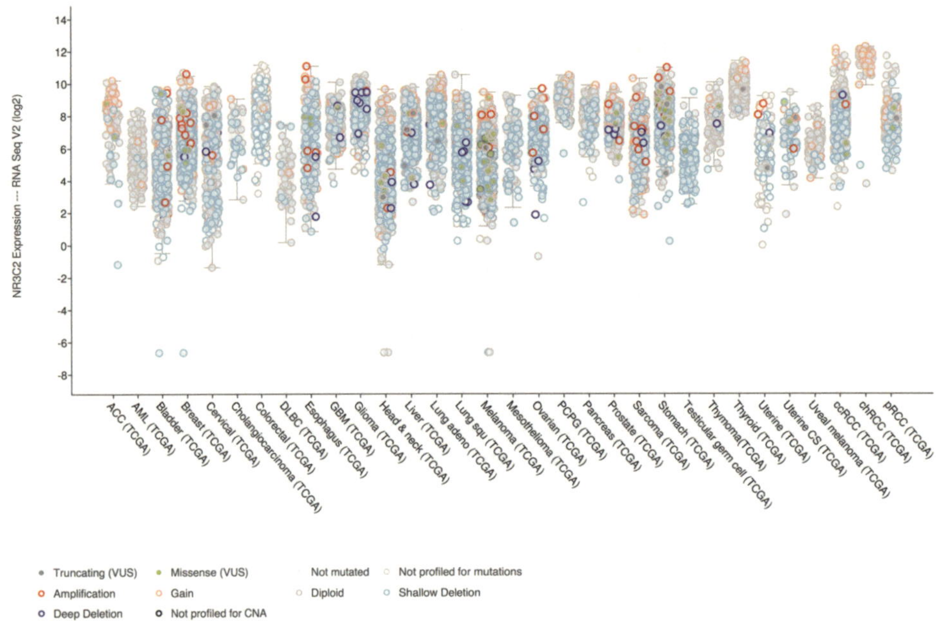


**Figure 1.**
*Boxplots of MR/NR3C2 expression across different TCGA provisional datasets obtained from cbioportal.org.*

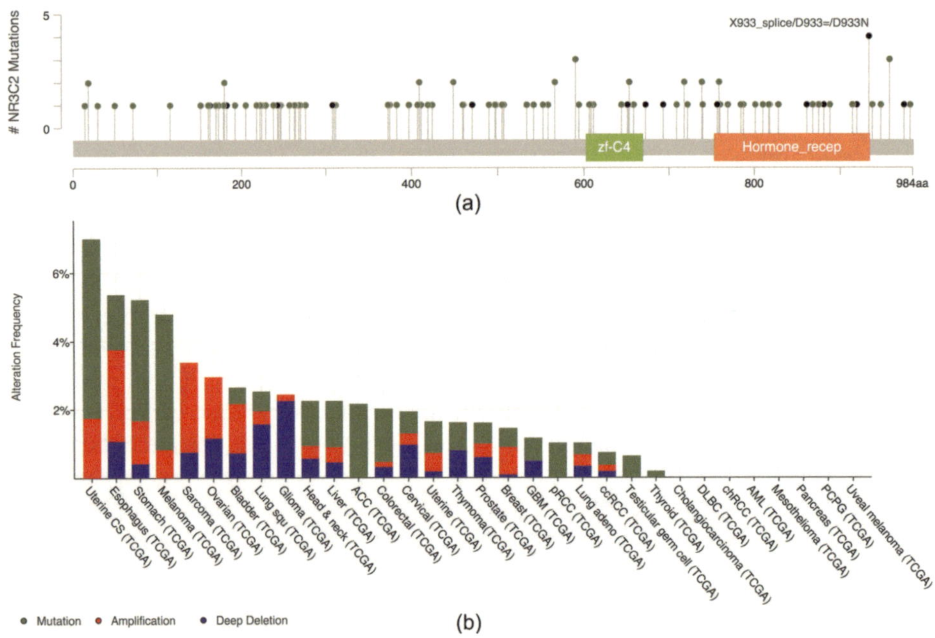


**Figure 2.**
*Mutation landscape and distribution of genetic alterations in MR. (a) Schema showing the location of MR mutations and the two functional domains of MR. (b) The bar graph showing the percentages of mutations, amplifications, and deletions in TCGA provisional datasets. Source: cbioportal.org.*

(zf-C4; 602–669), and ligand-binding domain of NR (753–934) (**Figure 2A**). However, it is important to note that TCGA datasets are dynamic in nature such that new samples as well as mutation/CNV annotations are continually being added. www.cbioportal.org webserver also offers two separate and large multi-cancer

| Sample ID | Cancer Type | Amino Acid | MutationAssessor | SIFT | Polyphen-2 |
|---|---|---|---|---|---|
| TCGA-32-2494-01 | Glioblastoma Multiforme | C606W | high | deleterious | probably_damaging |
| TCGA-QK-A8Z8-01 | Head and Neck Squamous Cell Carcinoma | C658G | high | deleterious | probably_damaging |
| TCGA-D3-A8GI-06 | Cutaneous Melanoma | M668I | high | deleterious | probably_damaging |
| TCGA-G3-A25W-01 | Hepatocellular Carcinoma | C658F | high | deleterious | probably_damaging |
| coadread_dfci_2016_3235 | Colorectal Adenocarcinoma | F626L | high | deleterious | probably_damaging |
| MM-0308 | Plasma Cell Myeloma | F626C | high | deleterious | probably_damaging |

**Table 1.**
*High-impact MR mutations based on MutationAssessor in curated TCGA and non-TCGA dataset collection (www.cbioportal.org).*

collections, i.e., TCGA PanCancer and curated TCGA/non-TCGA (curated set of non-redundant) datasets. Upon analysis of these two collections, the numbers of observed missense mutations in the MR gene increase to 193 and 281, and truncating mutations to 34 and 48, respectively. It is also possible to download functional annotations for these mutations that include scores showing the impact of mutations, e.g., analyzed through MutationAssessor.org [84, 85]. Accordingly, in the curated TCGA/non-TCGA dataset collection, we have identified, among all 334 mutations, 6 high-impact mutations, all of which are located in the zf-C4 domain (**Table 1**). Functional analysis of MR mutation landscape thus can help researchers select high-impact variants for future validation studies using MutationAssessor as well as other tools linked with www.cbioportal.org, e.g., SIFT [86] and PolyPhen-2 [87].

Moreover, using TCGA provisional datasets, we analyzed whether MR accumulated different rates of genetic alterations in different cancers (**Figure 2B**). The mean proportion of genetic alterations per cancer was 0.024 (0.017–0.031, 95% confidence interval, CI). The results in percentages showed that around 7% of uterine carcinosarcoma patients exhibited genomic alterations (mutation, amplification; 7.02% in 57 cases), while the second and third ranking cancers were those of esophageal carcinoma (5.38% in 186 cases) and stomach adenocarcinomas (5.23% in 478 cases) (**Figure 2B**). As mentioned above the ranking of these cancers in terms of percent genomic alterations can be dynamic depending on which data collection has been used. For example, when using TCGA PanCancer sample collection, which reports a more complete mutation/CNV annotation information, the first ranking cancer with the highest percentage of genetic alterations has become melanoma (8.71% out of 448 skin cutaneous melanoma) followed by uterine carcinomas (7.75% out of 529 uterine corpus endometrial carcinoma and 7.02% out of 57 uterine carcinosarcomas). Future studies may focus on uterine carcinomas and melanoma to address the mechanisms and effects of these observed alterations.

## 4. Investigating the role of MR in cancer patient stratification and prognosis using genomics resources

Survival analysis is often used for studying the association of an event of interest, e.g., death and disease recurrence, with another clinical or biological variable [88]. Analysis of TCGA-associated survival data (overall survival (OS) and/or relapse-free survival (RFS)) is available through several online webservers including GEPIA [89], OncoLnc [90], Kaplan–Meier Plotter [91], and KM-Express [92]. These tools help evaluate survival of cancer patients whose genomic/transcriptomic and clinical data are stored in TCGA, by using Cox coefficient statistics, hazard ratio (HR) and/or logrank tests, and Kaplan–Meier plots. GEPIA, which has previously been used in prognostic identification of several biomarkers in ACC [93, 94], performs survival statistics in addition to providing other functionalities such as co-expression analysis and diagnostic marker prediction. We analyzed data from all cancers available in GEPIA and showed that an NR3C2/MR expression higher than the median level predicted a significantly better prognosis (OS) and low HR in adrenocortical carcinoma (ACC), kidney renal clear cell carcinoma (KIRC), breast invasive carcinoma (BRCA), colon adenocarcinoma (COAD), brain lower-grade glioma (LGG), and liver hepatocellular carcinoma (LIHC) (logrank p-value <0.1; **Figure 3**).

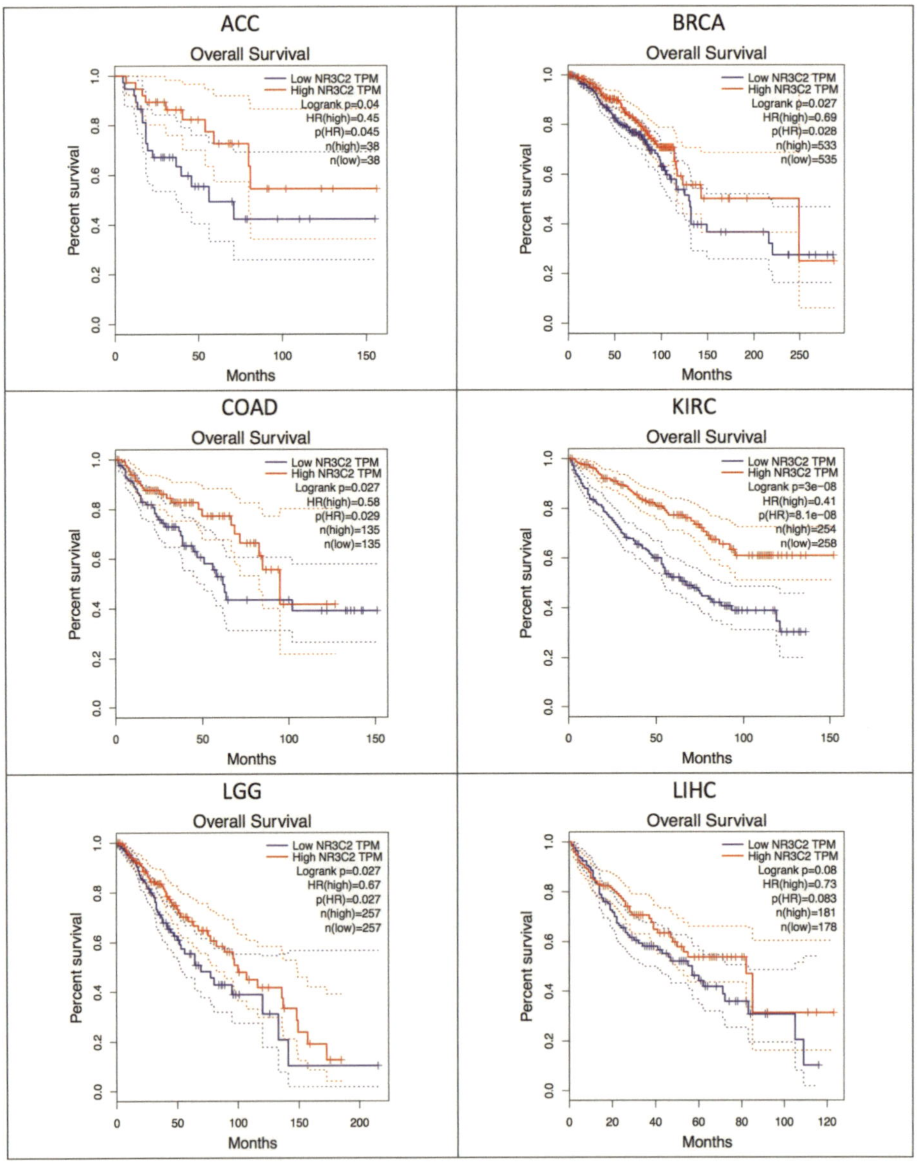


**Figure 3.**
*MR expression-based overall survival (OS) analyses performed using GEPIA. Adrenocortical carcinoma (ACC), breast invasive carcinoma (BRCA), colorectal adenocarcinoma (COAD), kidney renal clear cell carcinoma, low-grade glioma (LGG), and liver hepatocellular carcinoma (LIHC). The statistics and their associated p-values are shown on graphs, while groups (red and blue) are separated by the median expression level of MR.*

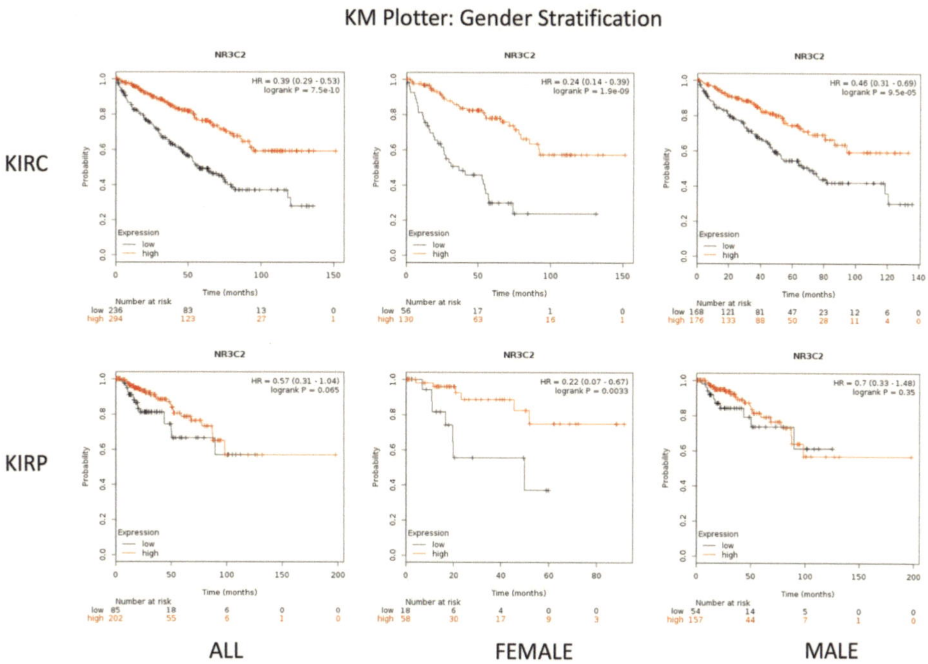


**Figure 4.**
*KM plotter analysis of kidney renal clear cell carcinoma (KIRC) and kidney renal papillary cell carcinoma (KIRP) for all, female and male patients, separately.*

Similar analyses can be performed using other webservers, such as KM plotter (http://kmplot.com/analysis/), which allows for auto-selection of an expression threshold that performs best in the logrank test. Recently, KM plotter has also made possible the stratification of TCGA PanCancer patient data according to different clinical and demographic variables including gender [95]. For example, we tested the significance of association between MR expression and OS using the best cutoff option separately for females and males, in renal cancers, KIRC and KIRP. Accordingly, we found that sexual dimorphism in MR expression can play a role in association with OS, warranting further investigation (**Figure 4**). Importantly, it is also possible to study MR expression and its role in RFS using the same tools. Our findings through GEPIA and KM plotter help confirm that downregulation of MR/NR3C2 expression can be significantly associated with cancer progress as has been previously reported in the literature. In conclusion, large-scale expression analysis in association with clinical data such as time to death or recurrence can thus reveal the importance of MR expression in epithelial and other solid tumors yet warrants further mechanistic studies.

## 5. Conclusion

A comprehensive look at the history of MR in cancer research strongly implicates the dysregulation of MR signaling in the development and progression of epithelial cancers. However, the interactions with its natural ligand aldosterone and/or with other potential ligands, such as tissue-specific progesterone as well as the growing evidence on the presence of receptor cross talk, complicate the "tumor suppressive" role often attributed to MR. MR's relatively well-established effects in renal tissue senescence, oxidative stress and DNA damage, as well as its emerging potential in the regulation of Warburg effect and fibrosis/regeneration in liver tissue represent novel avenues to pursue especially in the context of cancer therapy. In addition, the genome-wide availability of CNV, SNV, and mRNA expression profiles from cancer patients enables comparisons within and between different tumors providing an enhanced level of accessibility to researchers in the field of cancer biology. Indeed, online examination of the interaction between different data sources such as expression and patient survival data is now effectively possible for MR and can be extended to other genes participating in MR signaling. Generation of large-scale genome-wide data along with the development of tools that help analyze and integrate such data is likely to further enhance our understanding of MR in the development and progression of different cancers.

## Acknowledgements

This publication is based upon work from the EU COST Action ADMIRE BM1301 in Aldosterone and Mineralocorticoid Receptor Physiology and Pathophysiology (www.admirecosteu.com) and support from The Scientific and Technological Research Council of Turkey (TUBITAK) (research grant number, 114S226). We thank the anonymous reviewers for helpful suggestions.

## Author details

Ozlen Konu* and Seniye Targen
Department of Molecular Biology and Genetics, Bilkent University, Ankara, Turkey

*Address all correspondence to: konu@fen.bilkent.edu.tr

## References

[1] Weinstein JN, Collisson EA, Mills GB, Shaw KRM, Ozenberger BA, Ellrott K, et al. The cancer genome atlas pan-cancer analysis project. Nature Genetics. 2013;**45**:1113-1120. DOI: 10.1038/NG.2764

[2] Moons KGM, Royston P, Vergouwe Y, Grobbee DE, Altman DG. Prognosis and prognostic research: What, why, and how? British Medical Journal. 2009;**338**:b375. DOI: 10.1136/BMJ.B375

[3] Suzuki S, Suzuki T, Tsubochi H, Koike K, Tateno H, Krozowski ZS, et al. Expression of 11 beta-hydroxysteroid dehydrogenase type 2 and mineralocorticoid receptor in primary lung carcinomas. Anticancer Research. 2000;**20**:323-328

[4] Jeong Y, Xie Y, Xiao G, Behrens C, Girard L, Wistuba II, et al. Nuclear receptor expression defines a set of prognostic biomarkers for lung cancer. PLoS Medicine. 2010;**7**:e1000378. DOI: 10.1371/JOURNAL.PMED.1000378

[5] Bar J, Ding K, Zhao H, Han L, Laurie SA, Seymour L, et al. Angiotensin-converting enzyme and aldosterone serum levels as prognostic and predictive biomarkers for cediranib in NCIC clinical trials group study BR.24. Clinical Lung Cancer. 2015;**16**:e189-e201. DOI: 10.1016/J.CLLC.2015.05.002

[6] Di Fabio F, Alvarado C, Majdan A, Gologan A, Voda L, Mitmaker E, et al. Underexpression of mineralocorticoid receptor in colorectal carcinomas and association with VEGFR-2 overexpression. Journal of Gastrointestinal Surgery. 2007;**11**:1521-1528

[7] Tiberio L, Nascimbeni R, Villanacci V, Casella C, Fra A, Vezzoli V, et al. The decrease of mineralcorticoid receptor drives angiogenic pathways in colorectal cancer. PLoS One. 2013;**8**:e59410. DOI: 10.1371/JOURNAL.PONE.0059410

[8] Leung W-H, Vong QP, Lin W, Janke L, Chen T, Leung W. Modulation of NKG2D ligand expression and metastasis in tumors by spironolactone via RXRγ activation. The Journal of Experimental Medicine. 2013;**210**:2675-2692. DOI: 10.1084/JEM.20122292

[9] Morris DJ, Ridlon JM. Glucocorticoids and gut bacteria: "The GALF hypothesis" in the metagenomic era. Steroids. 2017;**125**:1-13. DOI: 10.1016/J.STEROIDS.2017.06.002

[10] Sasano H, Fukushima K, Sasaki I, Matsuno S, Nagura H, Krozowski ZS. Immunolocalization of mineralocorticoid receptor in human kidney, pancreas, salivary, mammary and sweat glands: A light and electron microscopic immunohistochemical study. Journal of Endocrinology. 1992;**132**:305-310. DOI: 10.1677/JOE.0.1320305

[11] Sasano H, Frost AR, Saitohi R, Matsunaga G, Nagura H, Krozowski ZS, et al. Localization of mineralocorticoid receptor and 11 beta-hydroxysteroid dehydrogenase type II in human breast and its disorders. Anticancer Research. 1997;**17**:2001-2007

[12] Conde I, Paniagua R, Fraile B, Lucio J, Arenas MI. Glucocorticoid receptor changes its cellular location with breast cancer development. Histology and Histopathology. 2008;**23**:77-85

[13] Ichinose RR, Nandi S. Influence of hormones on lobulo-alveolar differentiation of mouse mammary glands in vitro. The Journal of Endocrinology. 1966;**35**:331-340

[14] Wood BG, Washburn LL, Mukherjee AS, Banerjee MR. Hormonal regulation of lobulo alveolar growth,

functional differentiation and regression of whole mouse mammary gland in organ culture. The Journal of Endocrinology. 1975;**65**:1-6

[15] Hussain-Hakimjee EA, Peng X, Mehta RR, Mehta RG. Growth inhibition of carcinogen-transformed MCF-12F breast epithelial cells and hormone-sensitive BT-474 breast cancer cells by 1α-hydroxyvitamin D5. Carcinogenesis. 2006;**27**:551-559. DOI: 10.1093/CARCIN/BGI231

[16] Moore NL, Hickey TE, Butler LM, Tilley WD. Multiple nuclear receptor signaling pathways mediate the actions of synthetic progestins in target cells. Molecular and Cellular Endocrinology. 2012;**357**:60-70. DOI: 10.1016/J.MCE.2011.09.019

[17] Koyama K, Myles K, Smith R, Krozowski Z. Expression of the 11beta-hydroxysteroid dehydrogenase type II enzyme in breast tumors and modulation of activity and cell growth in PMC42 cells. Journal of Steroid Biochemistry and Molecular Biology. 2001;**76**:153-159. DOI: 10.1016/S0960-0760(00)00157-6

[18] Leo JC, Guo C, Woon CT, Aw SE, Lin VC. Glucocorticoid and mineralocorticoid cross-talk with progesterone receptor to induce focal adhesion and growth inhibition in breast cancer cells. Endocrinology. 2004;**145**:1314-1321

[19] Rigiracciolo DC, Scarpelli A, Lappano R, Pisano A, Santolla MF, Avino S, et al. GPER is involved in the stimulatory effects of aldosterone in breast cancer cells and breast tumor-derived endothelial cells. Oncotarget. 2016;7:94-111. DOI: 10.18632/ONCOTARGET.6475

[20] Nie H, Li J, Yang XM, Cao QZ, Feng MX, Xue F, et al. Mineralocorticoid receptor suppresses cancer progression and the Warburg effect by modulating the miR-338-3p-PKLR axis in hepatocellular carcinoma. Hepatology. 2015;**62**:1145-1159. DOI: 10.1002/HEP.27940

[21] Vander HMG, Cantley LC, Thompson CB. Understanding the Warburg effect: The metabolic requirements of cell proliferation. Science. 2009;**324**:1029-1033. DOI: 10.1126/SCIENCE.1160809

[22] Aydin MM, Akcali KC. Liver fibrosis. Turkish Journal of Gastroenterology. 2018;**29**:14-21. DOI: 10.5152/TJG.2018.18330

[23] Bataller R, Brenner DA. Liver fibrosis. The Journal of Clinical Investigation. 2005;**115**:209-218. DOI: 10.1042/BJ20071570

[24] Cox TR, Erler JT. Remodelling of the extracellular matrix: Implications for cancer. In: Schatten H, editor. Cell and Molecular Biology of Breast Cancer. New York: Springer; 2013. pp. 65-90. DOI: 10.1007/978-1-62703-634-4_4

[25] Rombouts K, Niki T, Wielant A, Hellemans K, Schuppan D, Kormoss N, et al. Effect of aldosterone on collagen steady state levels in primary and subcultured rat hepatic stellate cells. Journal of Hepatology. 2001;**34**:230-238. DOI: 10.1016/S0168-8278(00)00087-8

[26] Parlakgumus A, Colakoglu T, Kayaselcuk F, Colakoglu S, Ezer A, Calskan K, et al. Two drugs with paradoxical effects on liver regeneration through antiangiogenesis and antifibrosis: Losartan and spironolactone: A pharmacologic dilemma on hepatocyte proliferation. Journal of Surgical Research. 2013;**179**:60-65. DOI: 10.1016/J.JSS.2012.08.046

[27] Fuller PJ, Funder JW. Mineralocorticoid and glucocorticoid receptors in human kidney. Kidney International. 1976;**10**:154-157

[28] Matulich DT, Spindler BJ, Schambelan M, Baxter JD. Mineralocorticoid receptors in human kidney. The Journal of Clinical Endocrinology and Metabolism. 1976; **43**:1170-1174

[29] Yakirevich E, Morris DJ, Tavares R, Meitner PA, Lechpammer M, Noble L, et al. Mineralocorticoid receptor and 11β-hydroxysteroid dehydrogenase type II expression in renal cell neoplasms: A tissue microarray and quantitative RT-PCR study. American Journal of Surgical Pathology. 2008;**32**:874-883. DOI: 10.1097/PAS.0B013E31815F2362

[30] King S, Bray S, Galbraith S, Christie L, Fleming S. Evidence for aldosterone-dependent growth of renal cell carcinoma. International Journal of Experimental Pathology. 2014;**95**: 244-250. DOI: 10.1111/IEP.12074

[31] Feldman RD, Ding Q, Hussain Y, Limbird LE, Pickering JG, Gros R. Aldosterone mediates metastatic spread of renal cancer via the G protein-coupled estrogen receptor (GPER). FASEB Journal. 2016;**30**:2086-2096. DOI: 10.1096/FJ.15-275552

[32] Weikert S, Boeing H, Pischon T, Weikert C, Olsen A, Tjonneland A, et al. Blood pressure and risk of renal cell carcinoma in the European prospective investigation into cancer and nutrition. American Journal of Epidemiology. 2008;**167**:438-446. DOI: 10.1093/AJE/KWM321

[33] Sanfilippo KM, McTigue KM, Fidler CJ, Neaton JD, Chang Y, Fried LF, et al. Hypertension and obesity and the risk of kidney cancer in 2 large cohorts of US men and women. Hypertension. 2014;**63**:934-941. DOI: 10.1161/HYPERTENSIONAHA.113.02953

[34] Schupp N, Queisser N, Wolf M, Kolkhof P, Bärfacker L, Schäfer S, et al. Aldosterone causes DNA strand breaks and chromosomal damage in renal cells, which are prevented by mineralocorticoid receptor antagonists. Hormone and Metabolic Research. 2010;**42**:458-465. DOI: 10.1055/S-0029-1243253

[35] Schupp N, Kolkhof P, Queisser N, Gärtner S, Schmid U, Kretschmer A, et al. Mineralocorticoid receptor-mediated DNA damage in kidneys of DOCA-salt hypertensive rats. The FASEB Journal. 2011;**25**:968-978. DOI: 10.1096/FJ.10-173286

[36] Queisser N, Oteiza PI, Stopper H, Oli RG, Schupp N. Aldosterone induces oxidative stress, oxidative DNA damage and NF-KB-activation in kidney tubule cells. Molecular Carcinogenesis. 2011;**50**:123-135. DOI: 10.1002/MC.20710

[37] Queisser N, Schupp N, Schwarz E, Hartmann C, Mackenzie GG, Oteiza PI. Aldosterone activates the oncogenic signals ERK1/2 and STAT3 via redox-regulated mechanisms. Molecular Carcinogenesis. 2017;**56**:1868-1883. DOI: 10.1002/MC.22643

[38] Dimri GP. What has senescence got to do with cancer? Cancer Cell. 2005;**7**: 505-512. DOI: 10.1016/J.CCR.2005.05.025

[39] Serrano M, Lin AW, McCurrach ME, Beach D, Lowe SW. Oncogenic ras provokes premature cell senescence associated with accumulation of p53 and p16(INK4a). Cell. 1997;**88**:593-602. DOI: 10.1016/S0092-8674(00)81902-9

[40] Alcorta DA, Xiong Y, Phelps D, Hannon G, Beach D, Barrett JC. Involvement of the cyclin-dependent kinase inhibitor p16 (INK4a) in replicative senescence of normal human fibroblasts. Proceedings of the National Academy of Sciences. 1996;**93**: 13742-13747. DOI: 10.1073/PNAS.93.24.13742

[41] Westhoff JH, Hilgers KF, Steinbach MP, Hartner A, Klanke B, Amann K,

et al. Hypertension induces somatic cellular senescence in rats and humans by induction of cell cycle inhibitor p16INK4a. Hypertension. 2008;**52**:123-129. DOI: 10.1161/HYPERTENSIONAHA.107.099432

[42] Fan YY, Kohno M, Hitomi H, Kitada K, Fujisawa Y, Yatabe J, et al. Aldosterone/mineralocorticoid receptor stimulation induces cellular senescence in the kidney. Endocrinology. 2011;**152**:680-688. DOI: 10.1210/EN.2010-0829

[43] Kitada K, Nakano D, Hitomi H, Kobori H, Deguchi K, Mori H, et al. Aldosterone induces p21-regulated apoptosis via increased synthesis and secretion of tumour necrosis factor- α in human proximal tubular cells. Clinical and Experimental Pharmacology and Physiology. 2012;**39**:858-863. DOI: 10.1111/J.1440-1681.2012.12001.X

[44] Yang S, He P, Wang J, Schetter A, Tang W, Funamizu N, et al. A novel MIF signaling pathway drives the malignant character of pancreatic cancer by targeting NR3C2. Cancer Research. 2016;**76**:3838-3850. DOI: 10.1158/0008-5472.CAN-15-2841

[45] Nath N, Lakshmi V, Rosenthal JC. Presence of 11 β-hydroxysteroid dehydrogenase enzyme in the human prostate tumor cell line LNCaP. The Prostate. 1993;**23**:225-233. DOI: 10.1002/PROS.2990230305

[46] Pagé N, Warriar N, Govindan MV. 11β-Hydroxysteroid dehydrogenase and tissue specificity of androgen action in human prostate cancer cell LNCaP. The Journal of Steroid Biochemistry and Molecular Biology. 1994;**49**:173-181. DOI: 10.1016/0960-0760(94)90008-6

[47] Dovio A, Sartori M, De Francia S, Mussino S, Perotti P, Saba L, et al. Differential expression of determinants of glucocorticoid sensitivity in androgen-dependent and androgen-independent human prostate cancer cell lines. The Journal of Steroid Biochemistry and Molecular Biology. 2009;**116**:29-36

[48] Attard G, Reid AHM, Yap TA, Raynaud F, Dowsett M, Settatree S, et al. Phase I clinical trial of a selective inhibitor of CYP17, abiraterone acetate, confirms that castration-resistant prostate cancer commonly remains hormone driven. Journal of Clinical Oncology. 2008;**26**:4563-4571. DOI: 10.1200/JCO.2007.15.9749

[49] Kim W, Jones JO, Diamond M, Haqq C, Molina A, Small EJ, et al. Inhibition of the androgen receptor by mineralocorticoids at levels physiologically achieved in serum in patients treated with abiraterone acetate. Prostate Cancer and Prostatic Diseases. 2014;**17**:292-299. DOI: 10.1038/PCAN.2014.27

[50] Pia A, Vignani F, Attard G, Tucci M, Bironzo P, Scagliotti G, et al. Strategies for managing ACTH dependent mineralocorticoid excess induced by abiraterone. Cancer Treatment Reviews. 2013;**39**:966-973. DOI: 10.1016/J.CTRV.2013.03.003

[51] Auchus RJ, Yu MK, Nguyen S, Mundle SD. Use of prednisone with abiraterone acetate in metastatic castration-resistant prostate cancer. The Oncologist. 2014;**19**:1231-1240. DOI: 10.1634/THEONCOLOGIST.2014-0167

[52] Gill D, Gaston D, Bailey E, Hahn A, Gupta S, Batten J, et al. Efficacy of eplerenone in the management of mineralocorticoid excess in men with metastatic castration-resistant prostate cancer treated with abiraterone without prednisone. Clinical Genitourinary Cancer. 2017;**15**:e599-e602. DOI: 10.1016/J.CLGC.2016.12.008

[53] Isikbay M, Otto K, Kregel S, Kach J, Cai Y, Vander Griend DJ, et al. Glucocorticoid receptor activity contributes to resistance to

androgen-targeted therapy in prostate cancer. Hormones and Cancer. 2014;**5**: 72-89. DOI: 10.1007/S12672-014-0173-2

[54] Arora VK, Schenkein E, Murali R, Subudhi SK, Wongvipat J, Balbas MD, et al. Glucocorticoid receptor confers resistance to antiandrogens by bypassing androgen receptor blockade. Cell. 2013;**155**:1309-1322. DOI: 10.1016/J.CELL.2013.11.012

[55] Shiota M, Fujimoto N, Higashijima K, Imada K, Kashiwagi E, Takeuchi A, et al. Mineralocorticoid receptor signaling affects therapeutic effect of enzalutamide. The Prostate. 2018;**78**: 1045-1052. DOI: 10.1002/PROS.23661

[56] Santala EE, Rannikko A, Murtola TJ. Antihypertensive drugs and prostate cancer survival after radical prostatectomy in Finland—A nationwide cohort study. International Journal of Cancer. 2018;**144**:440-447. DOI: 10.1002/IJC.31802

[57] Terzolo M, Bovio S, Pia A, Reimondo G, Angeli A. Management of adrenal incidentaloma. Best Practice & Research: Clinical Endocrinology & Metabolism. 2009;**23**:233-243. DOI: 10.1016/J.BEEM.2009.04.001

[58] Crona J, Backman S, Welin S, Taïeb D, Hellman P, Stålberg P, et al. RNA-sequencing analysis of adrenocortical carcinoma, pheochromocytoma and paraganglioma from a pan-cancer perspective. Cancers. 2018;**10**:518. DOI: 10.3390/CANCERS10120518

[59] Conn JW, Knopf RF, Nesbit RM. Clinical characteristics of primary aldosteronism from an analysis of 145 cases. The American Journal of Surgery. 1964;**107**:159-172. DOI: 10.1016/0002-9610(64)90252-1

[60] Young WF. Primary aldosteronism: Renaissance of a syndrome. Clinical Endocrinology. 2007;**66**:607-618. DOI: 10.1111/J.1365-2265.2007.02775.X

[61] El Zein RM, Boulkroun S, Fernandes-Rosa FL, Zennaro MC. Molecular genetics of Conn adenomas in the era of exome analysis. La Presse Médicale. 2018;**47**:e151-e158. DOI: 10.1016/J.LPM.2018.07.006

[62] Peng KY, Chang HM, Lin YF, Chan CK, Chang CH, Chueh SCJ, et al. MiRNA-203 modulates aldosterone levels and cell proliferation by targeting wnt5a in aldosterone-producing adenomas. The Journal of Clinical Endocrinology and Metabolism. 2018; **103**:3737-3747. DOI: 10.1210/JC.2018-00746

[63] Zhang G, Zou X, Liu Q, Xie T, Huang R, Kang H, et al. MiR-193a-3p functions as a tumour suppressor in human aldosterone-producing adrenocortical adenoma by down-regulating CYP11B2. International Journal of Experimental Pathology. 2018;**99**:77-86. DOI: 10.1111/IEP.12267

[64] He J, Cao Y, Su T, Jiang Y, Jiang L, Zhou W, et al. Downregulation of miR-375 in aldosterone-producing adenomas promotes tumour cell growth via MTDH. Clinical Endocrinology. 2015;**83**: 581-589. DOI: 10.1111/CEN.12814

[65] Calissendorff J, Calissendorff F, Falhammar H. Adrenocortical cancer: Mortality, hormone secretion, proliferation and urine steroids—Experience from a single centre spanning three decades. BMC Endocrine Disorders. 2016;**16**:15. DOI: 10.1186/S12902-016-0095-9

[66] Lesouhaitier O, Chiappe A, Rossier MF. Aldosterone increases T-type calcium currents in human adrenocarcinoma (H295R) cells by inducing channel expression. Endocrinology. 2001;**142**:4320-4330. DOI: 10.1210/ENDO.142.10.8435

[67] Burton TJ, Cope G, Wang J, Sim JC, Azizan EAB, O'Shaughnessy KM, et al. Expression of the epithelial $Na^+$ channel

and other components of an aldosterone response pathway in human adrenocortical cells. European Journal of Pharmacology. 2009;**613**:176-181. DOI: 10.1016/J.EJPHAR.2009.04.005

[68] Mohan DR, Lerario AM, Else T, Mukherjee B, Almeida MQ, Vinco M, et al. Targeted assessment of G0S2 methylation identifies a rapidly recurrent, routinely fatal molecular subtype of adrenocortical carcinoma. Clinical Cancer Research. 2019;**25**:3276-3288. DOI: 10.1158/1078-0432.CCR-18-2693

[69] Liu S, Ding G, Zhou Z, Feng C. β-Catenin-driven adrenocortical carcinoma is characterized with immune exclusion. OncoTargets and Therapy. 2018;**11**:2029-2036. DOI: 10.2147/OTT.S159979

[70] James Kent W, Sugnet CW, Furey TS, Roskin KM, Pringle TH, Zahler AM, et al. The human genome browser at UCSC. Genome Research. 2002;**12**: 996-1006. DOI: 10.1101/GR.229102

[71] Karolchik D, Baertsch R, Diekhans M, Furey TS, Hinrichs A, Lu YT, et al. The UCSC genome browser database. Nucleic Acids Research. 2003;**31**:51-54. DOI: 10.1093/NAR/GKG129

[72] Hubbard T. The Ensembl genome database project. Nucleic Acids Research. 2002;**30**:38-41. DOI: 10.1093/NAR/30.1.38

[73] Stalker J, Gibbins B, Meidl P, Smith J, Spooner W, Hotz HR, et al. The Ensembl web site: Mechanics of a genome browser. Genome Research. 2004;**14**:951-955. DOI: 10.1101/GR.1863004

[74] Hede K. Superhighway or blind alley? The cancer genome atlas releases first results. Journal of the National Cancer Institute. 2008;**100**:1566-1569. DOI: 10.1093/JNCI/DJN424

[75] Mardis ER, Wilson RK. Cancer genome sequencing: A review. Human Molecular Genetics. 2009;**18**:R163-R168. DOI: 10.1093/HMG/DDP396

[76] McLendon R, Friedman A, Bigner D, Van Meir EG, Brat DJ, Mastrogianakis GM, et al. Comprehensive genomic characterization defines human glioblastoma genes and core pathways. Nature. 2008;**455**:1061-1068. DOI: 10.1038/NATURE07385

[77] Forbes SA, Bhamra G, Bamford S, Dawson E, Kok C, Clements J, et al. The catalogue of somatic mutations in cancer (COSMIC). Current Protocols in Human Genetics. 2008;**57**:10.11.1-10.11.26. DOI:10.1002/0471142905.HG1011S57

[78] Cerami E, Gao J, Dogrusoz U, Gross BE, Sumer SO, Aksoy BA, et al. The cBio cancer genomics portal: An open platform for exploring multidimensional cancer genomics data. Cancer Discovery. 2012;**2**:401-404. DOI: 10.1158/2159-8290.CD-12-0095

[79] Gao J, Aksoy BA, Dogrusoz U, Dresdner G, Gross B, Sumer SO, et al. Integrative analysis of complex cancer genomics and clinical profiles using the cBioPortal. Science Signaling. 2013;**6**: pl1. DOI: 10.1016/J.EXPNEUROL.2012.04.021

[80] Long MD, Campbell MJ. Pan-cancer analyses of the nuclear receptor superfamily. Nuclear Receptor Research. 2015;**2**:101182. DOI: 10.11131/2015/101182

[81] Zennaro MC, Fernandes-Rosa F. Mineralocorticoid receptor mutations. Journal of Endocrinology. 2017;**234**:T93-T106. DOI: 10.1530/JOE-17-0089

[82] Mohaupt MG, Frey FJ. Mineralocorticoid receptor malfunction: Further insights from rare forms of hypertension. Nephrology Dialysis Transplantation. 2002;**17**:539-542. DOI: 10.1093/NDT/17.4.539

[83] Hudson WH, Youn C, Ortlund EA. Crystal structure of the mineralocorticoid receptor DNA binding domain in complex with DNA. PLoS One. 2014;**9**:e107000. DOI: 10.1371/JOURNAL.PONE.0107000

[84] Reva B, Antipin Y, Sander C. Determinants of protein function revealed by combinatorial entropy optimization. Genome Biology. 2007;**8**: R232. DOI: 10.1186/GB-2007-8-11-R232

[85] Reva B, Antipin Y, Sander C. Predicting the functional impact of protein mutations: Application to cancer genomics. Nucleic Acids Research. 2011; **39**:e118. DOI: 10.1093/NAR/GKR407

[86] Sim NL, Kumar P, Hu J, Henikoff S, Schneider G, Ng PC. SIFT web server: Predicting effects of amino acid substitutions on proteins. Nucleic Acids Research. 2012;**40**:W452-W457. DOI: 10.1093/NAR/GKS539

[87] Adzhubei I, Jordan DM, Sunyaev SR. Predicting functional effect of human missense mutations using PolyPhen-2. Current Protocols in Human Genetics. 2013;**76**: 7.20.1-7.20.41. DOI: 10.1002/0471142905.HG0720S76

[88] Gray RJ. Flexible methods for analyzing survival data using splines, with applications to breast cancer prognosis. Journal of the American Statistical Association. 1992;**87**:942-951. DOI: 10.1080/01621459.1992.10476248

[89] Tang Z, Li C, Kang B, Gao G, Li C, Zhang Z. GEPIA: A web server for cancer and normal gene expression profiling and interactive analyses. Nucleic Acids Research. 2017;**45**: W98-W102. DOI: 10.1093/NAR/GKX247

[90] Anaya J. OncoLnc: Linking TCGA survival data to mRNAs, miRNAs, and lncRNAs. PeerJ Computer Science. 2016;**2**:e67. DOI: 10.7717/PEERJ-CS.67

[91] Lánczky A, Nagy Á, Bottai G, Munkácsy G, Szabó A, Santarpia L, et al. miRpower: A web-tool to validate survival-associated miRNAs utilizing expression data from 2178 breast cancer patients. Breast Cancer Research and Treatment. 2016;**160**:439-446. DOI: 10.1007/S10549-016-4013-7

[92] Chen X, Miao Z, DIvate M, Zhao Z, Cheung E. KM-express: An integrated online patient survival and gene expression analysis tool for the identification and functional characterization of prognostic markers in breast and prostate cancers. Database. 2018;**2018**:bay069. DOI: 10.1093/DATABASE/BAY069

[93] Xiao H, Xu D, Chen P, Zeng G, Wang X, Zhang X. Identification of five genes as a potential biomarker for predicting Progress and prognosis in adrenocortical carcinoma. Journal of Cancer. 2018;**9**:4484-4495. DOI: 10.7150/JCA.26698

[94] Yuan L, Qian G, Chen L, Wu CL, Dan HC, Xiao Y, et al. Co-expression network analysis of biomarkers for adrenocortical carcinoma. Frontiers in Genetics. 2018;**9**:328. DOI: 10.3389/FGENE.2018.00328

[95] Nagy Á, Lánczky A, Menyhárt O, Gyorffy B. Validation of miRNA prognostic power in hepatocellular carcinoma using expression data of independent datasets. Scientific Reports. 2018;**8**:9227. DOI: 10.1038/S41598-018-27521-Y

Chapter 10

# MR/GR Signaling in the Brain during the Stress Response

*Edo R. de Kloet and Onno C. Meijer*


## Abstract

This contribution is about mineralocorticoid receptors (MRs) in their capacity as mediators of glucocorticoid action in the brain. This paradox has evolved because MRs are promiscuous and bind with high-affinity cortisol and corticosterone as well as aldosterone, deoxycorticosterone, and progesterone. The MRs "see," however, predominantly glucocorticoids, because of their 100–1000-fold excess over aldosterone; bioavailability is further enhanced because of local regeneration of glucocorticoids by 11βOH-steroid dehydrogenase (HSD-1). In contrast to these *glucocorticoid-preferring* MR, the evolutionary later appearance of *aldosterone-selective* MR in epithelial cells depends on co-localization with the oxidase 11β-hydroxysteroid-dehydrogenase type 2 (HSD-2) in a few hundred neurons in the nucleus tractus solitarii (NTS), which innervate frontal brain regions to regulate cognitive, emotional, and motivational aspects of salt appetite. The glucocorticoid-MRs and classical glucocorticoid receptors (GRs) mediate in a complementary manner the glucocorticoid coordination of circadian events and mediate the regulation of stress coping and adaptation. If an individual is exposed to a threat, MRs are crucial for the selection of a particular coping style, which is via GR activation subsequently stored in the memory for future use. Our contribution is concluded with the notion that an imbalance in MR- and GR-mediated actions increases susceptibility to stress-related disorders.


**Keywords:** stress, brain, behavior, inflammation, glucocorticoid receptors, mineralocorticoid receptors

## 1. Introduction

The naturally occurring glucocorticoids, cortisol and corticosterone (the latter only in rodents), are secreted as end products of the hypothalamus-pituitary-adrenal (HPA) axis. The glucocorticoids have two modes of operation. Firstly, the hormones synchronize and coordinate circadian and sleep-related events. This action is based on hourly ultradian pulses with increasing amplitude toward the start of the active period with the goal to generate the necessary energy for the day to come. The hourly pulses maintain responsivity to the glucocorticoids. The frequency and amplitude of the glucocorticoid pulses may change as is the case during, e.g., inflammatory disorders and depression, or may become irregular as part of the aging process. High glucocorticoid concentrations prevent the onset of sleep [1–3].

Secondly, the glucocorticoids mediate the response to stress. A "stress reaction" can be due to physical stimuli such as pain, blood loss, and infection or can be psychogenic. Anticipation is an important component of the psychogenic stress reaction. Hence, the prediction of an upcoming event and the ability to exert control are essential for effective coping irrespective whether it concerns an adverse experience or a reward. Actually, stress is the "spice of life" and essential for adaptation and survival. However, the most severe stressor is characterized by inability to predict upcoming events and uncertainty during a threat. If uncertainty because of lack of control persists, the very same glucocorticoids that promote adaptation are now disruptive, facilitate breakdown of adaptation, reduce resilience, and enhance vulnerability to disease [4].

Glucocorticoid secretion from the adrenocortical zona fasciculata is under the control of pituitary adrenocorticotropic hormone (ACTH) that is cleaved from the large precursor molecule: pro-opiomelanocortin (POMC). The anterior pituitary synthesis of POMC is driven by corticotropin-releasing hormone (CRH) from neurosecretory cells of the paraventricular nucleus (PVN) in the hypothalamus; co-localized vasopressin amplifies the CRH-induced release of ACTH. Physical stressors directly activate CRH neurons via ascending neuronal projections of the brain stem. Psychological stressors are processed in higher brain regions for appraisal, decision-making, and choice of coping style to deal with the stressor. At last, the stress reaction dissipates and the experience is stored in the memory [5].

## 2. Corticosteroid receptors

The action of glucocorticoids is mediated by two types of corticosteroid receptors. One type is, surprisingly, the mineralocorticoid receptor (MR). This receptor was first identified in 1968 by Bruce McEwen: retention of $^{3}$H-labeled corticosterone was observed in hippocampal neurons at 1 hour after administration of the tracer to an adrenalectomized (ADX) rat [6]. $^{3}$H-aldosterone given to ADX animals showed essentially the same neuroanatomical distribution pattern as $^{3}$H-corticosterone. The MR was cloned: immunoreactive (ir) MR protein and MR gene expression showed the same distribution pattern as radioligand binding in the hippocampus [7, 8].

The GR was initially not detected by in vivo radioligand binding studies for two reasons. Firstly, the amount of radiolabeled corticosterone tracer was insufficient to occupy GR, because this receptor binds cortisol and corticosterone with a tenfold lower-affinity than the high-affinity MR. Second, our in vivo tracer studies with the high-affinity GR ligand, dexamethasone, did not provide a signal in the brain because the synthetic steroid was exported by multidrug resistance P-glycoprotein localized in the blood-brain barrier. When pure glucocorticoids became available, we managed to identify distinct populations of MR and GR in vitro. GR was found widely distributed in the brain and highly expressed in the typical stress centers. MR and GR are abundant and co-localized in limbic neurons [9, 10].

The MRs actually occur as glucocorticoid-preferring and aldosterone-selective variations in receptor function. Aldosterone-selectivity occurs solely in epithelial cells engaged in Na homeostasis. In a collaborative study with Edwards et al., we discovered in 1988 that aldosterone selectivity hinges on co-expression with the enzyme 11β-hydroxysteroid-dehydrogenase type 2 (HSD-2), which breaks down the naturally occurring glucocorticoids, cortisol and corticosterone, into their inactive 11-dehydro congeners [11]. The Australian group led by John Funder reached the same conclusion [12]. In the brain, the *aldosterone-selective* MRs involved in salt homeostasis are mostly restricted to neurons of the nucleus tractus solitarii (NTS) and the circumventricular organs. The MR-NTS neurons project to limbic forebrain regions, notably the locus coeruleus area involved in arousal and the bed nucleus of the stria terminalis (BNST). Via the BNST hub, the NTS neurons can affect emotions, memory performance, and reward processing [13–15].

A pharmacological amount of aldosterone, administered to rats, is anxiogenic and causes changes in coping with stress [16]. Such an effect can be explained by overstimulation of the aldosterone-responsive brain network. In fact, patients suffering from essential hypertension have an enhanced aldosterone secretion following stress exposure [17]. It would be of interest, therefore, to further explore this line of research, particularly in light of the persistent evidence of excess mineralocorticoids and aberrant MRs as risk factors for mood disorders [18, 19], also in patients with Conn's syndrome [20]. In addition, the brain aldosterone MRs were found to be causal in hypertension in case a high-salt diet was offered [21], see overview on aldosterone and mineralocorticoid receptors [22].

The majority of MRs that are abundantly expressed in limbic-frontocortical neurons were identified as *glucocorticoid-preferring*. This is because cortisol and corticosterone are present in a 100–1000-fold excess over aldosterone, thus competing out aldosterone binding, even though part of the circulating glucocorticoid is bound to corticosteroid-binding globulin (CBG). Accordingly, these glucocorticoid-preferring MRs predominantly "see" the naturally occurring glucocorticoids, cortisol and corticosterone. Moreover, glucocorticoid preference is further enhanced by co-expression with HSD-1, which regenerates locally bioactive glucocorticoids from the inactive 11-dehydro congener [23]. Finally, MRs are promiscuous in that they bind in addition to glucocorticoids and aldosterone also progesterone and deoxycorticosterone. This promiscuity may be related to the fact that evolutionary the MRs preceded the GRs, progesterone receptors and androgen receptors [24].

Thus, some 30 years ago, we felt as if we were "digging gold." We knew the precise localization of MR and GR in the brain and that these receptors did bind the same hormones—cortisol and corticosterone—but with an order of a magnitude difference in affinity. This was the start of a systematic search for their molecular, cellular, neuroendocrine, and behavioral function, together with the group of Marian Joëls in Amsterdam. This helped to define better the temporal, spatial, and contextual domains of the stress response that are so extremely important for understanding stress coping and adaptation [25–28]. Before discussing MR/GR function, we will first briefly summarize the main aspects of their role in the molecular and cellular mechanisms of glucocorticoids.

## 3. Molecular mechanisms of MR-/GR-mediated actions

The non-genomic effects notwithstanding (see Section 4) MR and GR are best understood as transcription factors involved in the regulation of gene expression. Classically, their differential effects have been related to (besides cell-specific expression) transcriptional effects that are independent of the highly homologous DNA-binding domain. For example, an important part of the anti-inflammatory actions of GR activation depends on interactions of GR monomers with pro-inflammatory transcription factors such as the "nuclear factor kappa-light-chain-enhancer of activated B cells" (NF-κB), a process called transrepression, and these interactions are much weaker for MR [29]. Recently, the interaction of the GR monomer with NF-κB was challenged with the discovery of GR binding to "cryptic" DNA sequences within the genomic NF-κB response elements (κBREs) that mediate GR-driven repression of inflammatory gene expression [30].

Recent studies that evaluated MR and GR binding to the DNA in the hippocampus indicate that the receptors interact with the DNA via their—homologous—DNA-binding domains [31–33]. MR and GR share 96% homology in their DNA-binding domain, and both recognize the same "GRE" sequence in the DNA to which they bind as homo- or heterodimers. Yet, they differ in other parts of the protein, in particular in their large N-terminal domain. The best known target genes that are shared between MR and GR are *FKBP5*, *Sgk1*, *GILZ*, and *PER1*. For these genes, GR activation seems to extend the MR-mediated action by an order of magnitude, as shown in dose-response studies.

Based on genome-wide profiling, many corticosterone-responsive hippocampal mRNAs—also in laser-dissected subregions—are known, allowing the identification of specific signaling pathways [34–37]. In other brain areas, information is more sparse, but likely will differ substantially, as patterns of MR and/or GR-responsive target genes overlap only partially between different cell types [38]. This cell specificity seems to be the consequence of a different chromatin organization and of cell-specific expression of coregulatory proteins that modulate the effects of MR and GR, once these are bound to the DNA [39, 40].

In view of their very different effects in the hippocampus, MR and GR should have unique target genes, and this assumption indeed recently has been materialized in three independent studies [31, 32, 41]. A unique signature of MR binding to DNA loci was discovered and found associated with the NeuroD transcription factor [33]. Also GR binding appeared associated to some extent with NeuroD, possibly as a result of heterodimer formation with MR [42]. Furthermore, current data suggest that NeuroD can interact with other unidentified proteins in the transcriptional complex that is formed upon MR binding to DNA. Such a MR-Neuro-D complex seems to confine specificity to cortisol action.

In spite of this progress in understanding receptor-specific cortisol actions, there is no single GR or MR target gene known to be responsible solely for circuit activation underlying a particular behavioral response during stress adaptation. Rather, MR and GR seem to be master regulators that mediate in complementary manner downstream regulatory networks in a cell- and context-specific fashion [37, 43]. Moreover, the transcriptional response of the hippocampal genome to corticosterone depends strongly on the recent past of the individual. About half of the significantly regulated mRNA's were found to be different between animals with a recent history of stress, as compared to control animals [37, 44].

## 4. Cellular mechanisms of MR-/GR-mediated action

In hippocampal CA1 neurons, in particular the membrane properties affected by norepinephrine (NE), serotonin (5HT), and glutamate are affected by corticosterone in a U-shaped dose-response curve [45, 46]. Thus, the activation of 5HT1A receptors produced during absence of corticosterone a large increase in conductance of an inwardly rectifying K-channel, causing the membrane to hyperpolarize. MR activation with a low concentration of corticosterone minimized the 5HT1A hyperpolarization response [47]. When corticosterone levels increased and gradually occupied GR, the hyperpolarization response returned, but not in $GR^{dim/dim}$ mutants [48], in which cannot dimerize because of point mutation in their DNA domain [49]. A similar U-shaped dose response was found for the accommodation of firing frequency upon steady depolarization of cells by NE and for the Ca influx via L-type voltage-dependent channels [46, 50–52].

The U-shaped dose-response curve is not a common phenomenon in the brain, since it is dependent on the presence of both receptor types. Even if both receptors are present, such as in the dentate gyrus, other membrane properties are affected than in the CA1 neurons. In the dentate gyrus MR activation increased the field potential, and the single cell response showed activation of glutamatergic receptors, and both responses were not further affected by additional GR activation

[46]. These cellular effects in CA1 and dentate gyrus have not been explained by transcriptional regulation. For instance, 5HT1A mRNA expression in CA1 cells was not affected by adrenalectomy, while it was in an MR-dependent fashion in dentate gyrus neurons [53].

The dentate gyrus is one of the two brain regions where neurogenesis occurs throughout life. In the absence of steroids, the turnover of these neurons increases, showing increased neurogenesis and apoptotic cell death. Both processes are normalized if the animals are replaced with low doses of corticosterone, just sufficient to occupy MR. Glucocorticoids suppress proliferation and migration of the newborn neurons via GRs. Lentiviral GR knockdown in the dentate progenitor cells accelerates neuronal differentiation and migration. The newborn neurons showed increased synaptic contacts and increased excitability and migrated further in establishing functional integration in the hippocampal circuitry. Accordingly, contextual fear-motivated behavior was impaired [54].

Regarding the non-genomic actions, MR mediates the rapid and transient increase of miniature excitatory postsynaptic currents (mEPSC) after treatment with corticosterone. The putative membrane MR is localized presynaptically and activates the release probability of glutamate. The rapid effects were eliminated after genetic deletion of the MR gene or with MR antagonists [55]. These effects are exerted by both aldosterone and corticosterone, and the dose-response curve suggests a lower affinity of steroid binding to the membrane than to nuclear MR. The membrane MR—in spite of much effort—has not been physically demonstrated yet [56–58] and likely is similar to the nuclear variant. The MR-enhanced increase of glutamate release downregulates the presynaptic metabotropic glutamate receptors ($mGluR_2$) [59].

The nature of the membrane-mediated MR effects shows, however, large regional differences in the brain. For instance, in contrast to the rapid transient rise in excitability, the excitation is long-lasting in basolateral amygdala (BLA) neurons due to cooperation with genomic GR-mediated actions. Moreover, the duration of BLA excitation is further prolonged if—as is the case during stress—these cells are also exposed to NE, which can be mimicked by the β-adrenergic agonist isoproterenol. Interestingly, such a prolonged increased excitability of the BLA protects against the effect of a second MR-mediated corticosterone pulse, probably via rapid endocannabinoid action linked to the membrane GR [60]. These composite cellular responses were defined as a manifestation of "corticosterone metaplasticity" and may explain why emotions are so strongly remembered [61, 62].

Thus, the data demonstrate that glucocorticoid actions may vary between cell groups. This variety in responses also has consequences for the influence of stress exposure and stress hormones on long-term potentiation (LTP), a cellular model of memory performance. It demonstrates that stress does not a priori disturb LTP, since the outcome depends on the context, the previous experiences, the phase of the stress response, and the analyzed brain regions [63]. In the hippocampus, MR is essential for neuronal viability and maintenance of excitatory transmission. If, with increasing corticosterone concentrations, GR becomes occupied, this receptor restores transiently raised excitability.

## 5. Functional cooperation of MR and GR

MRs and GRs cooperate in glucocorticoid regulation, and below we will distinguish four different phases of this cooperation in stress coping and adaptation (see **Figure 1**). This distinction is based on temporal and contextual features of membrane and genomic glucocorticoid actions. The conditional nature is an important

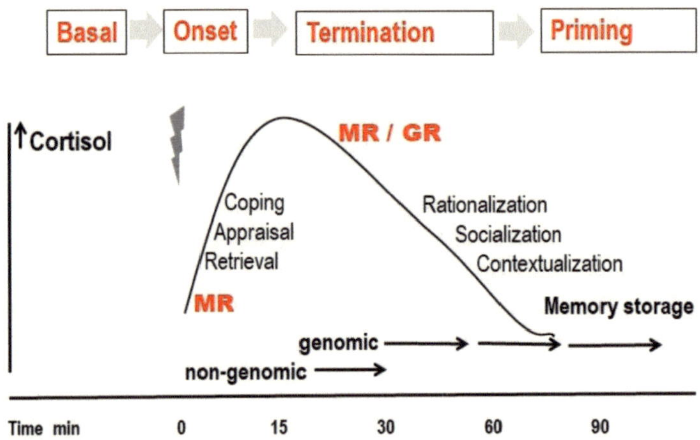


**Figure 1.**
*Four phases of MR/GR signaling in the brain during the stress response.* ***Phase 1****: "Basal" MR/GR signaling during ultradian/circadian activity is a determinant of the sensitivity of the stress response.* ***Phase 2****: "Onset" of the stress reaction non-genomic MR-mediated actions promotes appraisal processes, retrieval of previously stored information, selection of coping style, and encoding of the experience for learning, all directed to defend the "self."* ***Phase 3****: "Termination" is the negative feedback action of GR-mediated glucocorticoid action aimed to prevent defense reactions from overshooting. Via GR, the experience is contextualized in the hippocampus and rationalized in the prefrontal cortex, with more "altruistic" solutions that increase motivation to assign a valence to social solutions and rewards.* ***Phase 4****: "Priming" refers to memory storage of the experience for future use (adapted from [27, 28, 64, 65]).*

criterion, since it assigns a specificity to glucocorticoid action. The temporal action is also critical. The rapid non-genomic actions wax and wane in correspondence with glucocorticoid concentrations. The genomic actions develop minutes to hours after glucocorticoid exposure and may last for days or even a lifetime. The latter concerns aspects of programming of brain circuitry for later life by epigenetic processes at glucocorticoid targets or even the receptors themselves [66]. The following phases in glucocorticoid action can be distinguished:

***Phase 1—basal*** is the basal state in which during the circadian/ultradian cycle, mostly genomic MRs are occupied during the trough, and, subsequently, when glucocorticoid levels show their hourly increases, the hormone progressively activates additional GRs. The continuous MR activation is a determinant of the threshold or sensitivity of the stress response system. The transient GR activation by the hourly pulses maintains responsivity to sudden changes in glucocorticoid secretion as they occur in response to stress [3, 9, 67].

***Phase 2—onset*** is the onset of the stress reaction when a novel experience is anticipated or actually happens and triggers sympathetic activation and CRH release. Non-genomic MRs that are rapidly activated by a stress-induced increase in circulating glucocorticoids enhance attention and vigilance to optimize sensory processing in support of perception and appraisal of novel information [68]. MR activation promotes memory retrieval in the hippocampus to deploy the previously used strategy in stress coping and enhances in amygdala emotional expressions of fear and aggression [69, 70]. MR activation also facilitates the choice of coping style. For instance, under mild stress conditions, most individuals will opt for a coping strategy involving the hippocampus (thinking). However, when stressors become more severe and less controllable, increasingly an emotion-driven habitual amygdala-striatal stimulus-response coping strategy is preferred (doing). The switch from "thinking to doing" depends on limbic MR. Corticosterone administration promotes habit formation, while MR antagonists prevent the switch and the slower, costlier hippocampal cognitive strategy is maintained. Finally, via MRs the context of the experience and the selected coping style are encoded for learning [71–73].

***Phase 3—termination*** marks a further increase of glucocorticoid secretion and progressive activation of the lower-affinity membrane and genomic GRs, which are in limbic-frontocortical structures co-localized with MRs [25, 28]. The MRs are continuously involved in appraisal processes to monitor the outcome of the stress-coping strategy. GR function limits defense reactions to prevent these from over-shoot that may cause damage, if not dampened [74]. These defense mechanisms are now abolished, and it is time for *rationalization* and *contextualization* of the experience and for assessment of valence as occurs in *social interactions* [27, 75]. At the same time, GR activation drives via a mitochondrial mechanism energy allocation to cells and circuits in need to facilitate recovery from the stressor [76]. This is a life-sustaining action since complete GR knockouts do not survive, while $GR^{dim/dim}$ do. After all, lack of glucocorticoids is not compatible with life as is illustrated by adrenalectomy and in the case of Addison's disease. Phase 3 is also characterized by increased motivational arousal, emotional expressions, and reinforcement learning, accompanied by increased gene expression of key components in the amygdala (re: enhanced CRH expression) and ventral striatum—frontocortical circuitry (re: increased dopaminergic function) [77–81].

***Phase 4—priming*** GR activation in the limbic-frontocortical circuits promotes storage of contextual and emotional-loaded information in the memory. This consolidation process takes a couple of hours after the stressful experience [82]. Synaptic adaptations occur which can be measured with fMRI and are characterized by genome-wide transcriptional signatures [83–85]. Growth factors such as BDNF participate by acting in the dentate neurogenic niche; also growth factor actions in e.g. mPFC and mesolimbic dopaminergic systems [86, 87] are all involved. Hence, GR-activated memory storage prepares for the future, so that stored information can be retrieved again in the proper context. During phases 3 and 4, the individual's homeostasis is restored and behavioral adaptation is promoted [4].

Using optogenetics combined with neuroanatomical tracing, the top-down organization of the brain's coping circuitry is rapidly unraveled today. Accordingly, the prelimbic mPFC sends excitatory projections to the lateroventral (av)-BNST, which operates as an inhibitory GABAergic hub over downstream neuroendocrine, autonomic, and behavioral responses [88]. Stressors activate the excitatory output of the mPFC, which translates into BNST-dependent inhibition of CRH neurons in the PVN and results in suppression of the HPA axis response. In another group of CRH neurons, the BNST input attenuates the sympathetic output. A separate pathway of the BNST projects to the ventrolateral periaqueductal (vl-PAG) where passive coping is promoted at the expense of the initial active coping strategy [89, 90]. Active coping refers to fight or flight, which, when the situation is appraised as inescapable, causes a reorganization of prelimbic to infralimbic mPFC circuitry that is aimed to restrain the emotional and autonomic responses [91–94]. Passive conservation withdrawal behavior is promoted allowing recuperation and storage of energy resources [95, 96].

This coping circuit is modulated in function by contextual information from the hippocampus, by emotional- and fear-input from the amygdala, visceral and autonomous inputs from the brain stem, and motivational arousal associated with valence assessment from the ventral striatum. The coping circuit and its modulating inputs are all targets of the glucocorticoids that convey environmental and physiological information. This bottom-up control exerted by the glucocorticoids is mediated by the MR and GR in a complementary manner along the four different phases of stress coping and adaptation [64] (see **Figure 1**). The action of the glucocorticoid during stress coping and adaptation has led to the formulation of the MR/GR balance hypothesis, which states that "upon imbalance of the MR- and GR-mediated actions, the initiation and/or management of the stress response becomes compromised. At a certain threshold this may lead to a condition of neuro-endocrine dysregulation and impaired behavioral adaptation, which potentially can aggravate stress-related deterioration and promote vulnerability" [9, 25, 28, 97–99].

## 6. Implications for pathogenesis and treatment of stress-related diseases

Physical or psychogenic stressors promote activation of circuits that underlie appraisal and decision-making processes, which are important for selection of an appropriate coping style to support physiological and behavioral adaptations. The most severe psychogenic stressor is lack of control and inability to predict, with an uncertain fearful feeling [96, 100]. The brain can adapt to this situation by proliferation of the emotional amygdala and atrophy of the hippocampus, ventral striatum, and prefrontal cortex [101–104]. Glucocorticoid secretion remains elevated and energy resources are drained. Essential defense mechanisms become compromised, and when then confronted with a novel stressor, coping fails, breakdown of adaptation is facilitated, and vulnerability to mood and anxiety disorders increases [105, 106].

Adverse (early) life experience and unfavorable socioeconomic conditions are important predisposing factors for such stress-related disorders [107]. Also genetic variants and epigenetic modifications are increasingly recognized as biomarkers of susceptibility and vulnerability. For instance, for MR, two functional SNPs (rs2070951 and rs5522) constitute a block of four haplotypes. Haplotype 2 generates in vitro the highest MR-binding capacity and transactivation. Carriers of haplotype 2 display a preferential *habit* rather than *cognitive* strategy in coping with stress. Haplotype 2 (C/A frequency 35%) is associated with optimism and protection to depression and predicts a higher efficacy of antidepressants [73, 108–110]. Actually, the MR is a promising target to facilitate the action of antidepressants [111].

Progress is made in exploiting the relevance of the MR/GR balance for devising preventive or curative strategies in the treatment of mental health. For instance, it is recognized that patients under dexamethasone therapy have very low levels of endogenous circulating glucocorticoids. While dexamethasone is a potent GR ligand, the MR becomes depleted of endogenous hormone, because of suppression of the HPA axis. Refill of the MR with cortisol add-on largely eliminates the psychologic/psychiatric side effects of dexamethasone therapy [112–115]. Alternatively, the glucocorticoid/progesterone antagonist mifepristone is applied for treatment of hyperglycemia in patients suffering from Cushing's syndrome [116]. Recently, selective GR modulators (SGRMs) became available that can target metabolism but do not show side effects on pituitary ACTH release [117–119].

## 7. Concluding remarks

Glucocorticoids, acting via brain MRs and GRs, coordinate multiple functions over time with one single goal: to promote stress coping and adaptation. Imbalance in the MR-/GR-mediated signaling pathways increases susceptibility to stress-related mental and neurodegenerative disorders. These imbalances develop under conditions of chronic stress when top-down control exerted by the mPFC over the stress-coping circuitry is compromised and the cost of bottom-up glucocorticoid action exceeds its benefit. New SGRMs are being developed that target the tissue- and context-specific action of glucocorticoids in specific domains of cognition, emotion, and motivation and which may assist in targeted therapies of stress-related mental disorders.

## Acknowledgements

This publication is based upon the work from the EU COST Action ADMIRE BM1301 in Aldosterone and Mineralocorticoid Receptor (MR) Physiology and Pathophysiology (www.admirecosteu.com). The Royal Netherlands Academy of Arts and Sciences (ERdK), NWO, and ZONMW (OCM) are gratefully acknowledged.

## Conflict of interest

ERdK is on the Scientific Advisory Board of the DynaCorts Group and owns stock of Corcept Therapeutics. OCM receives funding from Corcept Therapeutics.

## Author details

Edo R. de Kloet* and Onno C. Meijer
Department of Internal Medicine, Division of Endocrinology, Leiden University Medical Center, Leiden, The Netherlands

*Address all correspondence to: erdekloet@gmail.com

## References

[1] Sarabdjitsingh RA, Isenia S, Polman A, Mijalkovic J, Lachize S, Datson N, et al. Disrupted corticosterone pulsatile patterns attenuate responsiveness to glucocorticoid signaling in rat brain. Endocrinology. 2010;**151**:1177-1186. DOI: 10.1210/en.2009-1119

[2] Lightman SL, Conway-Campbell BL. The crucial role of pulsatile activity of the HPA axis for continuous dynamic equilibration. Nature Reviews. Neuroscience. 2010;**11**:710-718. DOI: 10.1038/nrn2914

[3] Sarabdjitsingh RA, Jezequel J, Pasricha N, Mikasova L, Kerkhofs A, Karst H, et al. Ultradian corticosterone pulses balance glutamatergic transmission and synaptic plasticity. Proceedings of the National Academy of Sciences. 2014;**111**:14265-14270. DOI: 10.1073/pnas.1411216111

[4] de Kloet ER, Joëls M, Holsboer F. Stress and the brain: From adaptation to disease. Nature Reviews. Neuroscience. 2005;**6**:463-475. DOI: 10.1038/nrn1683

[5] Ulrich-Lai YM, Herman JP. Neural regulation of endocrine and autonomic stress responses. Nature Reviews. Neuroscience. 2009;**10**:397-409. DOI: 10.1038/nrn2647

[6] McEwen BS, Weiss JM, Schwartz LS. Selective retention of corticosterone by limbic structures in rat brain. Nature. 1968;**220**:911-912. DOI: 10.1038/220911a0

[7] Reul JM, de Kloet ER. Two receptor systems for corticosterone in rat brain: Microdistribution and differential occupation. Endocrinology. 1985;**117**:2505-2511. DOI: 10.1210/endo-117-6-2505

[8] Arriza JL, Weinberger C, Cerelli G, Glaser TM, Handelin BL, Housman DE, et al. Cloning of human mineralocorticoid receptor complementary DNA: Structural and functional kinship with the glucocorticoid receptor. Science. 1987;**237**:268-275. DOI: 10.1126/science.3037703

[9] De Kloet ER, Reul JMHM. Feedback action and tonic influence of corticosteroids on brain function: A concept arising from the heterogeneity of brain receptor systems. Psychoneuroendocrinology. 1987;**12**:83-105. DOI: 10.1016/0306-4530(87)90040-0

[10] Meijer OC, De Lange ECM, Breimer DD, De Boer AG, Workel JO, De Kloet ER. Penetration of dexamethasone into brain glucocorticoid targets is enhanced in mdr1A P-glycoprotein knockout mice. Endocrinology. 1998;**139**:1789-1793. DOI:10.1210/endo.139.4.5917

[11] Edwards CR, Stewart PM, Burt D, Brett L, McIntyre MA, Sutanto WS, et al. Localisation of 11 beta-hydroxysteroid dehydrogenase—Tissue specific protector of the mineralocorticoid receptor. Lancet (London, England). 1988;**2**:986-989. DOI: 10.1016/S0140-6736(88)90742-8

[12] Funder JW, Pearce PT, Smith R, Smith AI. Mineralocorticoid action: Target tissue specificity is enzyme, not receptor, mediated. Science. 1988;**242**:583-585. DOI: 10.1126/science.2845584

[13] Krause EG, Sakai RR. Richter and sodium appetite: From adrenalectomy to molecular biology. Appetite. 2007;**49**:353-367. DOI: 10.1016/j.appet.2007.01.015

[14] Geerling JC, Loewy AD. Aldosterone in the brain. AJP Renal Physiology. 2009;**297**:F559-F576. DOI: 10.1152/ajprenal.90399.2008

[15] Gasparini S, Resch JM, Narayan SV, Peltekian L, Iverson GN, Karthik S, et al. Aldosterone-sensitive HSD2 neurons in mice. Brain Structure & Function. 2019;**224**:387-417. DOI: 10.1007/s00429-018-1778-y

[16] Hlavacova N, Jezova D. Chronic treatment with the mineralocorticoid hormone aldosterone results in increased anxiety-like behavior. Hormones and Behavior. 2008;**54**:90-97. DOI: 10.1016/j.yhbeh.2008.02.004

[17] Markou A, Sertedaki A, Kaltsas G, Androulakis II, Marakaki C, Pappa T, et al. Stress-induced aldosterone hyper-secretion in a substantial subset of patients with essential hypertension. The Journal of Clinical Endocrinology and Metabolism. 2015;**100**:2857-2864. DOI: 10.1210/jc.2015-1268

[18] de Kloet ER, Joëls M. Brain mineralocorticoid receptor function in control of salt balance and stress-adaptation. Physiology & Behavior. 2017;**178**:13-20. DOI: 10.1016/j.physbeh.2016.12.045

[19] Murck H, Schüssler P, Steiger A. Renin-angiotensin-aldosterone system: The forgotten stress hormone system: Relationship to depression and sleep. Pharmacopsychiatry. 2012;**45**:83-95. DOI: 10.1055/s-0031-1291346

[20] Künzel HE, Apostolopoulou K, Pallauf A, Gerum S, Merkle K, Schulz S, et al. Quality of life in patients with primary aldosteronism: Gender differences in untreated and long-term treated patients and associations with treatment and aldosterone. Journal of Psychiatric Research. 2012;**46**:1650-1654. DOI: 10.1016/j.jpsychires.2012.08.025

[21] Evans LC, Ivy JR, Wyrwoll C, McNairn JA, Menzies RI, Christensen TH, et al. Conditional deletion of Hsd11b2 in the brain causes salt appetite and hypertension. Circulation. 2016;**133**:1360-1370. DOI: 10.1161/CIRCULATIONAHA.115.019341

[22] Jaisser F, Farman N. Emerging roles of the mineralocorticoid receptor in pathology: Toward new paradigms in clinical pharmacology. Pharmacological Reviews. 2016;**68**:49-75. DOI: 10.1124/pr.115.011106

[23] Chapman K, Holmes M, Seckl J. 11-Hydroxysteroid dehydrogenases: Intracellular gate-keepers of tissue glucocorticoid action. Physiological Reviews. 2013;**93**:1139-1206. DOI: 10.1152/physrev.00020.2012

[24] Baker ME, Funder JW, Kattoula SR. Evolution of hormone selectivity in glucocorticoid and mineralocorticoid receptors. The Journal of Steroid Biochemistry and Molecular Biology. 2013;**137**:57-70. DOI: 10.1016/j.jsbmb.2013.07.009

[25] de Kloet ER. Brain corticosteroid receptor balance and homeostatic control. Frontiers in Neuroendocrinology. 1991;**12**:95-164. DOI: 10.1080/09614520701469617

[26] Joëls M, de Kloet ER. 30 years of the mineralocorticoid receptor: The brain mineralocorticoid receptor: A saga in three episodes. The Journal of Endocrinology. 2017;**234**:T49-T66. DOI: 10.1530/JOE-16-0660

[27] Joëls M, Karst H, Sarabdjitsingh RA. The stressed brain of humans and rodents. Acta Physiologica (Oxford, England). 2018;**223**:e13066. DOI: 10.1111/apha.13066

[28] de Kloet ER, Meijer OC, de Nicola AF, de Rijk RH, Joëls M. Importance of the brain corticosteroid receptor balance in metaplasticity, cognitive performance and neuro-inflammation. Frontiers in Neuroendocrinology. 2018;**49**:124-145. DOI: 10.1016/j.yfrne.2018.02.003

[29] D. Pearce, K.R. Yamamoto, Mineralocorticoid and glucocorticoid receptor activities distinguished by nonreceptor factors at a composite response element, Science (New York, N.Y.). 259 (1993) 1161-1165. DOI: 10.1126/science.8382376

[30] Hudson WH, de Vera IMS, Nwachukwu JC, Weikum ER, Herbst AG, Yang Q, et al. Cryptic glucocorticoid receptor-binding sites pervade genomic NF-κB response elements. Nature Communications. 2018;**9**:1337. DOI: 10.1038/s41467-018-03780-1

[31] Polman JAE, de Kloet ER, Datson NA. Two populations of glucocorticoid receptor-binding sites in the male rat hippocampal genome. Endocrinology. 2013;**154**:1832-1844. DOI: 10.1210/en.2012-2187

[32] Pooley JR, Flynn BP, Grøntved L, Baek S, Guertin MJ, Kershaw YM, et al. Genome-wide identification of basic helix-loop helix and NF-1 motifs underlying GR binding sites in male rat hippocampus. Endocrinology. 2017;**158**:1486-1501. DOI: 10.1210/en.2016-1929

[33] van Weert LTCM, Buurstede JC, Mahfouz A, Braakhuis PSM, Polman JAE, Sips HCM, et al. NeuroD factors discriminate mineralocorticoid from glucocorticoid receptor DNA binding in the male rat brain. Endocrinology. 2017;**158**:1511-1522. DOI: 10.1210/en.2016-1422

[34] Datson NA, Van Der Perk J, De Kloet ER, Vreugdenhil E. Identification of corticosteroid-responsive genes in rat hippocampus using serial analysis of gene expression. The European Journal of Neuroscience. 2001;**14**:675-689. DOI: 10.1046/j.0953-816x.2001.01685.x

[35] Datson NA, Morsink MC, Meijer OC, de Kloet ER. Central corticosteroid actions: Search for gene targets. European Journal of Pharmacology. 2008;**583**:272-289. DOI: 10.1016/j.ejphar.2007.11.070

[36] Datson NA, Speksnijder N, Mayer JL, Steenbergen PJ, Korobko O, Goeman J, et al. The transcriptional response to chronic stress and glucocorticoid receptor blockade in the hippocampal dentate gyrus. Hippocampus. 2012;**22**:359-371. DOI: 10.1002/hipo.20905

[37] Datson NA, van den Oever JME, Korobko OB, Magarinos AM, De Kloet ER, Mcewen B. Prior history of chronic stress changes the transcriptional response to glucocorticoid challenge in the dentate gyrus region of the male rat hippocampus. Endocrinology. 2013;**154**:3261-3272. DOI: 10.1210/en.2012-2233

[38] S. John, P.J. Sabo, R.E. Thurman, M.-H. Sung, S.C. Biddie, T.A. Johnson, G.L. Hager, J.A. Stamatoyannopoulos, Chromatin accessibility pre-determines glucocorticoid receptor binding patterns TL-43, Nature Genetics. 2011;**43**:264-268. DOI: 10.1038/ng.759

[39] Mahfouz A, Lelieveldt BPF, Grefhorst A, van Weert LTCM, Mol IM, Sips HCM, et al. Genome-wide coexpression of steroid receptors in the mouse brain: Identifying signaling pathways and functionally coordinated regions. Proceedings of the National Academy of Sciences of the United States of America. 2016;**113**:2738-2743. DOI: 10.1073/pnas.1520376113

[40] Zalachoras I, Verhoeve SL, Toonen LJ, van Weert LTCM, van Vlodrop AM, Mol IM, et al. Isoform switching of steroid receptor co-activator-1 attenuates glucocorticoid-induced anxiogenic amygdala CRH expression. Molecular Psychiatry. 2016;**21**:1733-1739. DOI: 10.1038/mp.2016.16

[41] Polman JAE, Hunter RG, Speksnijder N, van den Oever JME,

Korobko OB, McEwen BS, et al. Glucocorticoids modulate the mTOR pathway in the hippocampus: Differential effects depending on stress history. Endocrinology. 2012;**153**: 4317-4327. DOI: 10.1210/en.2012-1255

[42] Mifsud KR, Reul JMHM. Acute stress enhances heterodimerization and binding of corticosteroid receptors at glucocorticoid target genes in the hippocampus. Proceedings of the National Academy of Sciences of the United States of America. 2016;**113**:11336-11341. DOI: 10.1073/pnas.1605246113

[43] Repunte-Canonigo V, Shin W, Vendruscolo LF, Lefebvre C, van der Stap L, Kawamura T, et al. Identifying candidate drivers of alcohol dependence-induced excessive drinking by assembly and interrogation of brain-specific regulatory networks. Genome Biology. 2015;**16**:68. DOI: 10.1186/s13059-015-0593-5

[44] Gray JD, Kogan JF, Marrocco J, McEwen BS. Genomic and epigenomic mechanisms of glucocorticoids in the brain. Nature Reviews. Endocrinology. 2017;**13**:661-673. DOI: 10.1038/nrendo.2017.97

[45] Joëls M, de Kloet ER. Control of neuronal excitability by corticosteroid hormones. Trends in Neurosciences. 1992;**15**:25-30. DOI: 10.1016/0166-2236(92)90345-9

[46] Joëls M. Corticosteroid effects in the brain: U-shape it. Trends in Pharmacological Sciences. 2006;**27**: 244-250. DOI: 10.1016/j.tips.2006.03.007

[47] Joels M, Hesen W, De Kloet ER. Mineralocorticoid hormones suppress serotonin-induced hyperpolarization of rat hippocampal CA 1 neurons. The Journal of Neuroscience. 1991;**11**:2288-2294. doi.org/10.1523/JNEUROSCI.11-08-02288

[48] Karst H, Karten YJ, Reichardt HM, de Kloet ER, Schutz G, Joels M. Corticosteroid actions in hippocampus require DNA binding of glucocorticoid receptor homodimers. Nature Neuroscience. 2000;**3**:977-978. DOI: 10.1038/79910

[49] Reichardt HM, Kaestner KH, Tuckermann J, Kretz O, Wessely O, Bock R, et al. DNA binding of the glucocorticoid receptor is not essential for survival. Cell. 1998;**93**:531-541. DOI: 10.1016/S0092-8674(00)81183-6

[50] Joëls M, de Kloet ER. Effects of glucocorticoids and norepinephrine on the excitability in the hippocampus. Science. 1989;**245**:1502-1505. DOI: 10.1126/science.2781292

[51] Joëls M, de Kloet ER. Mineralocorticoid receptor-mediated changes in membrane properties of rat CA1 pyramidal neurons in vitro. Proceedings of the National Academy of Sciences of the United States of America. 1990;**87**:4495-4498. DOI: 10.1073/pnas.87.12.4495

[52] Joëls M, Sarabdjitsingh RA, Karst H.Unraveling the time domains of corticosteroid hormone influences on brain activity: Rapid, slow, and chronic modes. Pharmacological Reviews. 2012;**64**:901-938. DOI: 10.1124/pr.112.005892

[53] Meijer OC, de Kloet ER. A role for the mineralocorticoid receptor in a rapid and transient suppression of hippocampal 5-HT1A receptor mRNA by corticosterone. Journal of Neuroendocrinology. 1995;7:653-657. DOI: 10.1111/j.1365-2826.1995.tb00804.x

[54] Fitzsimons CP, Van Hooijdonk LWA, Schouten M, Zalachoras I, Brinks V, Zheng T, et al. Knockdown of the glucocorticoid receptor alters functional integration of newborn neurons in the adult hippocampus

and impairs fear-motivated behavior. Molecular Psychiatry. 2013;**18**:993-1005. DOI: 10.1038/mp.2012.123

[55] Karst H, Berger S, Turiault M, Tronche F, Schutz G, Joels M. Mineralocorticoid receptors are indispensable for nongenomic modulation of hippocampal glutamate transmission by corticosterone. Proceedings of the National Academy of Sciences. 2005;**102**:19204-19207. DOI: 10.1073/pnas.0507572102

[56] Groeneweg FL, Karst H, de Kloet ER, Joëls M. Rapid non-genomic effects of corticosteroids and their role in the central stress response. The Journal of Endocrinology. 2011;**209**:153-167. DOI: 10.1530/JOE-10-0472

[57] Groeneweg FL, Karst H, de Kloet ER, Joëls M. Mineralocorticoid and glucocorticoid receptors at the neuronal membrane, regulators of nongenomic corticosteroid signalling. Molecular and Cellular Endocrinology. 2012;**350**:299-309. DOI: 10.1016/j.mce.2011.06.020

[58] Groeneweg FL, van Royen ME, Fenz S, Keizer VIP, Geverts B, Prins J, et al. Quantitation of glucocorticoid receptor DNA-binding dynamics by single-molecule microscopy and FRAP. PLoS ONE. 2014;**9**:e90532. DOI: 10.1371/journal.pone.0090532

[59] Nasca C, Zelli D, Bigio B, Piccinin S, Scaccianoce S, Nisticò R, et al. Stress dynamically regulates behavior and glutamatergic gene expression in hippocampus by opening a window of epigenetic plasticity. Proceedings of the National Academy of Sciences. 2015;**112**:14960-14965. DOI: 10.1073/pnas.1516016112

[60] Hill MN, Tasker JG. Endocannabinoid signaling, glucocorticoid-mediated negative feedback, and regulation of the hypothalamic-pituitary-adrenal axis. Neuroscience. 2012;**204**:5-16. DOI: 10.1016/j.neuroscience.2011.12.030

[61] Karst H, Berger S, Erdmann G, Schütz G, Joëls M. Metaplasticity of amygdalar responses to the stress hormone corticosterone. Proceedings of the National Academy of Sciences of the United States of America. 2010;**107**:14449-14454. DOI: 10.1073/pnas.0914381107

[62] Karst H, Joëls M. Severe stress hormone conditions cause an extended window of excitability in the mouse basolateral amygdala. Neuropharmacology. 2016;**110**:175-180. DOI: 10.1016/j.neuropharm.2016.07.027

[63] Joëls M, Krugers HJ. LTP after stress: Up or down? Neural Plasticity. 2007;**2007**:93202. DOI: 10.1155/2007/93202

[64] de Kloet ER, de Kloet SF, de Kloet CS, de Kloet AD. Top-down and bottom-up control of stress-coping. Journal of Neuroendocrinology. 2019;**31**:e12675. DOI: 10.1111/jne.12675

[65] Molendijk ML, de Kloet ER. Coping with the forced swim stressor: Current state-of-the-art. Behavioural Brain Research. 2019;**364**:1-10. DOI: 10.1016/j.bbr.2019.02.005

[66] Turecki G, Meaney MJ. Effects of the social environment and stress on glucocorticoid receptor gene methylation: A systematic review. Biological Psychiatry. 2016;**79**:87-96. DOI: 10.1016/j.biopsych.2014.11.022

[67] Sarabdjitsingh RA, Conway-Campbell BL, Leggett JD, Waite EJ, Meijer OC, De Kloet ER, et al. Stress responsiveness varies over the ultradian glucocorticoid cycle in a brain-region-specific manner. Endocrinology. 2010. DOI: 10.1210/en.2010-0832

[68] Cornelisse S, Joëls M, Smeets T. A randomized trial on mineralocorticoid

receptor blockade in men: Effects on stress responses, selective attention, and memory. Neuropsychopharmacology. 2011;**36**:2720-2728. DOI: 10.1038/npp.2011.162

[69] Korte SM, De Boer SF, De Kloet ER, Bohus B. Anxiolytic-like effects of selective mineralocorticoid and glucocorticoid antagonists on fear-enhanced behavior in the elevated plus-maze. Psychoneuroendocrinology. 1995;**20**:385-394. DOI: 10.1016/0306-4530(94)00069-7

[70] Kruk MR, Haller J, Meelis W, de Kloet ER. Mineralocorticoid receptor blockade during a rat's first violent encounter inhibits its subsequent propensity for violence. Behavioral Neuroscience. 2013;**127**:505-514. DOI: 10.1037/a0033553

[71] Oitzl MS, de Kloet ER. Selective corticosteroid antagonists modulate specific aspects of spatial orientation learning. Behavioral Neuroscience. 1992;**106**:62-71. DOI: 10.1037/0735-7044.106.1.62

[72] Schwabe L, Schächinger H, de Kloet ER, Oitzl MS. Corticosteroids operate as a switch between memory systems. Journal of Cognitive Neuroscience. 2010;**22**:1362-1372. DOI: 10.1162/jocn.2009.21278

[73] Wirz L, Reuter M, Wacker J, Felten A, Schwabe L. A haplotype associated with enhanced mineralocorticoid receptor expression facilitates the stress-induced shift from "cognitive" to "habit" learning. eNeuro. 2017;**4**. DOI: 10.1523/ENEURO.0359-17.2017

[74] Sapolsky RM, Romero LM, Munck AU. How do glucocorticoids influence stress responses? Integrating permissive, suppressive, stimulatory, and preparative actions. Endocrine Reviews. 2000;**21**:55-89. DOI: 10.1210/er.21.1.55

[75] Weger M, Sandi C. High anxiety trait: A vulnerable phenotype for stress-induced depression. Neuroscience and Biobehavioral Reviews. 2018;**87**:27-37. DOI: 10.1016/j.neubiorev.2018.01.012

[76] Hollis F, van der Kooij MA, Zanoletti O, Lozano L, Cantó C, Sandi C. Mitochondrial function in the brain links anxiety with social subordination. Proceedings of the National Academy of Sciences. 2015;**112**:15486-15491. DOI: 10.1073/pnas.1512653112

[77] Makino S, Gold PW, Schulkin J. Effects of corticosterone on CRH mRNA and content in the bed nucleus of the stria terminalis; comparison with the effects in the central nucleus of the amygdala and the paraventricular nucleus of the hypothalamus. Brain Research. 1994;**657**:141-149. DOI: 10.1016/0006-8993(94)90961-x

[78] Piazza PV, Le Moal ML. Pathophysiological basis of vulnerability to drug abuse: Role of an interaction between stress, glucocorticoids, and dopaminergic neurons. Annual Review of Pharmacology and Toxicology. 1996;**36**:359-378. DOI: 10.1146/annurev.pa.36.040196.002043

[79] Lachize S, Apostolakis EM, van der Laan S, Tijssen AMI, Xu J, de Kloet ER, et al. Steroid receptor coactivator-1 is necessary for regulation of corticotropin-releasing hormone by chronic stress and glucocorticoids. Proceedings of the National Academy of Sciences of the United States of America. 2009;**106**:8038-8042. DOI: 10.1073/pnas.0812062106

[80] Barik J, Marti F, Morel C, Fernandez SP, Lanteri C, Godeheu G, et al. Chronic stress triggers social aversion via glucococorticoid receptor in dopaminoceptive neurons. Science. 2013;**(80).339**:332-335. DOI: 10.1007/s13398-014-0173-7.2

[81] Bagot RC, Parise EM, Peña CJ, Zhang H-X, Maze I, Chaudhury D, et al. Ventral hippocampal afferents to the nucleus accumbens regulate susceptibility to depression. Nature Communications. 2015;**6**:7062. DOI: 10.1038/ncomms8062

[82] De Quervain D, Schwabe L, Roozendaal B. Stress, glucocorticoids and memory: Implications for treating fear-related disorders. Nature Reviews. Neuroscience. 2016;**18**:7-19. DOI: 10.1038/nrn.2016.155

[83] Datson NA, Morsink MC, Steenbergen PJ, Aubert Y, Schlumbohm C, Fuchs E, et al. A molecular blueprint of gene expression in hippocampal subregions CA1, CA3, and DG is conserved in the brain of the common marmoset. Hippocampus. 2009;**19**:739-752. DOI: 10.1002/hipo.20555

[84] Henckens MJAG, Pu Z, Hermans EJ, Van Wingen GA, Joëls M, Fernández G. Dynamically changing effects of corticosteroids on human hippocampal and prefrontal processing. Human Brain Mapping. 2012;**33**:2885-2897. DOI: 10.1002/hbm.21409

[85] Hermans EJ, Henckens MJ, Joels M, Fernandez G. Dynamic adaptation of large-scale brain networks in response to acute stressors. Trends in Neurosciences. 2014;**37**:304-314. DOI: 10.1016/j.tins.2014.03.006

[86] Krishnan V, Han M-H, Graham DL, Berton O, Renthal W, Russo SJ, et al. Molecular adaptations underlying susceptibility and resistance to social defeat in brain reward regions. Cell. 2007;**131**:391-404. DOI: 10.1016/j.cell.2007.09.018

[87] Lucassen PJ, Pruessner J, Sousa N, Almeida OFX, Van Dam AM, Rajkowska G, et al. Neuropathology of stress. Acta Neuropathologica. 2014;**127**:109-135. DOI: 10.1007/s00401-013-1223-5

[88] Radley JJ, Johnson SB. Anteroventral bed nuclei of the stria terminalis neurocircuitry: Towards an integration of HPA axis modulation with coping behaviors—Curt Richter Award Paper 2017. Psychoneuroendocrinology. 2018;**89**:239-249. DOI: 10.1016/j.psyneuen.2017.12.005

[89] Keay KA, Bandler R. Parallel circuits mediating distinct emotional coping reactions to different types of stress. Neuroscience and Biobehavioral Reviews. 2001;**25**:669-678. DOI: 10.1016/S0149-7634(01)00049-5

[90] Johnson SB, Emmons EB, Lingg RT, Anderson RM, Romig-Martin SA, LaLumiere RT, et al. Prefrontal-bed nucleus circuit modulation of a passive coping response set. The Journal of Neuroscience. 2019;**39**:1405-1419. DOI: 10.1523/JNEUROSCI.1421-18.2018

[91] Fiore VG, Mannella F, Mirolli M, Latagliata EC, Valzania A, Cabib S, et al. Corticolimbic catecholamines in stress: A computational model of the appraisal of controllability. Brain Structure & Function. 2015;**220**:1339-1353. DOI: 10.1007/s00429-014-0727-7

[92] McKlveen JM, Morano RL, Fitzgerald M, Zoubovsky S, Cassella SN, Scheimann JR, et al. Chronic stress increases prefrontal inhibition: A mechanism for stress-induced prefrontal dysfunction. Biological Psychiatry. 2016;**80**:754-764. DOI: 10.1016/j.biopsych.2016.03.2101

[93] Milad MR, Quirk GJ. Fear extinction as a model for translational neuroscience: Ten years of progress. Annual Review of Psychology. 2012;**63**:129-151. DOI: 10.1146/annurev.psych.121208.131631

[94] Wood M, Adil O, Wallace T, Fourman S, Wilson SP, Herman JP, et al. Infralimbic prefrontal cortex structural and functional connectivity with the limbic forebrain: A combined viral genetic and optogenetic analysis. Brain

Structure & Function. 2019;**224**:73-97. DOI: 10.1007/s00429-018-1762-6

[95] Henry J, Stephens P. Stress, Health and the Social Environment: A Sociobiological Approach. New York: Springer; 1977. DOI: https://doi.org/10.1007/978-1-4612-6363-

[96] de Boer SF, Buwalda B, Koolhaas JM. Untangling the neurobiology of coping styles in rodents: Towards neural mechanisms underlying individual differences in disease susceptibility. Neuroscience and Biobehavioral Reviews. 2017;**74**:401-422. DOI: 10.1016/j.neubiorev.2016.07.008

[97] De Kloet ER, Vreugdenhil E, Oitzl MS, Joëls M. Brain corticosteroid receptor balance in health and disease. Endocrine Reviews. 1998;**19**:269-301. DOI: 10.1210/edrv.19.3.0331

[98] Holsboer F. The corticosteroid receptor hypothesis of depression. Neuropsychopharmacology. 2000;**23**:477-501. DOI: 10.1016/S0893-133X(00)00159-7

[99] de Kloet ER. From receptor balance to rational glucocorticoid therapy. Endocrinology. 2014;**155**:2754-2769. DOI: 10.1210/en.2014-1048

[100] Peters A, McEwen BS, Friston K. Uncertainty and stress: Why it causes diseases and how it is mastered by the brain. Progress in Neurobiology. 2017;**156**:164-188. DOI: 10.1016/j.pneurobio.2017.05.004

[101] McEwen BS. Physiology and neurobiology of stress and adaptation: Central role of the brain. Physiological Reviews. 2007;**87**:873-904. DOI: 10.1152/physrev.00041.2006

[102] McEwen BS. Redefining neuroendocrinology: Epigenetics of brain-body communication over the life course. Frontiers in Neuroendocrinology. 2018;**49**:8-30. DOI: 10.1016/j.yfrne.2017.11.001

[103] Sousa N. The dynamics of the stress neuromatrix. Molecular Psychiatry. 2016;**21**:302-312. DOI: 10.1038/mp.2015.196

[104] Magalhães R, Barrière DA, Novais A, Marques F, Marques P, Cerqueira J, et al. The dynamics of stress: A longitudinal MRI study of rat brain structure and connectome. Molecular Psychiatry. 2018;**23**:1998-2006. DOI: 10.1038/mp.2017.244

[105] Karatsoreos IN, McEwen BS. Psychobiological allostasis: Resistance, resilience and vulnerability. Trends in Cognitive Sciences. 2011;**15**:576-584. DOI: 10.1016/j.tics.2011.10.005

[106] Picard M, McEwen BS, Epel ES, Sandi C. An energetic view of stress: Focus on mitochondria. Frontiers in Neuroendocrinology. 2018;**49**:72-85. DOI: 10.1016/j.yfrne.2018.01.001

[107] McEwen BS, Gianaros PJ. Stress- and Allostasis-induced brain plasticity. Annual Review of Medicine. 2011;**62**:431-445. DOI: 10.1146/annurev-med-052209-100430

[108] Klok MD, Giltay EJ, Van der Does AJW, Geleijnse JM, Antypa N, Penninx BWJH, et al. A common and functional mineralocorticoid receptor haplotype enhances optimism and protects against depression in females. Translational Psychiatry. 2011;**1**:e62. DOI: 10.1038/tp.2011.59

[109] de Kloet ER, Otte C, Kumsta R, Kok L, Hillegers MHJ, Hasselmann H, et al. Stress and depression: A crucial role of the mineralocorticoid receptor. Journal of Neuroendocrinology. 2016;**28**:8. DOI: 10.1111/jne.12379

[110] Kumsta R, Kliegel D, Linden M, DeRijk R, de Kloet ER. Genetic variation of the mineralocorticoid

receptor gene (MR, NR3C2) is associated with a conceptual endophenotype of "CRF-hypoactivity". Psychoneuroendocrinology. 2018. DOI: 10.1016/j.psyneuen.2018.09.036

[111] Otte C, Hinkelmann K, Moritz S, Yassouridis A, Jahn H, Wiedemann K, et al. Modulation of the mineralocorticoid receptor as add-on treatment in depression: A randomized, double-blind, placebo-controlled proof-of-concept study. Journal of Psychiatric Research. 2010;**44**:339-346. DOI: 10.1016/j.jpsychires.2009.10.006

[112] Born J, DeKloet ER, Wenz H, Kern W, Fehm HL. Gluco- and antimineralocorticoid effects on human sleep: A role of central corticosteroid receptors. The American Journal of Physiology. 1991;**260**:E183-E188

[113] Groch S, Wilhelm I, Lange T, Born J. Differential contribution of mineralocorticoid and glucocorticoid receptors to memory formation during sleep. Psychoneuroendocrinology. 2013;**38**:2962-2972. DOI: 10.1016/j.psyneuen.2013.08.006

[114] Warris LT, Van Den Heuvel-Eibrink MM, Aarsen FK, Pluijm SMF, Bierings MB, Den Van Bos C, et al. Hydrocortisone as an intervention for dexamethasone-induced adverse effects in pediatric patients with acute lymphoblastic leukemia: Results of a double-blind, randomized controlled trial. Journal of Clinical Oncology. 2016;**34**:2287-2293. DOI: 10.1200/JCO.2015.66.0761

[115] Meijer OC, de Kloet ER. A refill for the brain mineralocorticoid receptor: The benefit of cortisol add-on to dexamethasone therapy. Endocrinology. 2017;**158**:448-454. DOI: 10.1210/en.2016-1495

[116] Moraitis AG, Block T, Nguyen D, Belanoff JK. The role of glucocorticoid receptors in metabolic syndrome and psychiatric illness. The Journal of Steroid Biochemistry and Molecular Biology. 2017;**165**:114-120. DOI: 10.1016/j.jsbmb.2016.03.023

[117] Kroon J, Koorneef LL, van den Heuvel JK, Verzijl CRC, van de Velde NM, Mol IM, et al. Selective glucocorticoid receptor antagonist CORT125281 activates brown adipose tissue and alters lipid distribution in male mice. Endocrinology. 2018;**159**:535-546. DOI: 10.1210/en.2017-00512

[118] Nguyen ET, Streicher J, Berman S, Caldwell JL, Ghisays V, Estrada CM, et al. A mixed glucocorticoid/mineralocorticoid receptor modulator dampens endocrine and hippocampal stress responsivity in male rats. Physiology & Behavior. 2017;**178**:82-92. DOI: 10.1016/j.physbeh.2017.01.020

[119] Meijer OC, Koorneef LL, Kroon J. Glucocorticoid receptor modulators. Annales d'Endocrinologie. 2018;**79**:107-111. DOI: 10.1016/j.ando.2018.03.004

Chapter 11

# View on Aldosterone and the Brain Revisited

*Natasa Hlavacova and Damiela Jezova*


## Abstract

The mineralocorticoid hormone aldosterone has been investigated almost exclusively with respect to cardiovascular function, as the main effects of aldosterone are related to water-electrolyte balance and the control of the blood pressure. This overview is focused on less traditional and long-time neglected effects of aldosterone on the brain and behavior. Preclinical studies by our research group brought evidence on causal relationships between aldosterone and anxiety as well as aldosterone and depression-like behavior. Aldosterone was found to be anxiogenic and depressogenic in a rat model. Preclinical studies also indicate that aldosterone may be an early marker of depression onset. Aldosterone is known to be an important component of the stress response, and we have shown that its role is particularly important during early postnatal period in pups. Studies in patients with major depressive disorder revealed that an unfavorable therapy outcome is predicted by a higher salivary aldosterone/cortisol ratio. Our clinical studies showed that salivary aldosterone concentrations reflect the severity, duration of the depressive episode, and treatment outcome in patients with major depressive disorder. Moreover, the patients with depression fail to exert known daily rhythmicity of aldosterone release.


**Keywords:** aldosterone, anxiety, depression, stress, rhythm

## 1. Introduction

The mineralocorticoid hormone aldosterone is typically viewed as the principal regulator of sodium and potassium balance thus playing a major role in maintaining extracellular volume homeostasis. The classical genomic actions of aldosterone are mediated by mineralocorticoid receptor (MR). The MR and its kin, the glucocorticoid receptor (GR), evolved from an ancestral corticoid receptor in a cyclostome (jawless fish) throughout gene duplication and divergence. Distinct orthologs of the MR and GR initially appeared in cartilaginous fishes, such as sharks, skates, rays, and chimeras. Aldosterone first appears in lungfish, lobe-finned fish that are forerunners of terrestrial vertebrates [1, 2]. The evolution of the relationship between aldosterone and MR likely occurred in response to dramatic changes associated with transition from aquatic to terrestrial life. In the ocean, aquatic organisms had the burden of fighting constant salt loading, whereas the prospect of a terrestrial existence presented the opposite problem, preventing their emergence from the sea. It is likely that the aldosterone-MR relationship was a part of the solution to maintain ion balance during this transition from water to land [3]. Further sequence divergence of the MR and GR in terrestrial vertebrates led to emergence of aldosterone as a selective ligand for the MR [4]. The first studies with recombinant human MR yielded an unexpected discovery [5] that human MR has strong binding affinities for several corticosteroids (aldosterone, cortisol, corticosterone, and 11-deoxycorticosterone) and for progesterone. Although these steroids show similar affinity for human MR, transcriptional activation of human MR by these steroids is different. Compared to glucocorticoids, aldosterone is a stronger activator of the MR [6]. The ability of aldosterone to activate human, rat, and mouse MRs is complicated by the substantially higher concentration of glucocorticoids.

Given the fact the glucocorticoids circulate at much higher concentrations than aldosterone, glucocorticoids would be expected to predominantly occupy the MRs under most conditions [7]. In the peripheral epithelial tissues, the specificity of MR for aldosterone is achieved by the enzyme 11β-hydroxysteroid dehydrogenase type 2 (11β-HSD2) which converts glucocorticoids to inactive metabolites, thus allowing aldosterone to bind to the MR. In the brain, the situation is much more complicated. Central action of aldosterone via MR is limited due to almost negligible levels of 11β-HSD2 in the brain. The lack of 11β-HSD2 in MR-rich regions suggests that the majority of brain MRs are likely to be fully occupied by glucocorticoids [8]. From these reasons, possible central effects of aldosterone have been neglected for a long time. Nevertheless, over the last 20 years, there is growing body of evidence that certain brain areas contain MRs that bind preferentially mineralocorticoids. This was demonstrated in the nucleus tractus solitarius, the subcommissural organ, and the ventrolateral subdivision of the ventromedial nucleus of the hypothalamus [9–13]. Importantly, nonclassical effects of aldosterone mediated via nongenomic actions [14] and de novo synthesis of aldosterone within the brain should also be considered [15].

Studies by Ron De Kloet group published more than 30 years ago were not in favor of aldosterone effects on exploratory activity or forced extinction paradigm of a passive avoidance response in rats [16]. Pretreatment with aldosterone blocked the serotonin response to corticosterone [17]. It should be noted, however, that aldosterone was administered in a single injection to acutely adrenalectomized rats. The authors concluded that that the time interval between acute aldosterone administration and behavioral testing (1 hr) was too long for the appearance of behavioral effects of aldosterone. Until 2008, nothing was known about repeated or chronic aldosterone treatment on behavior related to anxiety or depression in normal intact rodents.

Writing this overview was motivated by the new evidence on atypical effects of aldosterone gathering during the last few years, when we have started our research on aldosterone and the brain. In spite of the generally accepted view on the absence of the central effect of aldosterone, we have decided to perform research in the field. The main focus of this mini-review is given on aldosterone action in the central nervous system from two points of view, namely, the pathophysiology of mood disorders from translational point of view and the significance of aldosterone during the development.

## 2. Nothing dared nothing won

The scientific work is based on testing the hypotheses formulated on the basis of thoroughly verified facts obtained in several laboratories using various experimental approaches. It might happen, however, that even not yet satisfactory confirmed evidence evokes the desire to lead the research in a new direction. This happened to us, and we have to formulate a hypothesis on anxiogenic and depressogenic action of aldosterone about 10 years ago. At that time, the arguments to formulate such a hypothesis were rather vague and certainly inadequate, but we were full of enthusiasm and courage.

Our scientific interest in atypical effects of aldosterone on mental functions was motivated by scattered data published 15 years ago by the authors Murck et al. [18] and Emanuele et al. [19]. In small groups of depressed patients, they observed increased plasma aldosterone concentrations. However, causal relationship between aldosterone and mood disorders has not been approached. Our first original data on this topic were obtained in animal studies.

In the first series of experiments, we have tested the hypothesis that prolonged elevation of circulating aldosterone induces increased anxiety-like behavior in rats. Subchronic treatment with aldosterone (2 μg/100 g body weight/day for 2 weeks) via subcutaneous osmotic minipumps was applied to induce a mild hyperaldosteronism. Rodents do not, of course, tell the researchers that they feel anxious, but there are behavioral tests in which anxiety level can be assessed. In these tests, we have shown that aldosterone-treated animals exhibited increased anxiety-like behavior [20]. Anxiogenic effect of aldosterone was manifested by a significantly reduced frequency of entries and time spent in the open arms in the elevated plus maze test as well as reduced number of entries and time spent in the central area of the open-field test in aldosterone-treated rats compared to controls. Aldosterone treatment negatively influenced both the conventional spatiotemporal measures of anxiety and the ethological parameters related to anxiety and risk assessment behavior [20].

The role of aldosterone in anxiety-like behavior was supported by the results obtained using a different approach, demonstrating an anxiolytic action of an aldosterone antagonist. As an aldosterone antagonist, the selective MR blocker eplerenone, a clinically used drug for the treatment of heart failure and hypertension, was used [21]. Mild anxiolytic effects were observed after a single administration of eplerenone at the dose of 100 mg/kg body weight [22]. Anxiolytic effects of MR blockade were completely demonstrated following repeated treatment with eplerenone [23]. Eplerenone administered for 11 days (50 mg/kg body weight twice daily) influenced ethological indicators of anxiety. More importantly, significant differences were found in classical spatiotemporal measures, as the eplerenone-treated rats entered more often and spent more time in the open arms of the elevated plus maze. Another original finding is the effect of subchronic MR blockade on hippocampal concentrations of brain-derived neurotrophic factor (BDNF), a marker of brain plasticity. Stress-induced alterations in BDNF have been identified as a strong candidate modulating stress-related pathology [24, 25]. On the contrary, chronic treatment with antidepressants was shown to increase BDNF levels [26]. We have demonstrated that eplerenone treatment prevented stress-induced decrease in hippocampal concentrations of BDNF, suggesting a positive influence of MR blockade on brain plasticity [23].

In the next series of experiments, we focused our attention on depression-like behavior. We have used the same rat model of hyperaldosteronism previously and assessed symptoms of depressive behavior using the sucrose preference test and the forced swim test. The results clearly demonstrated that the subchronic increase in circulating aldosterone exerts depressogenic effects [27]. Aldosterone treatment induced an anhedonic state manifested by decreased sucrose preference. Depressogenic action of aldosterone was confirmed also in the forced swimming test. Animals treated with aldosterone spent significantly longer time in immobility and showed significantly decreased latency to become immobile [27]. Our results on depression-like behavior induced by aldosterone treatment in rats were confirmed by the authors Bay-Richter et al. [28]. As a result of our collaboration with colleagues from the USA, we revealed that hyperaldosteronism induces changes in expression of genes that have been shown to be associated with a major depressive disorder in humans [27].

Supporting data on the role of aldosterone in the development of depressive behavior have also been obtained in another animal model of depression. We have established a new and novel animal model of depression based on diet-induced tryptophan depletion in female rats [29]. Diet-induced tryptophan depletion resulted in a significant reduction of brain serotonin and induction of depression-like behavior manifested by increased immobility in the forced swim test [30]. Interestingly, the depression-like state was associated with a significant increase in serum aldosterone concentrations. We showed that aldosterone secretion had increased already after 4 days of tryptophan depletion, prior to the rise in serum corticosterone. This finding suggests that aldosterone may be more important than corticosterone in the development of a depression-like state and aldosterone may constitute an early marker for the onset of depression-like behavior [30].

In a very recent study by Geerling et al. [13], the authors characterized a hallmark of aldosterone-sensitive HSD2 neurons in the nucleus of the solitary tract. They showed that axons of HSD2 neurons project to the parabrachial complex/pre-locus coeruleus and the ventrolateral bed nucleus of the stria terminalis, two neural hubs with a crucial function in salt appetite (salt hunger) and accompanying arousal. They suggested that downstream targets of HSD2 neurons promote sodium appetite, but they may also influence stress coping and mood circuits to produce dysphoric, anhedonic, and anorexic symptoms of hyperaldosteronism.

Our evidence of a causal relationship between hyperaldosteronism and anxiety- and depression-like behaviors in animals represents a breakthrough in the research on aldosterone action in the central nervous system and reveals a new area of research with potential clinical significance.

## 3. Translation of experimental data to clinical research

Animal models can be useful tools in biomedical research, but undoubtedly, it has frequently been observed that effects found in animal models cannot be translated to the clinic [31]. It is therefore essential that knowledge gained from animal studies should be carefully confirmed in human studies.

To be able to translate the knowledge obtained in animal models to clinical research, we have initially introduced a methodology to measure aldosterone concentrations in saliva [32]. Determination of steroids in saliva has become a valuable alternative due to the noninvasiveness and laboratory independence of sampling. While assays for salivary cortisol are widely used, the availability of assays for measurement of aldosterone in saliva has been limited. Concentrations of aldosterone in saliva represent approximately one-third of the total level in plasma, and they correlate well with plasma values [33, 34]. We have modified the methodology of aldosterone radioimmunoassay by concentrating the saliva and validated the method by a low-dose ACTH test and by confirmation of daily rhythm and sex differences [35].

We have provided the first original data on the relationship between aldosterone and trait anxiety in humans. We have shown that the relationship between aldosterone and trait anxiety is determined by sex and the phase of the menstrual cycle in women [32]. Negative correlation between salivary aldosterone concentrations and trait anxiety was observed in women in the luteal phase, while a positive association was found in women in the follicular phase of the menstrual cycle.

In recent years, we have performed several studies to clarify the role of aldosterone in depressive disorder. We have conducted a pilot study in patients with a major depressive disorder in collaboration with Marburg University, Germany. Biomarkers of MR function were examined in order to characterize their relationship to clinical treatment outcome after 6 weeks in 30 patients with major depression [36, 37]. Although the number of patients was not very high, there was a significant association between salivary aldosterone concentrations and the severity of depressive symptoms. A negative correlation between aldosterone concentrations in saliva and improvement in clinical state of patients was revealed. Interestingly, a higher ratio of aldosterone to cortisol concentrations at baseline was predictive for poorer clinical outcome after 6 weeks of treatment [36].

Supporting data came also from other researcher groups. In patients with primary hyperaldosteronism, a higher occurrence of anxiety and depressive symptoms compared to healthy volunteers was demonstrated [38–40]. A population study in humans revealed that the combination of the chronic stress of living alone and depressive symptomatology was accompanied by high levels of aldosterone [41]. On the other hand, Hallberg et al. [42] found lower concentrations of aldosterone in patients with major depression with suicidal behavior than suicidal patients without depression and non-suicidal depressive patients.

The most complete results so far have been obtained by examining 60 patients with major depressive disorder in a study performed in collaboration with clinical psychiatrists, particularly the Department of Psychiatry, Faculty of Medicine, Comenius University and University Hospital Bratislava, Slovakia [43]. The sample consisted of 37 postmenopausal women and 23 men suffering from major depressive disorder. Morning and evening samples of saliva were obtained during depressive episode (admission to the hospital) and after reaching clinical remission (discharge). Results showed several notable original findings. Salivary aldosterone concentrations were higher at the time of admission to the hospital than those at the time of discharge, i.e., after improvement of the clinical state. It is well known that aldosterone secretion shows a daily rhythm [35, 44, 45] with the highest values in the morning and the lowest at evening. The patients with depression failed to exert known daily rhythmicity of aldosterone release [43]. An intriguing finding was the observation of the relationship between morning aldosterone concentrations and the duration of the current depressive episode. When patients were stratified according to the length of the depressive episode, women with a shorter duration of the depressive episode (up to 12 weeks) exhibited significantly higher aldosterone concentrations than women with a longer episode (over 16 weeks). In men, this difference was not observed. We have also demonstrated that morning salivary aldosterone concentrations are particularly higher in patients with severe depressive episode than those with moderate depressive episode. These findings strongly support the role of aldosterone in the pathophysiology of depressive disorder. Concentrations of aldosterone in the saliva appear to reflect the clinical outcome, duration, and severity of depressive episode in a sex-dependent manner [43].

## 4. Aldosterone during the development

In pups, the main physiological role of the renin-angiotensin-aldosterone system is to maintain water-electrolyte balance, while the hypothalamic-pituitary-adrenocortical (HPA) axis regulates energy metabolism. Prenatal and early postnatal brain development is a very complex process that can be endangered by a number of endogenous and exogenous stimuli. This is a serious problem given the neurodevelopmental background of several psychiatric disorders [46, 47]. Environmental stimuli that may interfere with the normal development of the central nervous system include excessive exposure to stressful situations. Exposure to stressors at the time of brain development may cause a repeated elevation in concentrations of glucocorticoids which are known to exert negative effects. Of the stress hormones, the neurotoxic effect is attributed, in particular, to glucocorticoids. Increased levels of glucocorticoids adversely affect neurogenesis and brain plasticity [25].

As was already mentioned, animal models represent a useful tool in the research in the field of neurodevelopmental disorders. Long time ago, scientists have discovered that there is a physiological mechanism in the rodents protecting the developing brain from neurotoxic glucocorticoids. During the first 2 weeks of life (from about days 2–14), rat pups show reduced capacity to secrete corticosterone in response to several stimuli [48–50]. This period was called the stress non-responsive period. Later, after introducing more sophisticated analytical methods for plasma corticosterone analysis, it has been found that a small increase occurred and the period was renamed to stress hyporesponsive period. In this period, corticosterone response to stress stimuli is several times lower than that in adult rats. This phenomenon is associated with dramatically reduced corticosteroid-binding globulin (CBG) levels [51, 52]. This occurs as a result of reduced half-life of CBG in plasma and decreased CBG production by the liver in the neonates [53, 54]. Thus, corticosterone circulates mainly in the free form during the stress hyporesponsive period, since CBG levels are negligible. During the stress hyporesponsive period, the adrenal gland is hyporesponsive to adrenocorticotropic hormone. Numerous studies have demonstrated that maternal factors, such as maternal care and feeding, are critical for the regulation of the pup's HPA axis and the maintenance of the stress hyporesponsive period [50]. It has been demonstrated that maternal deprivation during the stress hyporesponsive period causes a rapid rise in corticosterone concentrations [50] and profoundly affects GR epigenetics [55]. This type of studies would be welcome for aldosterone and the MR as well, since these are understudied. No information on possible similar reduction of aldosterone in response to stressors during the stress hyporesponsive period was available.

In a joint project with the Institute of Experimental Medicine, Hungarian Academy of Sciences, we have demonstrated that 10-day rat pups showed increased rather than reduced response of aldosterone to several acute stress stimuli. Stress-induced rise in aldosterone concentrations was significantly higher in pups compared to that in adulthood as well as compared to the rise in corticosterone [56]. In adult rats, the response was quite opposite; the increase in stress-induced aldosterone concentrations was only mild, whereas the elevation of corticosterone was much more pronounced. The physiological significance of increased aldosterone secretion during stress in the early postnatal period is supported by our findings of altered expression of mineralocorticoid and glucocorticoid receptors in the hypothalamus, hippocampus, and prefrontal cortex and in particular by increased expression of 11β-HSD2 [56].

It may be suggested that the main physiological importance of higher aldosterone secretion in pups is related to the maintenance of water-electrolyte balance during the perinatal period. MRs are present in the heart, blood vessels, adipocytes, and macrophages. It is possible to assume that during the perinatal period, aldosterone takes over the regulatory role of glucocorticoids in certain cellular processes and molecular mechanisms. Experiments in vasopressin-deficient Brattleboro rats excluded the possible important role of vasopressin. It appears that the shift from a more pronounced aldosterone to corticosterone rise during stress occurs after 40 postnatal days [57]. It is therefore clear that during rodent development, aldosterone is the more important stress hormone of the adrenal cortex than corticosterone.

## Acknowledgements

This publication is based upon the work from the EU COST Action ADMIRE BM1301 in aldosterone and mineralocorticoid receptor (MR) physiology and pathophysiology (www.admirecosteu.com) and was partly supported by the grant of Slovak Research and Development Agency under the contract APVV-14-0840.

## Author details

Natasa Hlavacova and Damiela Jezova*
Institute of Experimental Endocrinology, Biomedical Research Center, Slovak Academy of Sciences, Bratislava, Slovakia

*Address all correspondence to: daniela.jezova@savba.sk

## References

[1] Baker ME, Funder JW, Kattoula SR. Evolution of hormone selectivity in glucocorticoid and mineralocorticoid receptors. The Journal of Steroid Biochemistry and Molecular Biology. 2013;**137**:57-70

[2] Baker ME, Katsu Y. 30 years of the mineralocorticoid receptor: Evolution of the mineralocorticoid receptor: Sequence, structure and function. Journal of Endocrinology. 2017;**234**(1):T1-T16

[3] Terker AS, Ellison DH. Renal mineralocorticoid receptor and electrolyte homeostasis. American Journal of Physiology. Regulatory, Integrative and Comparative Physiology. 2015;**309**(9):R1068-R1070

[4] Baker ME, Katsu Y. Evolution of the mineralocorticoid receptor. Vitamins and Hormones. 2019;**109**:17-36

[5] Arriza JL, Weinberger C, Cerelli G, Glaser TM, Handelin BL, Housman DE, et al. Cloning of human mineralocorticoid receptor complementary DNA: Structural and functional kinship with the glucocorticoid receptor. Science. 1987;**237**(4812):268-275

[6] Arriza JL, Simerly RB, Swanson LW, Evans RM. The neuronal mineralocorticoid receptor as a mediator of glucocorticoid response. Neuron. 1988;**1**(9):887-900

[7] Fuller PJ, Lim-Tio SS, Brennan FE. Specificity in mineralocorticoid versus glucocorticoid action. Kidney International. 2000;**57**(4):1256-1264

[8] De Kloet ER. Hormones, brain and stress. Endocrine Regulations. 2003;**37**:51-68

[9] Roland BL, Li KX, Funder JW. Hybridization histochemical localization of 11 beta-hydroxysteroid dehydrogenase type 2 in rat brain. Endocrinology. 1995;**136**(10):4697-4700

[10] Robson AC, Leckie CM, Seckl JR, Holmes MC. 11 Beta-hydroxysteroid dehydrogenase type 2 in the postnatal and adult rat brain. Brain Research-Molecular Brain Research. 1998;**61**(1-2):1-10

[11] Geerling JC, Loewy AD. Aldosterone in the brain. American Journal of Physiology. Renal Physiology. 2009;**297**:F559-F576

[12] Askew ML, Muckelrath HD, Johnston JR, Curtis KS. Neuroanatomical association of hypothalamic HSD2-containing neurons with ERalpha, catecholamines, or oxytocin: Implications for feeding? Frontiers in System Neurosciences. 2015;**9**:91

[13] Gasparini S, Resch JM, Narayan SV, Peltekian L, Iverson GN, Karthik S, et al. Aldosterone-sensitive HSD2 neurons in mice. Brain Structure and Function. 2019;**224**(1):387-417

[14] Wendler A, Albrecht C, Wehling M. Nongenomic actions of aldosterone and progesterone revisited. Steroids. 2012;**77**(10):1002-1006

[15] Gomez-Sanchez EP, Ahmad N, Romero DG, Gomez-Sanchez CE. Is aldosterone synthesized within the rat brain? American Journal of Physiology Endocrinology and Metabolism. 2005;**288**(2):E342-E346

[16] Veldhuis HD, De Kloet ER. Antagonistic effects of aldosterone on corticosterone-mediated changes in exploratory behavior of adrenalectomized rats. Hormones and Behavior. 1983;**17**(2):225-232

[17] De Kloet ER, Versteeg DH, Kovacs GL. Aldosterone blocks the response

to corticosterone in the raphe-hippocampal serotonin system. Brain Research. 1983;**264**(2):323-327

[18] Murck H, Held K, Ziegenbein M, Künzel H, Koch K, Steiger A. The renin-angiotensin-aldosterone system in patients with depression compared to controls: A sleep endocrine study. BMC Psychiatry. 2003;**29**(3):15

[19] Emanuele E, Geroldi D, Minoretti P, Coen E, Politi P. Increased plasma aldosterone in patients with clinical depression. Archives of Medical Research. 2005;**36**:544-548

[20] Hlavacova N, Jezova D. Chronic treatment with the mineralocorticoid hormone aldosterone results in increased anxiety-like behavior. Hormones and Behavior. 2008;**54**:90-97

[21] Stewart Coats AJ, Shewan L. Eplerenone's role in the management of complex cardiovascular disorders. International Journal of Cardiology. 2015;**200**:1-2

[22] Hlavacova N, Jezova D. Effect of single treatment with the antihypertensive drug eplerenone on hormone levels and anxiety-like behaviour in rats. Endocrine Regulations. 2008b;**42**:147-153

[23] Hlavacova N, Bakos J, Jezova D. Eplerenone, a selective mineral-ocorticoid receptor blocker, exerts anxiolytic effects accompanied by changes in stress hormone release. Journal of Psychopharmacology. 2010;**24**:779-786

[24] Bath KG, Schilit A, Lee FS. Stress effects on BDNF expression: Effects of age, sex, and form of stress. Neuroscience. 2013;**239**:149-156

[25] Numakawa T, Odaka H, Adachi N. Actions of brain-derived neurotrophic factor and glucocorticoid stress in neurogenesis. International Journal of Molecular Sciences. 2017;**18**(11)

[26] Kishi T, Yoshimura R, Ikuta T, Iwata N. Brain-derived neurotrophic factor and major depressive disorder: Evidence from meta-analyses. Frontiers of Psychiatry. 2018;**8**:308

[27] Hlavacova N, Wes PD, Ondrejcakova M, Flynn ME, Poundstone PK, Babic S, et al. Subchronic treatment with aldosterone induces depression-like behaviours and gene expression changes relevant to major depressive disorder. International Journal of Neuropsychopharmacology. 2012;**15**:247-265

[28] Bay-Richter C, Hallberg L, Ventorp F, Janelidze S, Brundin L. Aldosterone synergizes with peripheral inflammation to induce brain IL-1β expression and depressive-like effects. Cytokine. 2012;**60**(3):749-754

[29] Franklin M, Bermudez I, Hlavacova N, Babic S, Murck H, Schmuckermair C, et al. Aldosterone increases earlier than corticosterone in new animal models of depression: Is this an early marker? Journal of Psychiatry Research. 2012;**46**:1394-1397

[30] Franklin M, Hlavacova N, Babic S, Pokusa M, Bermudez I, Jezova D. Aldosterone signals the onset of depressive behaviour in a female rat model of depression along with SSRI treatment resistance. Neuroendocrinology. 2015;**102**:274-287

[31] Martić-Kehl MI, Schibli R, Schubiger PA. Can animal data predict human outcome? Problems and pitfalls of translational animal research. Eurupean Journal of Nuclear Medicine and Molecular Imaging. 2012;**39**(9):1492-1496

[32] Jezova D, Hlavacova N. Endocrine factors in stress and psychiatric disorders: Focus on anxiety and

salivary steroids. Annals of the New York Academy of Sciences. 2008;**1148**:495-503

[33] Atherden SM, Corrie JE, Jones DB, Al-Dujaili EA, Edwards CR. Development and application of a direct radioimmunoassay for aldosterone in saliva. Steroids. 1985;**46**(4-5):845-855

[34] Few JD, Wallis PJ, James VH. The relationship between salivary aldosterone and plasma free aldosterone concentrations. Clinical Endocrinology. 1986;**24**:119-126

[35] Hlavacova N, Kerlik J, Radikova Z, Izakova L, Jezova D. Measurement of salivary aldosterone: Validation by low-dose ACTH test and gender differences. Endocrine Regulations. 2013;**47**:201-204

[36] Büttner M, Jezova D, Greene B, Konrad C, Kircher T, Murck H. Target-based biomarker selection: mineralocorticoid receptor-related biomarkers and treatment outcome in major depression. Journal of Psychiatry Research. 2015;**66-67**:24-37

[37] Murck H, Braunisch MC, Konrad C, Jezova D, Kircher T. Markers of mineralocorticoid receptor function: Changes over time and relationship to response in patients with major depression. International Clinical Psychopharmacology. 2019;**34**(1):18-26

[38] Sonino N, Tomba E, Genesia ML, et al. Psychological assessment of primary aldosteronism: A controlled study. Journal of Clinical Endocrinology and Metabolism. 2011;**96**(6):E878-E883

[39] Apostolopoulou K, Künzel HE, Gerum S, et al. Gender differences in anxiety and depressive symptoms in patients with primary hyperaldosteronism: A cross-sectional study. World Journal of Biological Psychiatry. 2014;**15**(1):26-35

[40] Reincke M. Anxiety, depression, and impaired quality of life in primary aldosteronism: Why we shouldn't ignore it. Journal of Clinical Endocrinology and Metabolism. 2018;**103**(1):1-4

[41] Häfner S, Baumert J, Emeny RT, Lacruz ME, Bidlingmaier M, Reincke M, et al., MONICA/KORA study investigators. To live alone and to be depressed, an alarming combination for the renin-angiotensin-aldosterone-system (RAAS). Psychoneuroendocrinology. 2012;**37**:230-237

[42] Hallberg L, Westrin A, Isaksson A, Janelidze S, Träskman-Bendz L, Brundin L. Decreased aldosterone in the plasma of suicide attempters with major depressive disorder. Psychiatry Research. 2011;**187**:135-139

[43] Segeda V, Izakova L, Hlavacova N, Bednarova A, Jezova D. Aldosterone concentrations in saliva reflect the duration and severity of depressive episode in a sex dependent manner. Journal of Psychiatry Reserch. 2017;**91**:164-168

[44] Lightman SL, James WHT, Linsell C, Mullen PE, Peart WS, Sever PS. Studies of diurnal changes in plasma renin activity and plasma noradrenaline, aldosterone and cortisol concentrations in man. Clinical Endocrinology. 1981;**14**(3):213-223

[45] Leppaluoto J, Ruskoaho H. Atrial natriuretic peptide, renin activity, aldosterone, urine volume and electrolytes during a 24-h sleep-wake cycle in man. Acta Physiologica Scandinavica. 1990;**139**(1):47-53

[46] Gao Y, Glenn AL, Schug RA, Yang Y, Raine A. The neurobiology of psychopathy: A neurodevelopmental perspective. Canadian Journal of Psychiatry. 2009;**54**(12):813-823

[47] Mastrototaro G, Zaghi M, Sessa A. Epigenetic mistakes in

neurodevelopmental disorders. Journal of Molecular Neuroscience. 2017;**61**(4):590-602

[48] Sapolsky RM, Meaney MJ. Maturation of the adrenocortical stress response: Neuroendocrine control mechanisms and the stress hyporesponsive period. Brain Research. 1986;**396**:64-76

[49] Levine S. Primary social relationships influence the development of the hypothalamic–pituitary–adrenal axis in the rat. Physiology and Behavior. 2001;**73**:255-260

[50] Levine S. Regulation of the hypothalamic-pituitary-adrenal axis in the neonatal rat: The role of maternal behavior. Neurotoxicology Research. 2002;**4**:557-564

[51] Henning S. Plasma concentrations of total and free corticosterone during development in the rat. American Journal of Physiology. 1989;**235**:E451-E456

[52] Schroeder RJ, Henning SJ. Roles of plasma clearance and corticosteroid-binding globulin in the developmental increase of circulating corticosterone in infant rats. Endocrinology. 1989;**124**:2612-2618

[53] Smith CL, Hammond GL. Ontogeny of corticosteroid-binding globulin biosynthesis in the rat. Endocrinology. 1991;**128**:983-988

[54] Viau V, Sharma S, Meaney MJ. Changes in plasma adrenocorticotropin, corticosterone, corticosteroid-binding globulin, and hippocampal glucocorticoid receptor occupancy/translocation in rat pups in response to stress. Journal of Neuroendocrinology. 1996;**8**(1):1-8

[55] Park SW, Lee JG, Seo MK, Ly NN, Lee CH, Cho HY, et al. Epigenetic modification of glucocorticoid receptor promoter I(7) in maternally separated and restraint-stressed rats. Neuroscience Letters. 2017;**650**:38-44

[56] Varga J, Ferenczi S, Kovács KJ, Garafova A, Jezova D, Zelena D. Comparison of stress-induced changes in adults and pups: Is aldosterone the main adrenocortical stress hormone during the perinatal period in rats? PLoS ONE. 2013;**8**(9):e72313

[57] Varga J, Ferenczi S, Kovács KJ, Csáno Á, Prokopova B, Jezova D, et al. Dissociation of adrenocorticotropin and corticosterone as well as aldosterone secretion during stress of hypoglycemia in vasopressin-deficient rats. Life Sciences. 2016;**166**:66-74

Chapter 12

# Transcriptional Regulation and Epigenetics in Cardiovascular Cells: Role of the Mineralocorticoid Receptor

*Lisa Deng, Lutz Hein and Achim Lother*

## Abstract

The mineralocorticoid receptor (MR), a ligand-activated transcription factor, plays an important role in the pathophysiology of cardiovascular disease. Epigenetic mechanisms such as DNA methylation or histone modifications in addition to the DNA sequence are decisive regulators of cell type-specific transcriptional activity and gene expression by controlling chromatin accessibility. In this review, we summarise the current knowledge about the impact of MR on gene expression in cardiovascular cells. We discuss studies investigating the interaction of MR with epigenetic mechanisms or other transcription factors and their implications for the cardiovascular system. Finally, we compare mechanisms of transcriptional regulation by MR and other nuclear transcription factors. In conclusion, MR is an important regulator of gene expression in cardiovascular cells. Potential mechanisms of cell type-specific transcriptional regulation by MR include interaction with other transcription factors or co-regulators, tethering and post-translational modifications of the MR. Further studies will be needed to clarify the interplay of MR and epigenetic mechanisms.

**Keywords:** mineralocorticoid receptor, epigenetics, chromatin, gene expression, cell types

## 1. Introduction

Mineralocorticoid receptor (MR) antagonists are a cornerstone in the current pharmacological therapy of chronic heart failure [1, 2]. MR in renal epithelial cells plays an important role for ion homeostasis and blood pressure control, but MR is also expressed in extrarenal tissue including different cell types of the heart and the vasculature [3]. This understanding has subsequently triggered intense research on the molecular basis of MR activity in the cardiovascular system. The MR is a member of the nuclear receptor (NR) family, which consists of different DNA-binding transcription factors [4]. As a ligand-activated transcription factor, MR controls the expression of its target genes. Despite increasing evidence for rapid, non-genomic effects of MR, regulation of gene expression is still regarded as a key feature of MR action. The MR holds a unique position among steroid-activated nuclear receptors as it binds two ligands, aldosterone as the main ligand as well as cortisol (corticosterone in rodents) with similar affinity. Indeed, progesterone which acts as an antagonist at the human MR [5] and, according to recent studies, has also activating properties at chicken and zebrafish MR [6] could also be seen as a third ligand to the MR. Despite their diverse range of action, nuclear receptors share a common, highly conserved structure [7]. A ligand-induced conformational change of the ligand-binding domain (LDB) leads to the activation of the receptor. Upon translocation into the nucleus, NR modulates transcription by interacting with specific DNA sequences. Eukaryote DNA is not linear but wrapped up in a complex with histones forming the chromatin. Histones are subjected to a variety of reversible post-translational modifications, which, in turn, can change chromatin density, accessibility and high-order chromatin structure and thereby determine transcription factor binding and gene expression [8].

Epigenetics is an emerging topic in cardiovascular research. The heart and the vasculature are composed of numerous different cell types including cardiac myocytes, endothelial cells, vascular smooth muscle cells, fibroblasts, immune cells and others [9]. These different cell types show marked heterogeneity in their specific transcriptomes [10–13]. Transcriptome analyses of different cell types of the heart revealed transcriptional changes during development and disease [12, 13], and these changes were associated with distinct alterations in the epigenome. For example, dysregulation of histone modifications or DNA methylation has been linked to numerous diseases of the cardiovascular system, such as atherosclerosis [14–16], hypertension [17, 18] or heart failure [19–22]. Based on these findings pharmacological targeting of epigenetic modifiers has been proposed for treatment of cardiovascular disease and successfully tested in preclinical models [23, 24].

Epigenetic modifications, such as histone modifications or DNA methylation, have been identified as decisive regulators of transcription factor activity, as chromatin compaction determines the cell-specific accessibility of DNA [4]. Vice versa, NR can alter the chromatin structure through recruitment of cofactors, which act as chromatin remodelers [25]. Chromatin immunoprecipitation (ChIP) assays with subsequent deep sequencing represent a powerful technique for genome-wide analysis of histone modifications or other DNA-associated proteins [26]. The combination of different histone modifications, often referred to as the histone code, gives information on proximal and distal regulatory DNA elements, including promoters and enhancers. Promoters are often located in close proximity to the transcription start site (TSS) and associated with monomethylation of histone 3 at lysin 4 (H3K4me1), while enhancers are usually distal to TSS and marked by trimethylation of H3K4 (H3K4me3). Active promoter or enhancer sites are marked by acetylation of histone 3 at lysin 27 (H3K27ac); in contrast, H3K9me3 and H3K27me3 mark heterochromatic or repressed regions [27]. Epigenetic modifications are reversible, being recognised, established or removed by reader, writer and eraser proteins. For example, acetylation of histones is regulated by two counteracting enzymes which add (histone acetyltransferases, HAT) acetyl groups to lysine residues or remove them (histone deacetylases HDAC) [28].

DNA methylation of CpGs is the only known epigenetic mechanism directly targeting the DNA and plays an important role in gene silencing when being recognised by reader proteins such as methyl-CpG-binding protein 2 (MeCP2) that act as transcriptional repressors [29]. DNA methylation is established and maintained during mitosis by DNA methyltransferases (DNMT) [29]. Oxidation of methylcytosines to hydroxylmethylcytosines, which is an intermediate step towards demethylation, is mediated by members of the ten-eleven translocation (TET) enzyme family. This occurs predominantly in promoter and enhancer regions with low CpG density, resulting in low methylated regions and can be used to identify active regulatory regions [29, 30]. CpG-rich regions, also referred to as CpG islands, in the promoter of constitutively active genes are typically unmethylated [29]. This allows to use DNA methylation as a stable mark of cell lineage during development [31]. Analysis of the DNA methylome of murine cardiomyocytes revealed distinct DNA methylation pattern during cardiomyocyte development and disease [32]. Demethylation of cardiac gene bodies correlated with active histone marks and increased gene expression. Interestingly, by comparison of the DNA methylome of healthy and failing cardiomyocytes, the DNA methylation pattern of failing cardiomyocytes was bearing a partial resemblance to foetal cardiomyocytes; however, changes were not major [32]. A similar result could be observed in human failing cardiac myocytes. Pathological gene expression in heart failure was accompanied by changes in active histone marks, whereas the DNA methylation pattern remained mostly the same [33]. Similarly, changes in the transcriptome of cardiac myocytes following myocardial infarction were accompanied by altered accessibility of chromatin [12].

Given the important role of epigenetics in transcriptional regulation, interaction of MR with epigenetic modifications; with epigenetic reader, writer or eraser proteins; or with other transcription factors might control the cell type-specific impact of MR on gene expression and function. In this review article, we will summarise what is known about MR-dependent gene expression, epigenetic mechanisms and their interaction with MR in cardiovascular cells.

## 2. Impact of aldosterone and MR on gene expression in the cardiovascular system

A series of experimental studies during the past years revealed distinct MR functions in cardiac myocytes, fibroblasts, endothelial cells, vascular smooth muscle cells and immune cells [3, 34, 35]. These studies provided evidence that the beneficial effect of MR antagonists in heart failure is directly related to MR in cardiovascular cells and independent from MR in renal epithelial cells. Several attempts have been made to understand the downstream signalling events following MR activation and to identify direct MR target genes in different cells or tissues of the cardiovascular system.

Early studies on cultured fibroblasts revealed an upregulation of collagen by aldosterone [36, 37] and by this suggested MR-dependent gene expression in cardiovascular cells. Later studies applied microarray or RNA-sequencing techniques to systematically detect MR-responsive genes. Similar to fibroblasts, aldosterone induced the expression of collagen types I and III in cultured smooth muscle cells from the coronary artery [38]. In mouse aorta, aldosterone regulated the expression of genes related to vascular function, such as oxidative stress, extracellular matrix and angiogenesis [39]. Treatment of EAhy926 endothelial cells expressing MR after retroviral transfection with aldosterone leads to regulation of only 17 transcripts [40]. In contrast, 133 genes were found up- or downregulated by aldosterone in human umbilical vein endothelial cells with naïve MR expression but not after MR knockdown [41]. These genes were associated leukocyte migration and angiogenesis. Interestingly, aldosterone treatment had opposing effects on endothelial cell gene expression when compared to treatment with vascular endothelial cell growth factor, a potent pro-angiogenic factor [41].

In a H9C2 cardiac myocyte cell line stably expressing MR, 53 transcripts were detected to be differentially regulated after treatment with aldosterone, the majority of them being upregulated [42]. Among the upregulated transcripts were genes related to extracellular matrix deposition such as *Adamts1* (A disintegrin and metalloprotease with thrombospondin motifs), *Pai-1* (plasminogen-activator inhibitor 1) or *Tnx* (tenascin-X) [42]. Studies using selective MR or GR antagonists confirmed MR-dependent expression of these genes in H9C2 cells [43, 44]. In heart tissue from untreated mice overexpressing MR in cardiac myocytes, microarray analysis revealed 24 transcripts upregulated and 22 transcripts downregulated. Again, the expression of *Adamts1* and *Pai-1* was induced by MR overexpression [43]. Vice versa, MR deletion from cardiac myocytes leads to differential regulation of 158 genes in heart tissue, including upregulation of *Nppa* (atrial natriuretic peptide type A); however, there was no clear reduction of genes related to collagen synthesis in this study [45]. In doxorubicin-treated mice, MR deletion from cardiac myocytes prevented the repressive effect of doxorubicin on gene expression, likely by a post-transcriptional mechanism [46]. One well-investigated gene that is upregulated in heart tissue by cardiac myocyte MR overexpression or aldosterone treatment is neutrophil-gelatinase-associated lipocalin (*Ngal*) [47]. Interestingly, *Ngal* was upregulated by aldosterone in endothelial cells and vascular smooth muscle cells as well [47].

Taken together, there is an overlap of several genes that were similarly regulated by MR in different cardiovascular cells or tissues including *Sgk1* [41–43, 45], *Tsc22d3* [40, 41], *Adamts1* [41–43], *Fkbp5* [40, 41, 43], *Klf9* [39–41], *Ngal* [47] or *Per1* [41, 48, 49], indicating a common signature of MR-regulated genes. Interestingly, these genes are well-related to the pathophysiological impact of MR on fibrosis and inflammation in the cardiovascular system.

## 3. Regulation of MR transcriptional activity

Transcriptional activity of MR is regulated at different levels: ligand binding, nuclear translocation, chromatin state and MR-DNA interaction. The main focus of this article will be on chromatin state and MR-DNA interaction; however, some specificities of cardiovascular cell types should be noticed: First, as MR binds to aldosterone or glucocorticoids with similar affinity, different mechanisms exist that allow ligand-specificity of MR. One of them is co-expression of 11β-hydroxysteroid dehydrogenase type 2 (11βHSD2), an enzyme converting glucocorticoids to derivates that are inactive at the MR (for review, see [50]). In the cardiovascular system, 11βHSD2 is highly expressed in endothelial cells, low expressed in cardiac myocytes and smooth muscle cells and probably absent in immune cells [51]. Second, while in most cell types unliganded MR is predominantly located at the cytoplasm and shuttles into the nucleus upon ligand binding, MR has been described to be constitutively located at the nucleus in cardiac myocytes [52]. Immunohistochemical analysis of heart tissue revealed nuclear localization of the MR, and subfractional analysis showed that the vast majority of MR was chromatin-bound irrespective of plasma aldosterone or glucocorticoid levels. The subcellular distribution depended on the balance of heat shock protein 90 expression and the synergy of two nuclear localization signals. Interestingly, transcriptional activation of chromatin-bound MR nevertheless required the presence of a ligand [52].

## 4. Validation of MR-responsive genes

To further elucidate the role of MR in transcriptional regulation, it has been aimed to identify genes that are direct MR targets by proofing MR binding to a corresponding regulatory region by ChIP experiments. In a human embryonic kidney cell line (HEK293) stably transfected with myc-tagged hMR, *Cnksr3* was identified as a novel MR target gene containing MR binding sites (MBS) upstream of the transcription start site using ChIP in conjunction with microarray analysis (ChIP-chip). *Cnksr3* was described as highly expressed in response to aldosterone, mediating ENaC activity and thereby influencing transepithelial $Na^+$ transport in renal collecting duct cells [53]. Ueda et al. combined ChIP with high-throughput sequencing for a genome-wide analysis of MR target genes in renal distal convoluted tubular cells and identified 1113 MR binding sites associated with 1414 genes [54]. Combining data from a microarray study 186 genes were considered to be aldosterone-responsive, showing an increase in mRNA expression levels after aldosterone stimulation and a decrease in expression by inhibitory treatment with spironolactone. Interestingly, only 25 genes showed an overlap between both assays and were thus classified as MR target genes, among those the well-known target genes *Sgk1*, *Fkbp5* and *Tsc22d3* [54]. Of note, strong enrichment of MR does not necessarily translate into increased expression of target genes. In another study, analysis of renal MR target genes revealed four commonly acknowledged target of MR signalling in renal cells such as *Scnn1a*, *Fkbp5*, *Zbtb16* and *Per1* and nine other genes not associated with MR signalling before [55]. MR target genes could be subcategorized according to their different kinetics of MR-dependent activation of gene expression into early, intermediate and late response genes [55]. However, molecular mechanisms of MR signalling are highly cell-specific, as distinct target genes could be found in one experiment but not reproduced in another [54, 55], whereas other MR target genes seem to be independent from tissue or cell type such as *Fkbp5* or *Per1* [54–57].

MR binding sites seem to be widespread across the genome, an equal proportion (almost 40%) of all identified peaks were located either within introns or intergenic. Surprisingly, only 40 of all approximately 1000 MBS were found within promoter regions and 11% within enhancer regions [55]. Among the 13 genes correlating to the highest MR binding peak scores in human renal cells, *LINC00963* was not regulated by MR, despite high aldosterone-induced MR recruitment. As the MR binding site was located far from the nearest TSS, the involvement of this remote MBS in transcriptional regulation of another gene through long-range chromatin interactions is possible [55, 58].

For cardiovascular cells, available studies are restricted to MR binding in the promoter region of certain target genes. $Ca_v1.2$, a voltage-gated calcium channel, could be identified as an MR target in the cardiovascular system using mutational and in silico analysis. An aldosterone-dependent recruitment of MR to the alternative cardiac *Cacna1c* P1-promoter was observed, subsequently regulating expression of cardiac $Ca_v1.2$ transcripts in cardiac myocytes as well as in vascular smooth muscle cells, underlining the importance of aldosterone signalling in vascular reactivity and regulation of blood pressure [59]. In a similar approach, MR-dependent regulation of *Icam1* in cultured endothelial cells was demonstrated using a reporter assay with different promoter fragments [60].

## 5. Mineralocorticoid receptor response elements

The canonical GRE DNA motif consists of two inverted palindromic half sites, separated by a 3 bp spacer [AGAACAnnnTGTTCT (**Figure 1**)] [61]. Different variations of this motif exist in human renal cells with the bases C5 and G11 remaining essential for MR binding. Strong sequence degeneration of the classic consensus motif correlated with low MR enrichment and therefore disrupted MR interaction [55]. A small percentage of 7.4% MBS contained the classic consensus MRE motif; the larger part of all identified MRE consisted of half sites or a combination out of palindromic sequences and half-MREs [55]. Of note, not all MR binding sites

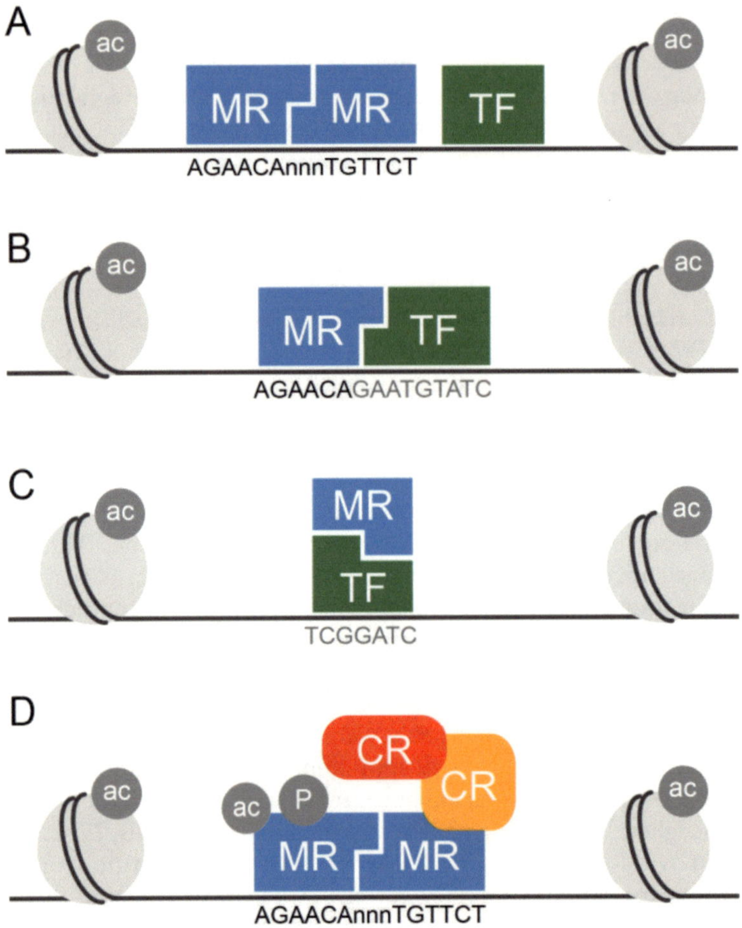


**Figure 1.**
*Proposed modes of MR-DNA interaction. Mineralocorticoid receptors can directly bind to MR response elements consisting of a 15 bp palindromic DNA sequence (A) or to composite elements when interacting with a neighbouring transcription factor (B). Indirect MR-DNA interaction can be facilitated by tethering to another transcription factor (C). MR-DNA interaction is modulated by co-regulatory transcription factors or post-translational modifications of the MR (D). MR, mineralocorticoid receptor; TF, transcription factor; CR, co-regulator; ac, acetylation; P, phosphorylation.*

contain an MRE consensus motif. The majority of peaks lacked the MRE implying interaction of MR with the DNA directly by binding to specific DNA sequences different from the consensus motif, indirectly via protein–protein interactions or possibly through tethering as known for GR (**Figure 1**) [55, 62, 63]. Indeed, an aldosterone-dependent *trans*-activation of AP-1 could recently be proven in human cells, underlining this hypothesis [64]. Interestingly, all MBS in rat hippocampal tissue contained an MRE [57], suggesting that the mode of MR-DNA interaction might be cell- or tissue-specific.

When analysing MRE it has to be taken into account that MR and GR share a common consensus sequence. Both receptors are simultaneously expressed in various tissues and interact with each other. For example, MR and GR are able to form homodimers as well as heterodimers in rat hippocampal tissue after acute stress challenges [56]. The binding of homodimers of the respective receptors or MR/GR heterodimers seems to be gene-specific. Using a tandem ChIP approach, it could be pointed out that MR and GR mainly bind as MR/MR and GR/GR homodimers at the GRE of *Sgk1*, whereas MR/GR heterodimer formation could be proven for the

*Per1* GRE in addition to homodimers of both receptors. Notably, at the *Fkbp5* GRE MR seems to bind only in a heterocomplex with GR [56], indicating distinct mechanisms controlling binding of receptors to GRE, such as local chromatin accessibility or interactions with co-regulators [65]. Interactions of MR/GR heterodimers with the *Per1* promoter in response to aldosterone or cortisol stimulation could also be detected in a human renal cell line [49]. In an extensive time-course ChIP-qPCR study, the authors provide evidence for different dynamics in MR or GR recruitment to the promoter region of a given target gene. MR recruitment kinetics onto the *Per1* promoter was ligand-dependent. Aldosterone induces a distinct kinetic pattern differing from MR-GR recruitment kinetics [49], suggesting different dynamics as mechanisms for receptor selectivity. MR/GR heterodimer show distinct dissociating rates differing from MR/MR or GR/GR homodimers [66], resulting in a stronger GRE binding and a synergistic effect on controlling transcriptional activity of each receptor [49, 56]. However, contrasting results have been reported. MR/GR heterodimers either enhanced [56] or inhibited [67] transcription of given target genes when compared to respective homodimers. In cardiac myocytes, *Per1* was upregulated by both cortisol and aldosterone. The impact of aldosterone was enhanced in the presence of the CLOCK transcription factor, suggesting a cooperative effect of both transcription factors on *Per1* expression [48]. Meinel et al. demonstrated an interaction of MR with the transcription factor specificity protein 1 (SP1) leading to the binding of an alternative MRE in the promoter region of epidermal growth factor receptor (EGFR) gene. The SP-1-dependent transactivation of EGFR through MR could also be demonstrated in cultured smooth vascular cells [68].

Comparison of GR-ChIP data with MR-ChIP data from rat hippocampal tissue revealed 918 MR-specific binding sites, 1450 GR-specific and 475 binding sites shared by MR and GR, all containing the GRE motif [57]. In all MR-exclusive binding sites, an additional motif, corresponding to the Atoh1 binding sequence, was present, and the protein was not expressed in hippocampal tissue. However, in Atoh1 belonging to the basic helix–loop–helix (bHLH) family of transcription factors, the brain-specific NeuroD family members could be identified as potential candidates for interaction with MR, thus ensuring MR specificity at MR-exclusive binding sites [57]. Different studies point at a role of differences in the nucleotide sequence of GREs in mediating distinct transcriptional activity of MR and GR [56, 59, 68], as some GRE do not enhance binding of the receptors [56], other GRE sequences favouring MR binding [69] or exclusively binding MR [68]. The ability to bind negative glucocorticoid response elements (nGRE) and therefore repressing transcription of given target genes is restricted to GR signalling and not shared with other steroid receptors [70]. Despite having a common ancestral with the capacity of binding nGRE, the ability was lost in the MR due to different mutations at independent timepoints and enhanced in the GR lineage, resulting and contributing to the capability of MR and GR to show specific and distinct transcriptional signatures even though being highly homologous. Nevertheless, repressing effects on transcriptional activities are not unique for GR as MR are likewise able to *trans*-repress NFκB signalling through tethering effects without interfering with DNA binding of the complex, putting an interesting angle to the pro- and antiinflammatory effects of MR and GR. However, *trans*-repressing effects of MR are notably weaker than those of GR [64]. Of note, in addition to the beforementioned activating protein-protein interactions of MR on inflammatory AP-1 signalling, suppressing effects on AP-1 activities in a DNA-sequence-specific manner—and therefore target gene-specific—could also be elucidated, stressing out the necessity of identifying cell type-specific target genes of MR in order to dissect augmenting effects of MR from repressing effects for the development of potential new MR antagonists [64].

## 6. Co-regulators of MR activity

MR transcriptional activity in the nucleus is finely controlled by a variety of different mechanisms, including the recruitment of co-regulators, a heterogeneous group of non-receptor proteins (**Figure 1**) [71]. Co-regulators modulate the transcriptional activity of the receptor by either acting as coactivators or as corepressors [72]. They predominantly interact at specific regions in the NTD and at the LBD. The NTD represents the least conserved region across the steroid receptor family and thereby harbouring most potential for differential recruitment of co-regulators [73]. The LDB is conserved between different species and harbours a ligand-dependent activation function site (AF-2), which is exposed upon conformational changes induced by ligand binding of the receptor [74]. AF-2 as a docking platform is essential for co-regulator binding. Many co-regulator molecules interact via an LxxLL (L stands for a leucine, x for any other amino acid) motif with the AF-2 region [50], e.g. the first identified and well-characterised NR co-regulator steroid receptor coactivator-1 (SRC-1) [73]. Among the over 400 putative co-regulators discovered in screening assays, a few MR-specific interaction partners could be characterised such as the elongation factor eleven-nineteen lysine-rich leukaemia (ELL). ELL is able to differentially regulate MR and GR, selectively enhancing MR transcriptional activity and repressing GR-mediated transactivation [75]. GEMIN4 represents an MR corepressor, attenuating MR transcriptional activity in a cell- and gene-specific manner, as a repressive effect could be demonstrated in human embryonic kidney cells but not in a rat cardiomyocyte cell line [76]. However, GEMIN4 actions are not restricted to MR, leaving NF-YC as the only described MR-specific corepressor [77]. Just recently, a specific MR cofactor modulation has been proposed as a molecular mechanism for the differential antifibrotic properties of the novel nonsteroidal MR antagonist finerenone when compared to steroidal MR antagonists [78].

## 7. Post-translational modification of the MR

Post-translational modifications such as phosphorylation, ubiquitination, sumoylation or acetylation are described to influence MR transactivation [79]. Phosphorylation of MR has contrasting effects, as it has reported early that phosphorylation of MR is necessary for aldosterone binding and enhancing the DNA-binding ability of MR [80, 81]. On the other hand, phosphorylation of MR on serine and threonine residues mediated by cyclin-dependent kinase 5 (CDK5) was shown to attenuate MR transcriptional activity, whereas nuclear receptor accumulation was not altered, suggesting impaired interaction of MR with co-regulators [82]. Recently, the ubiquitously expressed casein kinase 2 (CK2) was identified as a positive modulator of MR transcriptional activity by direct phosphorylation of the receptor and potentially by changing the phosphorylation status of other MR-co-regulators [83]. Interestingly, phosphorylation of MR is also implied as a cell type-specific mechanism, modulating MR activity. Hyperkalaemia was found to increase MR phosphorylation at S843 and subsequently prevent ligand-binding and receptor activation, a phosphorylation site specific in renal intercalated cells [84]. Intriguingly, the phosphorylation of MR can also regulate the ubiquitylation state and the subsequent degradation of the protein [85].

The epigenetic writer proteins HDACs are generally perceived as corepressors of nuclear receptors [86]. The attenuating effects on gene transcription of the earliest described corepressors, nuclear receptor corepressor (NCoR) and silencing mediator of retinoid and thyroid receptor corepressor (SMRT) rely on the subsequent recruitment of HDACs [72]. Different studies could reveal that increased acetylation of MR, induced by HDAC inhibition, interferes with MR recruitment onto the DNA and attenuates transactivation of MR target genes [87, 88]. HDAC3 is acting as a coactivator in this context, as deacetylation of MR in the hinge region restores transcriptional activities of the receptor [88]. The treatment with HDAC inhibitors has also been linked to reduced antifibrotic effects in DOCA-salt-induced hypertensive rats and decreased expression of inflammatory markers in spontaneously hypertensive rats [17, 88, 89].

## 8. Summary

In summary, the distinct biological effects of MR in different cardiovascular cells are associated with changes in gene expression. Epigenetic modifications and modifying enzymes have been identified as crucial regulators of gene expression and cellular function in the cardiovascular system; however, presently available data on MR-dependent gene expression in the cardiovascular system is predominantly derived from experiments on cultured cells, in some cases after artificial overexpression of the MR, or tissue analysis. Analyses of complex tissues consisting of a dynamically changing mixture of multiple cell types can lead to ambiguous results. To date there is no ChIP-seq data published describing genome-wide MR-DNA interactions in cardiovascular cells. Studies in renal epithelial cells or brain tissue indicate that MR-DNA interaction can occur in promoter regions as well as at distal enhancer sites, but it remains speculative whether the insights from renal epithelial cells can be applied to the cardiovascular system as well.

This implies the necessity to perform cell type-specific studies from primary cardiovascular cells in homeostasis and different states of disease in order to identify distinct changes in gene expression and (epigenetic) mechanisms regulating MR activity in a given cell type (**Figure 2**). Utilisation of cell type-specific bulk or single-cell RNA-sequencing as well as integrated analysis of locus-specific histone modifications and DNA methylation, spatial organisation of the chromatin, MR-DNA binding and MR post-translational modification would allow a comprehensive insight into regulation of transcription by MR in cardiovascular cells and might lead to novel concepts for selective MR-targeting therapeutics.

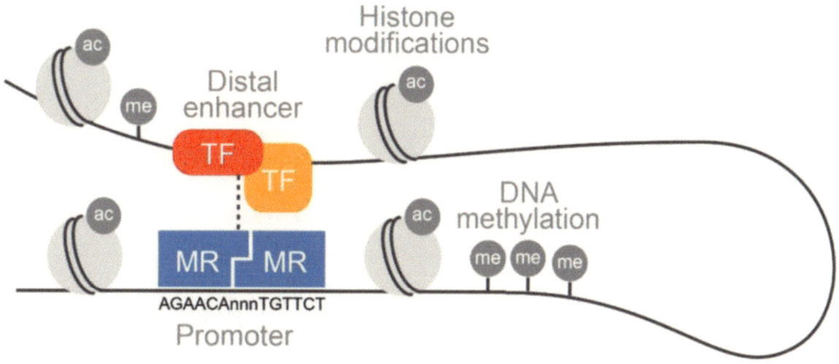


**Figure 2.**
*Proposed epigenetic determents of MR transcriptional activity. Transcriptional activity of the mineralocorticoid receptor is determined by DNA methylation and histone modifications governing chromatin accessibility and activation status of promoter and distal enhancer regions. Transactivation of MR-bound promoter or enhancer regions involves spatial chromatin organisation and other transcription factors. MR, mineralocorticoid receptor; TF, transcription factor; ac, acetylation; me, methylation.*

## Acknowledgements

This publication is based upon work from the EU COST Action ADMIRE BM1301 in Aldosterone and Mineralocorticoid Receptor (MR) Physiology and Pathophysiology www.admirecosteu.com and was supported by the Else-Kröner-Fresenius-Stiftung (2016_ A163 to A. Lother).

## Author details

LisaDeng[1], Lutz Hein[1] and Achim Lother[1,2]*

1 Institute of Experimental and Clinical Pharmacology and Toxicology, Faculty of Medicine, University of Freiburg, Germany

2 Heart Center Freiburg University, Department of Cardiology and Angiology I, Faculty of Medicine, University of Freiburg, Germany

*Address all correspondence to: achim.lother@universitaets-herzzentrum.de

## References

[1] Ponikowski P, Voors AA, Anker SD, Bueno H, Cleland JG, Coats AJ, et al. 2016 ESC guidelines for the diagnosis and treatment of acute and chronic heart failure: The task force for the diagnosis and treatment of acute and chronic heart failure of the european Society of Cardiology (ESC) developed with the special contribution of the heart failure association (HFA) of the ESC. European Heart Journal. 2016;**37**(27):2129-2200

[2] Lother A, Hein L. Pharmacology of heart failure: From basic science to novel therapies. Pharmacology & Therapeutics. 2016;**166**:136-149

[3] Lother A, Moser M, Bode C, Feldman RD, Hein L. Mineralocorticoids in the heart and vasculature: New insights for old hormones. Annual Review of Pharmacology and Toxicology. 2015;**55**:289-312

[4] Gadaleta RM, Magnani L. Nuclear receptors and chromatin: An inducible couple. Journal of Molecular Endocrinology. 2014;**52**(2):13-0170

[5] Fuller PJ. Novel interactions of the mineralocorticoid receptor. Molecular and Cellular Endocrinology. 2015;**408**:33-37

[6] Katsu Y, Oka K, Baker ME. Evolution of human, chicken, alligator, frog, and zebrafish mineralocorticoid receptors: Allosteric influence on steroid specificity. Science Signaling. 2018;**11**(537)

[7] Sever R, Glass CK. Signaling by nuclear receptors. Cold Spring Harbor Perspectives in Biology. 2013;**5**(3)

[8] Kouzarides T. Chromatin modifications and their function. Cell. 2007;**128**(4):693-705

[9] Pinto AR, Ilinykh A, Ivey MJ, Kuwabara JT, D'Antoni ML, Debuque R, et al. Revisiting cardiac cellular composition. Circulation Research. 2016;**118**(3):400-409

[10] Preissl S, Schwaderer M, Raulf A, Hesse M, Gruning BA, Kobele C, et al. Deciphering the epigenetic code of cardiac myocyte transcription. Circulation Research. 2015;**117**(5):413-423

[11] Lother A, Bergemann S, Deng L, Moser M, Bode C, Hein L. Cardiac endothelial cell transcriptome. Arteriosclerosis, Thrombosis, and Vascular Biology. 2018;**38**(3):566-574

[12] Quaife-Ryan GA, Sim CB, Ziemann M, Kaspi A, Rafehi H, Ramialison M, et al. Multicellular transcriptional analysis of mammalian heart regeneration. Circulation. 2017;**136**(12):1123-1139

[13] DeLaughter DM, Bick AG, Wakimoto H, McKean D, Gorham JM, Kathiriya IS, et al. Single-cell resolution of temporal gene expression during heart development. Developmental Cell. 2016;**39**(4):480-490

[14] Dunn J, Qiu H, Kim S, Jjingo D, Hoffman R, Kim CW, et al. Flow-dependent epigenetic DNA methylation regulates endothelial gene expression and atherosclerosis. The Journal of Clinical Investigation. 2014;**124**(7):3187-3199

[15] Jiang YZ, Jimenez JM, Ou K, McCormick ME, Zhang LD, Davies PF. Hemodynamic disturbed flow induces differential DNA methylation of endothelial kruppel-like factor 4 promoter in vitro and in vivo. Circulation Research. 2014;**115**(1):32-43

[16] Zampetaki A, Zeng L, Margariti A, Xiao Q, Li H, Zhang Z, et al. Histone deacetylase 3 is critical in endothelial survival and atherosclerosis

development in response to disturbed flow. Circulation. 2010;**121**(1):132-142

[17] Cardinale JP, Sriramula S, Pariaut R, Guggilam A, Mariappan N, Elks CM, et al. HDAC inhibition attenuates inflammatory, hypertrophic, and hypertensive responses in spontaneously hypertensive rats. Hypertension. 2010;**56**(3):437-444

[18] Kato N, Loh M, Takeuchi F, Verweij N, Wang X, Zhang W, et al. Trans-ancestry genome-wide association study identifies 12 genetic loci influencing blood pressure and implicates a role for DNA methylation. Nature Genetics. 2015;**47**(11):1282-1293

[19] Cao DJ, Wang ZV, Battiprolu PK, Jiang N, Morales CR, Kong Y, et al. Histone deacetylase (HDAC) inhibitors attenuate cardiac hypertrophy by suppressing autophagy. Proceedings of the National Academy of Sciences of the United States of America. 2011;**108**(10):4123-4128

[20] Aune SE, Herr DJ, Mani SK, Menick DR. Selective inhibition of class I but not class IIb histone deacetylases exerts cardiac protection from ischemia reperfusion. Journal of Molecular and Cellular Cardiology. 2014;**72**:138-145

[21] Gusterson RJ, Jazrawi E, Adcock IM, Latchman DS. The transcriptional co-activators CREB-binding protein (CBP) and p300 play a critical role in cardiac hypertrophy that is dependent on their histone acetyltransferase activity. The Journal of Biological Chemistry. 2003;**278**(9):6838-6847

[22] Zhang CL, McKinsey TA, Chang S, Antos CL, Hill JA, Olson EN. Class II histone deacetylases act as signal-responsive repressors of cardiac hypertrophy. Cell. 2002;**110**(4):479-488

[23] van der Harst P, de Windt LJ, Chambers JC. Translational perspective on epigenetics in cardiovascular disease. Journal of the American College of Cardiology. 2017;**70**(5):590-606

[24] McKinsey TA. Therapeutic potential for HDAC inhibitors in the heart. Annual Review of Pharmacology and Toxicology. 2012;**52**:303-319

[25] Biddie SC, John S. Minireview: Conversing with chromatin: The language of nuclear receptors. Molecular Endocrinology. 2014;**28**(1):3-15

[26] Pepke S, Wold B, Mortazavi A. Computation for ChIP-seq and RNA-seq studies. Nature Methods. 2009;**6** (11 Suppl):S22-S32

[27] Shlyueva D, Stampfel G, Stark A. Transcriptional enhancers: From properties to genome-wide predictions. Nature Reviews Genetics. 2014;**15**(4):272-286

[28] Stratton MS, McKinsey TA. Acetyl-lysine erasers and readers in the control of pulmonary hypertension and right ventricular hypertrophy. Biochemistry and Cell Biology. 2015;**93**(2):149-157

[29] Smith ZD, Meissner A. DNA methylation: Roles in mammalian development. Nature Reviews Genetics. 2013;**14**(3):204-220

[30] Burger L, Gaidatzis D, Schubeler D, Stadler MB. Identification of active regulatory regions from DNA methylation data. Nucleic Acids Research. 2013;**41**(16):e155

[31] Jones PA. Functions of DNA methylation: Islands, start sites, gene bodies and beyond. Nature Reviews Genetics. 2012;**13**(7):484-492

[32] Gilsbach R, Preissl S, Gruning BA, Schnick T, Burger L, Benes V, et al. Dynamic DNA methylation orchestrates cardiomyocyte development, maturation and disease. Nature Communications. 2014;**5**(5288)

[33] Gilsbach R, Schwaderer M, Preissl S, Gruning BA, Kranzhofer D, Schneider P, et al. Distinct epigenetic programs regulate cardiac myocyte development and disease in the human heart in vivo. Nature Communications. 2018;**9**(1):017-02762

[34] Cole TJ, Young MJ. 30 Years of the mineralocorticoid receptor: Mineralocorticoid receptor null mice: Informing cell-type-specific roles. The Journal of Endocrinology. 2017;**234**(1):T83-T92

[35] Lother A, Hein L. Vascular mineralocorticoid receptors: Linking risk factors, hypertension, and heart disease. Hypertension. 2016;**68**(1):6-10

[36] Brilla CG, Zhou G, Matsubara L, Weber KT. Collagen metabolism in cultured adult rat cardiac fibroblasts: Response to angiotensin II and aldosterone. Journal of Molecular and Cellular Cardiology. 1994;**26**(7):809-820

[37] Bunda S, Liu P, Wang Y, Liu K, Hinek A. Aldosterone induces elastin production in cardiac fibroblasts through activation of insulin-like growth factor-I receptors in a mineralocorticoid receptor-independent manner. The American Journal of Pathology. 2007;**171**(3):809-819

[38] Jaffe IZ, Mendelsohn ME. Angiotensin II and aldosterone regulate gene transcription via functional mineralocortocoid receptors in human coronary artery smooth muscle cells. Circulation Research. 2005;**96**(6):643-650

[39] Newfell BG, Iyer LK, Mohammad NN, McGraw AP, Ehsan A, Rosano G, et al. Aldosterone regulates vascular gene transcription via oxidative stress-dependent and -independent pathways. Arteriosclerosis, Thrombosis, and Vascular Biology. 2011;**31**(8):1871-1880

[40] Sekizawa N, Yoshimoto T, Hayakawa E, Suzuki N, Sugiyama T, Hirata Y. Transcriptome analysis of aldosterone-regulated genes in human vascular endothelial cell lines stably expressing mineralocorticoid receptor. Molecular and Cellular Endocrinology. 2011;**341**(1-2):78-88

[41] Lother A, Deng L, Huck M, Fürst D, Kowalski J, Esser JS, et al. Endothelial cell mineralocorticoid receptors oppose VEGF-induced gene expression and angiogenesis. The Journal of Endocrinology. 2019;**240**(1):15-26

[42] Fejes-Toth G, Naray-Fejes-Toth A. Early aldosterone-regulated genes in cardiomyocytes: Clues to cardiac remodeling? Endocrinology. 2007; **148**(4):1502-1510

[43] Latouche C, Sainte-Marie Y, Steenman M, Castro Chaves P, Naray-Fejes-Toth A, Fejes-Toth G, et al. Molecular signature of mineralocorticoid receptor signaling in cardiomyocytes: From cultured cells to mouse heart. Endocrinology. 2010;**151**(9):4467-4476

[44] Grune J, Beyhoff N, Smeir E, Chudek R, Blumrich A, Ban Z, et al. Selective mineralocorticoid receptor cofactor modulation as molecular basis for finerenone's antifibrotic activity. Hypertension. 2018;**71**(4):599-608

[45] Lother A, Berger S, Gilsbach R, Rosner S, Ecke A, Barreto F, et al. Ablation of mineralocorticoid receptors in myocytes but not in fibroblasts preserves cardiac function. Hypertension. 2011;**57**(4):746-754

[46] Lother A, Bergemann S, Kowalski J, Huck M, Gilsbach R, Bode C, et al. Inhibition of the cardiac myocyte mineralocorticoid receptor ameliorates doxorubicin-induced cardiotoxicity. Cardiovascular Research. 2018;**114**(2):282-290

[47] Latouche C, El Moghrabi S, Messaoudi S, Nguyen Dinh Cat A, Hernandez-Diaz I, Alvarez de la Rosa D, et al. Neutrophil gelatinase-associated lipocalin is a novel mineralocorticoid target in the cardiovascular system. Hypertension. 2012;**59**(5):966-972

[48] Fletcher EK, Morgan J, Kennaway DR, Bienvenu LA, Rickard AJ, Delbridge LMD, et al. Deoxycorticosterone/salt-mediated cardiac inflammation and fibrosis are dependent on functional CLOCK signaling in male mice. Endocrinology. 2017;**158**(9):2906-2917

[49] Le Billan F, Amazit L, Bleakley K, Xue QY, Pussard E, Lhadj C, et al. Corticosteroid receptors adopt distinct cyclical transcriptional signatures. FASEB Journal: Official Publication of the Federation of American Societies for Experimental Biology. 2018;**32**(10):5626-5639. DOI: 10.1096/fj.201800391RR

[50] Fuller PJ, Yao Y, Yang J, Young MJ. Mechanisms of ligand specificity of the mineralocorticoid receptor. The Journal of Endocrinology. 2012;**213**(1):15-24

[51] Chapman K, Holmes M, Seckl J. 11beta-hydroxysteroid dehydrogenases: Intracellular gate-keepers of tissue glucocorticoid action. Physiological Reviews. 2013;**93**(3):1139-1206

[52] Hernandez-Diaz I, Giraldez T, Arnau MR, Smits VA, Jaisser F, Farman N, et al. The mineralocorticoid receptor is a constitutive nuclear factor in cardiomyocytes due to hyperactive nuclear localization signals. Endocrinology. 2010;**151**(8):3888-3899

[53] Ziera T, Irlbacher H, Fromm A, Latouche C, Krug SM, Fromm M, et al. Cnksr3 is a direct mineralocorticoid receptor target gene and plays a key role in the regulation of the epithelial sodium channel. The FASEB Journal. 2009;**23**(11):3936-3946

[54] Ueda K, Fujiki K, Shirahige K, Gomez-Sanchez CE, Fujita T, Nangaku M, et al. Genome-wide analysis of murine renal distal convoluted tubular cells for the target genes of mineralocorticoid receptor. Biochemical and Biophysical Research Communications. 2014;**445**(1):132-137

[55] Le Billan F, Khan JA, Lamribet K, Viengchareun S, Bouligand J, Fagart J, et al. Cistrome of the aldosterone-activated mineralocorticoid receptor in human renal cells. FASEB Journal: Official Publication of the Federation of American Societies for Experimental Biology. 2015;**29**(9):3977-3989

[56] Mifsud KR, Reul JM. Acute stress enhances heterodimerization and binding of corticosteroid receptors at glucocorticoid target genes in the hippocampus. Proceedings of the National Academy of Sciences of the United States of America. 2016;**113**(40):11336-11341

[57] van Weert L, Buurstede JC, Mahfouz A, Braakhuis PSM, Polman JAE, Sips HCM, et al. NeuroD factors discriminate mineralocorticoid from glucocorticoid receptor DNA binding in the male rat brain. Endocrinology. 2017;**158**(5):1511-1522

[58] Mifsud B, Tavares-Cadete F, Young AN, Sugar R, Schoenfelder S, Ferreira L, et al. Mapping long-range promoter contacts in human cells with high-resolution capture Hi-C. Nature Genetics. 2015;**47**(6):598-606

[59] Mesquita TR, Auguste G, Falcon D, Ruiz-Hurtado G, Salazar-Enciso R, Sabourin J, et al. Specific activation of the alternative cardiac promoter of Cacna1c by the mineralocorticoid receptor. Circulation Research. 2018;**122**(7):e49-e61

[60] Marzolla V, Armani A, Mammi C, Moss ME, Pagliarini V, Pontecorvo L,

et al. Essential role of ICAM-1 in aldosterone-induced atherosclerosis. International Journal of Cardiology. 2017;**232**:233-242

[61] Del Monaco M, Covello SP, Kennedy SH, Gilinger G, Litwack G, Uitto J. Identification of novel glucocorticoid-response elements in human elastin promoter and demonstration of nucleotide sequence specificity of the receptor binding. The Journal of Investigative Dermatology. 1997;**108**(6):938-942

[62] Starick SR, Ibn-Salem J, Jurk M, Hernandez C, Love MI, Chung HR, et al. ChIP-exo signal associated with DNA-binding motifs provides insight into the genomic binding of the glucocorticoid receptor and cooperating transcription factors. Genome Research. 2015;**25**(6):825-835

[63] Ratman D, Vanden Berghe W, Dejager L, Libert C, Tavernier J, Beck IM, et al. How glucocorticoid receptors modulate the activity of other transcription factors: A scope beyond tethering. Molecular and Cellular Endocrinology. 2013;**380**(1-2):41-54

[64] Dougherty EJ, Elinoff JM, Ferreyra GA, Hou A, Cai R, Sun J, et al. Mineralocorticoid receptor (MR) trans-activation of inflammatory AP-1 signaling: Dependence on DNA sequence, MR conformation, and AP-1 family member expression. The Journal of Biological Chemistry. 2016;**291**(45):23628-23644

[65] Mifsud KR, Reul J. Mineralocorticoid and glucocorticoid receptor-mediated control of genomic responses to stress in the brain. Stress 2018;**21**(5):389-402

[66] Trapp T, Rupprecht R, Castren M, Reul JM, Holsboer F. Heterodimerization between mineralocorticoid and glucocorticoid receptor: A new principle of glucocorticoid action in the CNS. Neuron. 1994;**13**(6):1457-1462

[67] Ou XM, Storring JM, Kushwaha N, Albert PR. Heterodimerization of mineralocorticoid and glucocorticoid receptors at a novel negative response element of the 5-HT1A receptor gene. The Journal of Biological Chemistry. 2001;**276**(17):14299-14307

[68] Meinel S, Ruhs S, Schumann K, Stratz N, Trenkmann K, Schreier B, et al. Mineralocorticoid receptor interaction with SP1 generates a new response element for pathophysiologically relevant gene expression. Nucleic Acids Research. 2013;**41**(17):8045-8060

[69] Kolla V, Robertson NM, Litwack G. Identification of a mineralocorticoid/glucocorticoid response element in the human Na/K ATPase alpha1 gene promoter. Biochemical and Biophysical Research Communications. 1999;**266**(1):5-14

[70] Hudson WH, Kossmann BR, de Vera IM, Chuo SW, Weikum ER, Eick GN, et al. Distal substitutions drive divergent DNA specificity among paralogous transcription factors through subdivision of conformational space. Proceedings of the National Academy of Sciences of the United States of America. 2016;**113**(2):326-331

[71] Yang J, Young MJ. The mineralocorticoid receptor and its coregulators. Journal of Molecular Endocrinology. 2009;**43**(2):53-64

[72] Yang J, Fuller PJ. Interactions of the mineralocorticoid receptor—Within and without. Molecular and Cellular Endocrinology. 2012;**350**(2):196-205

[73] Fuller PJ, Yang J, Young MJ. 30 Years of the mineralocorticoid receptor: Coregulators as mediators of

mineralocorticoid receptor signalling diversity. The Journal of Endocrinology. 2017;**234**(1):T23-T34

[74] Gomez-Sanchez E, Gomez-Sanchez CE. The multifaceted mineralocorticoid receptor. Comprehensive Physiology. 2014;**4**(3):965-994

[75] Pascual-Le Tallec L, Simone F, Viengchareun S, Meduri G, Thirman MJ, Lombes M. The elongation factor ELL (eleven-nineteen lysine-rich leukemia) is a selective coregulator for steroid receptor functions. Molecular Endocrinology. 2005;**19**(5):1158-1169

[76] Yang J, Fuller PJ, Morgan J, Shibata H, Clyne CD, Young MJ. GEMIN4 functions as a coregulator of the mineralocorticoid receptor. Journal of Molecular Endocrinology. 2015;**54**(2):149-160

[77] Murai-Takeda A, Shibata H, Kurihara I, Kobayashi S, Yokota K, Suda N, et al. NF-YC functions as a corepressor of agonist-bound mineralocorticoid receptor. The Journal of Biological Chemistry. 2010;**285**(11):8084-8093

[78] Grune J, Beyhoff N, Smeir E, Chudek R, Blumrich A, Ban Z, et al. Selective mineralocorticoid receptor cofactor modulation as molecular basis for finerenone's antifibrotic activity. Hypertension. 2018;**71**(4):599-608

[79] Faresse N. Post-translational modifications of the mineralocorticoid receptor: How to dress the receptor according to the circumstances? The Journal of Steroid Biochemistry and Molecular Biology. 2014;**143**:334-342

[80] Galigniana MD. Native rat kidney mineralocorticoid receptor is a phosphoprotein whose transformation to a DNA-binding form is induced by phosphatases. The Biochemical Journal. 1998;**333**(Pt 3):555-563

[81] Le Moellic C, Ouvrard-Pascaud A, Capurro C, Cluzeaud F, Fay M, Jaisser F, et al. Early nongenomic events in aldosterone action in renal collecting duct cells: PKCalpha activation, mineralocorticoid receptor phosphorylation, and cross-talk with the genomic response. Journal of the American Society of Nephrology. 2004;**15**(5):1145-1160

[82] Kino T, Jaffe H, Amin ND, Chakrabarti M, Zheng YL, Chrousos GP, et al. Cyclin-dependent kinase 5 modulates the transcriptional activity of the mineralocorticoid receptor and regulates expression of brain-derived neurotrophic factor. Molecular Endocrinology. 2010;**24**(5):941-952

[83] Ruhs S, Stratz N, Quarch K, Masch A, Schutkowski M, Gekle M, et al. Modulation of transcriptional mineralocorticoid receptor activity by casein kinase 2. Scientific Reports. 2017;**7**(1):017-15418

[84] Shibata S, Rinehart J, Zhang J, Moeckel G, Castaneda-Bueno M, Stiegler AL, et al. Mineralocorticoid receptor phosphorylation regulates ligand binding and renal response to volume depletion and hyperkalemia. Cell Metabolism. 2013;**18**(5):660-671

[85] Faresse N, Vitagliano JJ, Staub O. Differential ubiquitylation of the mineralocorticoid receptor is regulated by phosphorylation. FASEB Journal: Official Publication of the Federation of American Societies for Experimental Biology. 2012;**26**(10):4373-4382

[86] Pascual-Le Tallec L, Lombes M. The mineralocorticoid receptor: A journey exploring its diversity and specificity of action. Molecular Endocrinology. 2005;**19**(9):2211-2221

[87] Lee HA, Lee DY, Cho HM, Kim SY, Iwasaki Y, Kim IK. Histone deacetylase inhibition attenuates transcriptional activity of mineralocorticoid

receptor through its acetylation and prevents development of hypertension. Circulation Research. 2013;**112**(7):1004-1012

[88] Kang SH, Lee HA, Lee E, Kim M, Kim I. Histone deacetylase inhibition, but not a mineralocorticoid receptor antagonist spironolactone, attenuates atypical transcription by an activating mutant MR (MRS 810L). Clinical and Experimental Pharmacology & Physiology. 2016;**43**(10):995-1003

[89] Iyer A, Fenning A, Lim J, Le GT, Reid RC, Halili MA, et al. Antifibrotic activity of an inhibitor of histone deacetylases in DOCA-salt hypertensive rats. British Journal of Pharmacology. 2010;**159**(7):1408-1417

Chapter 13

# MicroRNAs in Aldosterone Production and Action

*Scott M. MacKenzie, Josie van Kralingen, Hannah Martin and Eleanor Davies*

## Abstract

The secretion of aldosterone by the adrenal cortex is a tightly regulated process. Loss of this control can result in severe hypertension and end-organ damage, so detailed understanding of the various mechanisms by which the body regulates aldosterone biosynthesis is key. The emergence of microRNAs (miRNAs) as negative regulators of numerous physiological processes has naturally led to their study in the context of aldosterone production. We summarise several studies that have demonstrated a significant role for microRNAs in aldosterone biosynthesis and action, thereby presenting a possible therapeutic role in the treatment of common forms of hypertension such as primary aldosteronism. Furthermore, the presence of microRNAs in the circulation offers the prospect of accessible and informative biomarkers that may simplify the currently protracted and technically difficult diagnosis of such conditions.

**Keywords:** aldosterone, microRNA, hypertension, adrenal cortex

## 1. Introduction

High blood pressure, or hypertension, is a major risk factor for coronary disease, heart failure and stroke. Hypertension is a contributing factor in over 7 million deaths per year, which provides strong motivation to understand the systems regulating normal blood pressure and how such control can be lost. Our own studies have focused on the role of the hormone aldosterone, a key determinant of blood pressure, and the various factors regulating its secretion from the adrenal gland.

Aldosterone is synthesised in the adrenal cortex and acts on specific mineralocorticoid receptors (MR), principally in epithelial tissue, to regulate fluid balance, electrolyte homeostasis and blood pressure. Excess secretion of aldosterone, as in primary aldosteronism (PA), leads to severe hypertension with markedly increased risk of myocardial infarction, stroke and left ventricular hypertrophy [1]. Originally believed to be a rare condition (principally due to practical difficulties in accurate diagnosis), the reported frequency of PA in all hypertensives has risen steadily over the years and is now generally regarded to lie somewhere between 10 and 20%; PA is therefore the single most common form of secondary hypertension [2]. Independent of its effects on blood pressure, excess aldosterone also has detrimental effects on various target organs including the renal and cardiovascular systems [3]. Such negative effects are not necessarily confined to PA; even when present in minimal excess, aldosterone associates with higher blood pressure and substantial cardiovascular morbidity [4]. Although major advances have been made in understanding aldosterone and its regulation in the 60 years since its discovery, many aspects remain incompletely understood. New factors capable of regulating aldosterone secretion are still emerging, and evidence generated by ourselves and others indicate that we must add microRNA (miRNA) to this list.

In this article we summarise the major findings to date regarding miRNA and its effects on aldosterone secretion and action. We also anticipate the future direction and outcomes of such studies—including the possible role for miRNA in the accurate diagnosis of PA and other subtypes of hypertension—and related therapeutic strategies that could be employed to modify hormone production and action in such patients to yield major health benefits.

## 2. Aldosterone biosynthesis

Aldosterone biosynthesis is confined to the adrenocortical zona glomerulosa (ZG) and in normal circumstances is principally controlled by the renin-angiotensin system (RAS) and potassium status. Synthesis consists of a series of enzymatic reactions commencing with the conversion of cholesterol by the side-chain cleavage enzyme, CYP11A1. The terminal reactions in aldosterone biosynthesis are catalysed by the enzyme aldosterone synthase, the product of the *CYP11B2* gene, which is expressed only in the ZG. Its expression is principally controlled by angiotensin II (AngII) and potassium through transcription factor binding of its 5′ regulatory region [5]. The key second messenger in this process is calcium; influx of $Ca^{2+}$ through channels in the ZG cell membrane raises aldosterone production by various means that include stimulation of *CYP11B2* transcription and increased availability of the cofactor NADH. Extensive study of the *CYP11B2* gene has shown it to be highly polymorphic, with multiple genetic sequence variations present across its introns and in the untranslated regions (UTRs) lying to the 5′ and 3′ ends of the locus. Certain of these 5′ and intronic variants associate with altered gene activity and also with raised plasma aldosterone, increased urinary excretion of aldosterone metabolites and high blood pressure, demonstrating that relatively subtle changes in expression of this gene can have significant cardiovascular effects. The discovery of microRNAs and their role in post-transcriptional repression of specific genes, principally through sites located in the 3’ UTR, has now focused interest on that region of *CYP11B2*.

## 3. MicroRNA

miRNAs are a class of endogenous, small (~20–25 nucleotides), single-stranded non-coding RNA molecules which act to post-transcriptionally regulate expression of specific target mRNAs. They are often regarded as having only subtle ‘fine-tuning’ roles in gene expression but are nevertheless capable of significant effects including roles in human disease, including numerous cancers [6, 7].

Synthesis of miRNA is a multistep process (see **Figure 1**), beginning with the transcription in the nucleus from miRNA genes located mainly in intergenic or intronic chromosomal regions of chromosomes, although some are also present in exons [8, 9]. This produces primary transcripts (pri-miRNA), which are processed by Drosha endonuclease into pre-miRNAs ~70 nucleotides in size. Due to self-complementary nucleotide binding, these pre-miRNAs have distinctive ‘hairpin loop’ structures and are transported by Exportin-5 from the nucleus to the cytoplasm, where they are processed further by Dicer to form a miRNA duplex.

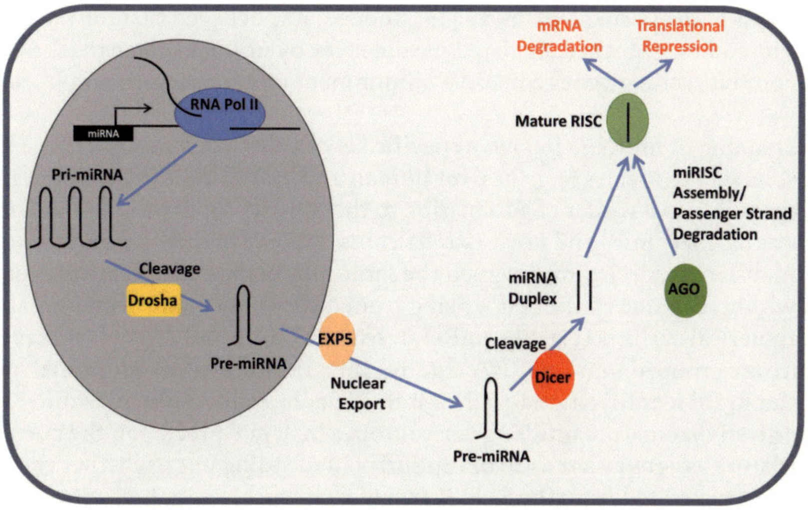


**Figure 1.**
*Overview of miRNA biogenesis and post-transcriptional repression mechanisms. MicroRNA genes are transcribed in the nucleus as primary transcripts (pri-miRNA) before being processed into ~70 nucleotide pre-miRNAs by Drosha endonuclease. The pre-miRNA is transported from the nucleus into the cytoplasm by Exportin-5 where it is processed further by dicer. The mature miRNA (red) is then loaded into Argonaute 1–4 and assembled into the miRNA-induced silencing complex (miRISC), which is subsequently guided to the 3'UTR of the target mRNA. mRNA translation is inhibited by miRISC through one or more repressive mechanisms, including mRNA cleavage, degradation and translational repression.*

The strand of the miRNA duplex with lower thermodynamic stability (usually the 3′ arm) is termed the passenger strand; this is removed, resulting in the formation of the mature miRNA [10]. It was initially thought that the passenger strand had no biological function and was automatically targeted for degradation, but recent studies show that passenger strands can have a functional role in mRNA regulation, prompting their study in current miRNA research [11, 12]. The mature miRNA then recruits a ribonucleoprotein complex called the miRNA-induced silencing complex (miRISC). At the core of the mammalian miRISC is one of the four Argonaute proteins (AGO1–4) and a 182 kDa protein, GW182. While the miRNA sequence determines which mRNAs are targeted for repression, it is the miRISC proteins that actually mediate the silencing [13]. The miRISC post-transcriptionally represses gene expression by initiating decay of target mRNAs and/or inhibiting their translation. It achieves this by recognising and binding to specific sequences on the target mRNA, usually in its 3'UTR, that is complementary to the miRNA seed site (located at nucleotides 2–8 of the miRNA, at its 5′ end). If the mRNA is sufficiently complementary to the miRNA, it will be cleaved by the slicer AGO and these cleaved mRNA fragments targeted for degradation [14, 15]. If binding is imperfect, AGO is unable to cleave the mRNA. However, complementary binding beyond the seed sequence can also initiate silencing; in this case the GW182 protein recruits deadenylation factors which destabilise the mRNA through the removal of its polyadenylated tail, again targeting it for degradation. Although the majority of miRNA-controlled gene silencing is achieved by mRNA cleavage or destabilisation, translation can also be repressed. This mechanism is less well understood but is thought to involve miRNA interaction with factors essential to the initiation of translation, such as cytoplasmic poly(A)-binding protein (PABPC) and cap-binding complex eIF4F [16].

While miRNA-mediated regulation is typically mild in nature, individual miRNAs can have significant and diverse biological effect due to their ability to target numerous different mRNA species within the same cell [17] and even several components within a single pathway [18]. Indeed, it is believed that the majority of protein-coding genes are regulated in some way by miRNAs given that >60% of human protein-coding genes contain a minimum of one conserved miRNA-binding site [19].

The naming of miRNAs follows a specific set of rules. Each miRNA name identifies first its source species (e.g. 'hsa' for human and 'mmu' for mouse) and is numbered according to its order of submission to the miRNA database [20], with mature sequences labelled 'miR' and precursor hairpins 'mir' [21]. Identical sequences found in different species are assigned the same numbers, while identical sequences found within the same species but arising from different genomic locations are given numerical suffixes (e.g. hsa-miR-1-1, hsa-miR-1-2). miRNAs of similar sequence are grouped into a miRNA 'family' and are allocated an additional lower-case letter to aid identification (e.g. hsa-miR-320a, hsa-miR-320b, hsa-miR-320c). Finally, given that mature miRNAs derive from a 'hairpin' precursor, the current nomenclature assigns either a -5p or -3p suffix, depending upon whether the miRNA was generated from the 5′ or 3′ arm of that hairpin (e.g. hsa-miR-34c-5p and hsa-miR-34c-3p).

## 4. Extracellular microRNAs

In addition to acting within the cell where they are transcribed, miRNAs can be released from those cells and have been detected in various bodily fluids, including the bloodstream. This has raised interest in the potential utility of circulating miRNAs as disease biomarkers [22, 23]. The majority of miRNAs within the circulation are associated with AGO2 in nuclease-resistant complexes. miRNAs also circulate within exosomes, which are small membrane vesicles that form within multivesicular bodies and are secreted upon fusion with the plasma membrane. Exosomes contain specific miRNAs rather than the complete spectrum of miRNAs of a cell, indicating as yet unknown mechanisms for their recognition, packaging and secretion. miRNAs may also be incorporated into high-density lipoprotein and low-density lipoprotein particles although this process is again not fully understood. Secreted miRNAs can, in principle, be transferred from one tissue to another through the circulation, but it is unclear whether a miRNA species taken up by a cell in this way can achieve sufficient levels to inhibit its target transcripts significantly. This mechanism of action raises the intriguing possibility that extracellular miRNAs participate in long-range signalling between tissues, in a manner analogous to endocrine systems. In this regard, miRNAs have been reported to act as agonists of Toll-like receptors and to trigger downstream pathway activation in target cells [24]. Distinctive expression patterns of extracellular miRNAs have also been associated with a variety of cardiovascular disorders, including atherosclerosis, myocardial infarction, heart failure, hypertension and type 2 diabetes [22]. However, whether these miRNAs participate in the disease process or simply serve as markers of disease progression has not been established. Greater patient cohorts will be needed to reach firm conclusions regarding the diagnostic and prognostic power of extracellular miRNAs.

## 5. MicroRNAs and corticosteroid production

Various studies have demonstrated the importance of microRNAs to adrenal development and maintenance in animal models [25, 26], but their effects on the human adrenal gland are less well defined. As far as secretion of corticosteroids such as aldosterone is concerned, miRNAs could have direct influence through the post-transcriptional repression of corticosteroidogenic or other related genes, which has been investigated. In 2008, Romero et al. identified miR-21 as a key modulator of aldosterone production. Overexpression of miR-21 in vitro significantly increased aldosterone production and cell proliferation in the H295R human adrenocortical carcinoma cell line [27]. These findings supported a role for miR-21 in both corticosteroid production and oncogenesis but possible target genes of miR-21 or a regulatory mechanism by which it increases aldosterone production and cell proliferation were not described. However, subsequent studies have demonstrated that miRNAs target numerous stages of the aldosterone biosynthesis pathway.

We have carried out comprehensive analysis of miRNA effects on aldosterone and cortisol production, as well as identifying and confirming target genes. We used a siRNA approach to knock down expression of Dicer, the protein essential to miRNA maturation, in H295R cells and studied its effects on cellular levels of steroidogenic mRNAs. Interestingly, only those encoding cytochrome P450 enzymes in the pathway (*CYP11A1*, *CYP21A1*, *CYP17A1*, *CYP11B1*, *CYP11B2*) were significantly increased in the absence of miRNA [28, 29]. Steroid production was also correspondingly changed, with levels of the end products aldosterone and cortisol—as well as many intermediate compounds in their biosynthesis—all increased relative to control cells (DOC, corticosterone, 18-OH corticosterone).

We then used a combination of bioinformatic prediction and experimental in vitro experimentation in H295R cells to confirm miRNA-24 as a direct regulator of *CYP11B1* and *CYP11B2* expression via sites in the mRNA 3'UTRs. We also observed changes in aldosterone and cortisol production rates that correlated with miRNA-altered levels of *CYP11B1* (11β-hydroxylase) and *CYP11B2* (aldosterone synthase). These experimental results were consistent with canonical miRNA action, whereby reduced levels of the mature miRNA result in less target mRNA degradation and therefore more abundant steroid product due to higher gene expression. These data therefore demonstrated a significant regulatory role for miRNAs in human steroidogenesis. Furthermore, other studies show miR-24 to be upregulated following MR activation in the kidney, leading to the proposal that it might form part of a feedback loop to the adrenal gland, repressing *CYP11B2* expression when aldosterone levels are high [30].

Subsequent studies have expanded the array of miRNAs known to regulate directly the expression of late enzymes in this pathway: Nusrin and colleagues showed that miR-10b also negatively regulates both *CYP11B1* and *CYP11B2* expressions in H295R cells, subsequently modulating aldosterone and cortisol production [31]. We found that miRNAs -125a-5p and -125b-5p modulate *CYP11B2* (but not *CYP11B1*) in H295R cells [29], as did Maharjan et al. with miR-766 [32], although either study determined the effect of this on aldosterone production or whether cortisol remains unaffected. Looking to steroidogenic enzymes earlier in the pathway, we demonstrated a direct regulatory effect of miR-320a-3p on *CYP11A1* and *CYP17A1* in H295R cells [29]. Furthermore, Hu and colleagues reported that miR-132 regulates steroidogenesis by inhibiting StAR protein expression, thereby inhibiting basal progestin production and stimulating 20α-OHP production in Y1 mouse adrenocortical cells [33]. They also demonstrated a secondary method of miR-132 regulation in Y1 cells, through which miRNA overexpression reduces methyl-DNA-binding (MECP2) protein and alters levels of 3β-HSD and 20α-HSD; this stimulates the conversion of progesterone to its inactive metabolite, 20α-OHP {Hu:2017iz}. The same group also showed negative regulation of HDL cholesteryl ester uptake and HDL-stimulated progesterone production by miR-125a and miR-455, acting via scavenger receptor class B type I (SR-B1), although this work was primarily carried out in Leydig testicular cells {Hu:2012by}. It is therefore clear that miRNAs—including those mentioned above and likely many more, as yet undiscovered—regulate steroidogenesis within the adrenal cortex, at many different points, although the full impact of these individual regulatory miRNAs acting concurrently across the entirety of the corticosteroid pathway is yet to be assessed.

Studies have also expanded to examine non-steroidogenic genes with regulatory influence. Decreased expression of TWIK-related acid-sensitive $K^+$ (TASK-2) channels is associated with increased *CYP11B2* and StAR expression and with raised aldosterone levels; miR-34 and miR-23 reduce TASK-2 expression by direct binding of its mRNA 3'UTR [34]. Regulation of RAS genes by the miRNA has also been shown, with miR-181a and miR-663 both binding the 3'-UTR of the renin transcript [35]. The same study showed both of these miRNAs to be downregulated in the renal cortex of hypertensive subjects relative to normotensives, providing a possible mechanistic factor. Separately, miR-483 has been shown to repress four RAS components, including angiotensinogen [18]. Furthermore, angiotensin II (AngII) causes downregulation of miR-483 itself in vascular smooth muscle cells, implying that RAS activation could derepress itself through reduction of miR-483.

In addition to understanding which miRNAs target which elements of corticosteroid production and regulation, if miRNA-mediated control is to be fully understood, then we must improve our understanding of how production of the individual miRNAs is itself regulated. It is intuitively obvious that levels of these miRNAs should fluctuate in response to physiological demands and there are plentiful instances of this from various studies. Of the miRNAs already mentioned here, it is known that miR-21 expression is increased in H295R cells following angiotensin II stimulation [27], that miR-10b levels increase in response to hypoxia in H295R cells [31] and that miR-212 and miR-132 are more abundant in adrenal cells in vitro and the adrenal gland in vivo in response, respectively, to cAMP and ACTH stimulation [33].

## 6. Adrenal microRNAs

Numerous studies have profiled circulating or adrenal tissue miRNA expression in patients with adrenal carcinoma and/or aldosterone-producing adenoma (APA), confirming that miRNA expression is altered by these conditions relative to healthy controls [28, 29, 34, 36–51].

Notably, of the 11 miRNAs that have been shown to regulate corticosteroid biosynthesis in adrenal tissue (above), 8 are dysregulated in patients with benign adenoma or adrenal carcinoma: miRNAs -10b, –24 and -125a are downregulated in APA tissue [28, 29]; miR-125b is downregulated in carcinoma vs. benign adrenal tumour tissue [43]; miR-21, miR-320a-3p and miR-34 are significantly increased in adenoma tissue [28, 29, 41] and miR-21 is further increased in carcinoma tissue [41]; serum levels of miR-34a are raised in patients with adrenocortical carcinoma relative to patients with benign adrenocortical neoplasm [42]. TASK-2 expression is reduced in APA tissue relative to healthy adrenal tissue and negatively correlates with miR-23 and miR-34 levels [34]. Given that APA increases aldosterone secretion, it is perhaps unsurprising that miRNAs known to modulate corticosteroid biosynthesis, such as miR-24, show altered expression. Interestingly, one of the two genomic locations from which miR-24 is transcribed is a cluster on chromosome 9, where miR-24 is produced alongside miR-23b and miR-27b; our studies show all three to be downregulated in APA, which is consistent with this clustering and implies that many and diverse biological effects could result from the change in regulation to all three microRNAs [28]. Overall, existing studies of miRNA changes in adrenal tumours add weight to the hypothesis that miRNA targeting of transcription is a common feature of such conditions and is likely to be of relevance to adrenal pathology generally.

Expression of several other miRNAs has also been found to be altered in multiple independent studies of adrenal disease. Most notably miR-483 is increased in tumour [36, 38, 41, 43, 47] and circulating (i.e. plasma or extracellular vesicle) [38, 42, 44, 48] samples from patients with adrenocortical carcinoma when compared to samples from patients with adrenocortical adenomas or healthy controls. miR-210 [37, 41, 48, 49] and miR-184 [48, 49] levels are also increased in tumour and plasma samples from patients with adrenocortical carcinoma in comparison to patients with adrenocortical adenoma or healthy controls and in some cases are increased in adrenocortical adenoma vs. healthy controls [41]. Other miRNAs are downregulated in tumour and serum samples of patients with adrenocortical carcinoma or adrenocortical adenoma relative to patients with adrenocortical adenoma or to healthy controls, respectively: these include miR-195 [38, 41, 43, 47] and miR-335 [38, 47]. However, little work has been done to assess the biological impact of these miRNAs on the regulation of corticosteroid biosynthesis in the context of these diseases, and this remains an obvious priority area of future study. Clearly defined miRNA profiles that are specific to certain tumour types clearly have the potential to facilitate and expedite the differential diagnosis of adrenocortical tumours and enhance our understanding of disease pathogenesis (reviewed by Singh et al.) [52].

## 7. MicroRNA and the mineralocorticoid receptor

As the nuclear receptor to which aldosterone binds in all aldosterone-responsive tissues, the mineralocorticoid receptor is clearly a key factor in mediating the hormone's effects and is itself subject to miRNA regulation. In silico analysis predicts the *NR3C2* gene, which encodes the MR and contains between 23 and 411 distinct miRNA-binding sites in its 3'UTR, depending on the prediction algorithm utilised. Of these predicted miRNAs, five were selected for further experimental validation; two—miRNA-124 and miRNA-135a—were subsequently confirmed to bind the *NR3C2* 3'UTR, as evidenced by a reduction in luciferase activity following *NR3C2* 3′UTR luciferase reporter and miRNA expression vector cotransfection. Neither miRNA decreased *NR3C2* mRNA level, suggesting miRNA-124 and miRNA-135a are involved solely in translational inhibition of MR [53]. Interestingly, miRNA-124 has also been identified as a regulator of the glucocorticoid receptor (GR), associated with cortisol action [54]. Given its brain-specific expression [55], miRNA-124 cannot directly influence aldosterone biosynthesis but may have a role in the regulation of its production and action through centrally mediated systems. It is currently the subject of much investigation in light of its apparently beneficial effects post-stroke [56–59]. A role in neuronal differentiation has been proposed, and it is possible that the beneficial effects of miRNA-124 are achieved through downregulation of MR expression or activation, mirroring the beneficial effects of MR antagonists.

In addition to demonstrating that MR is regulated by miRNA, other studies identify MR as a mediator of miRNA expression. For example, aldosterone treatment of aortal or vascular smooth muscle cells (SMCs) causes downregulation of miRNA-29b, but this effect can be prevented through MR blockade with the antagonist eplerenone [60]. Interestingly, this MR-regulated change does not occur in mouse endothelial cells, which demonstrates the cell specificity of this MR effect in the vasculature. As with miRNA-124, the benefits of miRNA-29b delivery to the brain post-stroke is currently being investigated [61, 62], although other reports suggest it may actually promote neuronal cell death [63].

Another key factor in MR action is the enzyme 11β-hydroxysteroid dehydrogenase type 2 (11β-HSD2). As cortisol is capable of binding MR and circulates at levels far higher than aldosterone, 11β-HSD2 effectively confers aldosterone selectivity on tissues where it is expressed (such as the renal tubule), by converting cortisol to inactive cortisone; this leaves aldosterone free to bind MR without significant competition. 11β-HSD2 activity is therefore important, and its loss can result in salt-sensitive hypertension. Although direct inhibition of 11β-HSD2 expression by miRNAs targeting the 3'UTR of its mRNA has been demonstrated in rats, the existence and importance of such regulation in human aldosterone-selective tissues is yet to be confirmed [64].

Despite the various inconsistencies and gaps in our current knowledge, such ongoing studies of miRNA targeting, action and expression are likely to provide valuable insights into aldosterone action in the future.

## 8. MicroRNAs as biomarkers and therapeutic targets in endocrine pathologies

Excessive aldosterone production and the consequent activation of MR are now generally accepted to be important and common factors in the pathogenesis of hypertension and a number of related comorbidities. Given that specific changes in miRNA expression and regulation are associated with certain disease states and that miRNAs can be released into extracellular fluids, the potential exists to use circulating microRNAs as biomarkers for conditions that are otherwise difficult to diagnose. This includes various endocrine pathologies, including PA, where the difficulty of accurately identifying and distinguishing aldosterone-producing adenoma and bilateral adrenal hyperplasia (BAH) is acknowledged to have restricted diagnosis and effective treatment. Given that miRNAs are known to regulate corticosteroid biosynthesis and that adrenal miRNA expression is altered in cases of adrenal pathology, it is reasonable to hypothesise that changes in the array of circulating miRNAs might result from diseases affecting corticosteroid regulation or other forms of adrenal function. A current ongoing initiative in this regard—which arose in part from the COST ADMIRE network—is the ENS@T-HT study. This is an EU-funded Horizon 2020 research and innovation project designed to define specific 'omics' for various forms of endocrine hypertension, including PA, Cushing's syndrome and phaeochromocytoma. Our particular focus as part of this project has been the profiling of circulating miRNAs in patient plasma, with the aim of identifying signature miRNAs of diagnostic value. Initial miRNA profiling has now been completed in archived samples, and analysis is under way to develop a signature for testing in a new study population. This study is part of a wave of current diagnostic initiatives aiming to improve diagnosis and better target patient treatment through a stratified medicine approach. MicroRNA is likely to be a focus of many such projects which share the implicit assumption that if miRNA profile is altered by disease, then manipulation of miRNA might also form part of an effective treatment. The longer-term aspiration of such studies— including ENS@T-HT—is therefore the progression from diagnostic applications to therapeutics.

The therapeutic potential of miRNAs is derived from the ability to inhibit miRNA function with antimiRs. These are small oligonucleotides that can be delivered subcutaneously or intravenously and inhibit the interaction of miRNAs with their targets by binding the miRNA seed site with high affinity [65]. Pharmacokinetic and pharmacodynamic studies of antimiR action suggest they are taken up from the circulation by endocytosis and accumulate within endosomes or multivesicular bodies, but much remains unknown about the precise mechanisms of action and cellular handling of antimiRs. In contrast to classical drugs, the action of antimiRs appears to be delayed, often taking several days to exert an effect. This reflects the time required to rebalance the proteome of a target cell as a consequence of the relatively modest changes in numerous miRNA targets. Conversely, the actions of antimiRs are long-lived, owing to their high stability and accumulation within intracellular depots from which they are slowly released. They show efficacy at doses acceptable for therapeutic development, and further chemical modifications may enhance their uptake, stability and/or action.

An additional challenge with respect to the development of miRNA-based drugs is the inability to correlate target engagement with mechanism and therapeutic efficacy. Because of their many targets and the summation of relatively small repressive effects that contribute to the therapeutic actions of miRNAs, it is difficult or impossible to directly ascribe the activity of an antimiR to a specific target. An individual miRNA may have a beneficial activity in one tissue and an adverse activity in another. Therefore local delivery systems are likely to be useful in reducing off-target effects. While the sustained activity of antimiRs allows for effective treatment, the long-term consequences of antimiR accumulation in different tissues and the inability to rapidly reverse their activity or eliminate the presence of a toxic antimiR raise obvious concerns. AntimiRs accumulate predominantly in the liver and kidney, necessitating substantially higher doses to achieve efficacy in other tissues. This poses challenges with respect to achieving sufficient intracellular concentrations that evoke a therapeutic effect without causing liver and renal toxicity.

Of course, miRNAs may also play beneficial rather than pathogenic roles so strategies for elevating their levels are also required, including the administration of miRNA mimics. These are double-stranded synthetic oligonucleotides that are processed into single-stranded miRNAs when introduced into cells. However, the delivery of miRNA mimics still requires significant optimisation [66]. Lipid formulations for enhancing uptake may help in this regard, while adenoviral delivery methods may assist targeting to the tissue of choice. As with antimiRs, though, it is crucial to avoid repression of nontarget mRNAs or toxic accumulation of mimics.

Finally, a further factor needs to be considered regarding miRNA and its role in the personalisation or stratification of diagnosis and therapy: genetic polymorphisms. Although single-nucleotide polymorphisms that occur in protein-encoding or upstream regulator regions of genes are commonly accepted to contribute—sometimes dramatically—to disease phenotype, it is increasingly recognised that polymorphisms in miRNA genes themselves or in those transcribed but untranslated regions of the genes that they target might contribute to interindividual phenotypic variability and possibly predispose to disease [67]. This may become a major factor in the future 'personalisation' of medicine and effective targeting of therapeutic agents.

## 9. Conclusion

MiRNAs are providing us with fresh insights into aldosterone regulation, action and pathology while offering the prospect of new diagnostic and therapeutic approaches. It is apparent that miRNAs are important regulators of adrenal function and have the ability to regulate the expression of multiple enzymes within the corticosteroidogenic pathway, modifying the steroid profile as a result. Consistent changes in miRNA expression in APA or adrenocortical carcinoma tissue relative to healthy controls imply a role in the pathogenesis of these diseases and/or their resulting dysregulation. While the effect of each individual miRNA may be small, as numerous miRNAs can target the steroidogenic pathway in the adrenal cortex and are altered in disease, the sum of multiple small individual effects could result in significant changes to corticosteroid synthesis within the adrenal cortex. The specificity with which miRNAs target their effect is potentially mirrored by the specificity with which dysregulated miRNAs might themselves be therapeutically targeted. The ability to do so raises the tantalising possibility of a new generation of therapeutic 'magic bullets'. However, much remains to be learned about the precise mechanisms by which an individual miRNA affects different physiological pathways within single and different tissues and cell types. This may add significantly to the complexity and consequences of manipulating miRNA for therapeutic ends. A deeper understanding as well as a 'systems biology' approach is required to fully explain miRNA activity under conditions of homeostasis and disease. Despite these challenges and uncertainties, it seems likely that some of the numerous miRNAs currently implicated in cardiovascular disease will eventually emerge as viable biomarkers and possibly drug targets, although the timescale and the reach of such miRNA-based approaches cannot yet be predicted.

## Acknowledgements

This publication is based upon the work from the EU COST Action ADMIRE BM1301 in Aldosterone and Mineralocorticoid Receptor Physiology and Pathophysiology (www.admirecosteu.com). SM, JvK and ED are supported by an EU Horizon 2020 award to the ENS@T-HT programme; HM is funded by a British Heart Foundation PhD studentship.

## Author details

Scott M. MacKenzie, Josie van Kralingen, Hannah Martin and Eleanor Davies*
Institute of Cardiovascular and Medical Sciences, University of Glasgow, United Kingdom

*Address all correspondence to: eleanor.davies@glasgow.ac.uk

## References

[1] Connell JMC, MacKenzie SM, Freel EM, Fraser R, Davies E. A lifetime of aldosterone excess: Long-term consequences of altered regulation of aldosterone production for cardiovascular function. Endocrine Reviews. 2008;**29**(2):133-154

[2] Piaditis G, Markou A, Papanastasiou L, Androulakis II, Kaltsas G. Progress in aldosteronism: A review of the prevalence of primary aldosteronism in pre-hypertension and hypertension. European Journal of Endocrinology. 2015;**172**(5):R191-R203

[3] Tesch GH, Young MJ. Mineralocorticoid receptor Signaling as a therapeutic target for renal and cardiac fibrosis. Frontiers in Pharmacology. 2017;**8**:313

[4] Vasan RS, Evans JC, Larson MG, Wilson PWF, Meigs JB, Rifai N, et al. Serum aldosterone and the incidence of hypertension in nonhypertensive persons. The New England Journal of Medicine. 2004;**351**(1):33-41

[5] Connell JMC, Davies E. The new biology of aldosterone. The Journal of Endocrinology. 2005;**186**(1):1-20

[6] Lu J, Getz G, Miska EA, Alvarez-Saavedra E, Lamb J, Peck D, et al. MicroRNA expression profiles classify human cancers. Nature. 2005;**435**(7043):834-838

[7] Suzuki HI, Yamagata K, Sugimoto K, Iwamoto T, Kato S, Miyazono K. Modulation of microRNA processing by p53. Nature. 2009;**460**(7254):529-533

[8] Lau NC, Lim LP, Weinstein EG, Bartel DP. An abundant class of tiny RNAs with probable regulatory roles in Caenorhabditis elegans. Science. 2001;**294**(5543):858-862

[9] Rodriguez A, Griffiths-Jones S, Ashurst JL, Bradley A. Identification of mammalian microRNA host genes and transcription units. Genome Research. 2004;**14**(10A):1902-1910

[10] Kawamata T, Seitz H, Tomari Y. Structural determinants of miRNAs for RISC loading and slicer-independent unwinding. Nature Structural & Molecular Biology. 2009;**16**(9):953-960

[11] Tsang FH-C, Au SL-K, Wei L, Fan DN-Y, Lee JM-F, Wong CC-L, et al. MicroRNA-142-3p and microRNA-142-5p are downregulated in hepatocellular carcinoma and exhibit synergistic effects on cell motility. Frontiers in Medicine. 2015;**9**(3):331-343

[12] Shan SW, Fang L, Shatseva T, Rutnam ZJ, Yang X, Du W, et al. Mature miR-17-5p and passenger miR-17-3p induce hepatocellular carcinoma by targeting PTEN, GalNT7 and vimentin in different signal pathways. Journal of Cell Science. 2013;**126**(Pt 6): 1517-1530

[13] Fabian MR, Sonenberg N. The mechanics of miRNA-mediated gene silencing: A look under the hood of miRISC. Nature Structural & Molecular Biology. 2012;**19**(6):586-593

[14] Lewis BP, Shih I-H, Jones-Rhoades MW, Bartel DP, Burge CB. Prediction of mammalian microRNA targets. Cell. 2003;**115**(7):787-798

[15] Parker R, Song H. The enzymes and control of eukaryotic mRNA turnover. Nature Structural & Molecular Biology. 2004;**11**(2):121-127

[16] Huntzinger E, Izaurralde E. Gene silencing by microRNAs: Contributions of translational repression and mRNA decay. Nature Reviews. Genetics. 2011 Feb;**12**(2):99-110

[17] Selbach M, Schwanhäusser B, Thierfelder N, Fang Z, Khanin R, Rajewsky N. Widespread changes in protein synthesis induced by microRNAs. Nature. 2008;**455**(7209):58-63

[18] Kemp JR, Unal H, Desnoyer R, Yue H, Bhatnagar A, Karnik SS. Angiotensin II-regulated microRNA 483-3p directly targets multiple components of the renin-angiotensin system. Journal of Molecular and Cellular Cardiology. 2014;**75**:25-39

[19] Friedman RC, Farh KK-H, Burge CB, Bartel DP. Most mammalian mRNAs are conserved targets of microRNAs. Genome Research. 2009;**19**(1):92-105

[20] Ambros V, Bartel B, Bartel DP, Burge CB, Carrington JC, Chen X, et al. A uniform system for microRNA annotation. RNA. 2003;**9**(3):277-279

[21] Griffiths-Jones S. miRBase: The microRNA sequence database. Methods in Molecular Biology. 2006;**342**:129-138

[22] Creemers EE, Tijsen AJ, Pinto YM. Circulating microRNAs: Novel biomarkers and extracellular communicators in cardiovascular disease? Circulation Research. 2012;**110**(3):483-495

[23] Kinet V, Halkein J, Dirkx E, Windt LJD. Cardiovascular extracellular microRNAs: Emerging diagnostic markers and mechanisms of cell-to-cell RNA communication. Frontiers in Genetics. 2013;**4**:214

[24] Fabbri M, Paone A, Calore F, Galli R, Croce CM. A new role for microRNAs, as ligands of toll-like receptors. RNA Biology. 2013;**10**(2):169-174

[25] Bernstein E, Kim SY, Carmell MA, Murchison EP, Alcorn H, Li MZ, et al. Dicer is essential for mouse development. Nature Genetics. 2003;**35**(3):215-217

[26] Huang C-CJ, Yao HHC. Inactivation of Dicer1 in steroidogenic factor 1-positive cells reveals tissue-specific requirement for Dicer1 in adrenal, testis, and ovary. BMC Developmental Biology. 2010;**10**(1):66

[27] Romero DG, Plonczynski MW, Carvajal CA, Gomez-Sanchez EP, Gomez-Sanchez CE. Microribonucleic acid-21 increases aldosterone secretion and proliferation in H295R human adrenocortical cells. Endocrinology. 2008;**149**(5):2477-2483

[28] Robertson S, MacKenzie SM, Alvarez-Madrazo S, Diver LA, Lin J, Stewart PM, et al. MicroRNA-24 is a novel regulator of aldosterone and cortisol production in the human adrenal cortex. Hypertension. 2013;**62**(3):572-578

[29] Robertson S, Diver LA, Alvarez-Madrazo S, Livie C, Ejaz A, Fraser R, et al. Regulation of Corticosteroidogenic genes by MicroRNAs. International Journal of Endocrinology. 2017;**2017**(6):2021903-2021911

[30] Butterworth MB. MicroRNAs and the regulation of aldosterone signaling in the kidney. American Journal of Physiology. Cell Physiology. 2015;**308**(7):C521-C527

[31] Nusrin S, Tong SKH, Chaturvedi G, Wu RSS, Giesy JP, Kong RYC. Regulation of CYP11B1 and CYP11B2 steroidogenic genes by hypoxia-inducible miR-10b in H295R cells. Marine Pollution Bulletin. 2014;**85**(2):344-351

[32] Maharjan S, Mopidevi B, Kaw MK, Puri N, Kumar A. Human aldosterone synthase gene polymorphism promotes miRNA binding and regulates gene expression. Physiological Genomics. 2014;**46**(24):860-865. DOI: 10.1152/physiolgenomics.00084.2014

[33] Hu Z, Shen W-J, Kraemer FB, Azhar S. Regulation of adrenal and

ovarian steroidogenesis by miR-132. Journal of Molecular Endocrinology. 2017;**59**(3):269-283

[34] Lenzini L, Caroccia B, Campos AG, Fassina A, Belloni AS, Seccia TM, et al. Lower expression of the TWIK-related acid-sensitive K+ channel 2 (TASK-2) gene is a hallmark of aldosterone-producing adenoma causing human primary aldosteronism. The Journal of Clinical Endocrinology and Metabolism. 2014;**99**(4):E674-E682

[35] Marques FZ, Campain AE, Tomaszewski M, Zukowska-Szczechowska E, Yang YHJ, Charchar FJ, et al. Gene expression profiling reveals renin mRNA overexpression in human hypertensive kidneys and a role for microRNAs. Hypertension. 2011;**58**(6):1093-1098

[36] Assié G, Letouzé E, Fassnacht M, Jouinot A, Luscap W, Barreau O, et al. Integrated genomic characterization of adrenocortical carcinoma. Nature Genetics. 2014;**46**(6):607-612

[37] Bimpaki EI, Iliopoulos D, Moraitis A, Stratakis CA. MicroRNA signature in massive macronodular adrenocortical disease and implications for adrenocortical tumourigenesis. Clinical Endocrinology. 2010;**72**(6):744-751

[38] Chabre O, Libé R, Assie G, Barreau O, Bertherat J, Bertagna X, et al. Serum miR-483-5p and miR-195 are predictive of recurrence risk in adrenocortical cancer patients. Endocrine-Related Cancer. 2013;**20**(4):579-594

[39] He J, Cao Y, Su T, Jiang Y, Jiang L, Zhou W, et al. Downregulation of miR-375 in aldosterone-producing adenomas promotes tumor cell growth via MTDH. Clinical Endocrinology. 2015;**83**(4):581-589

[40] Iliopoulos D, Bimpaki EI, Nesterova M, Stratakis CA. MicroRNA signature of primary pigmented nodular adrenocortical disease: Clinical correlations and regulation of Wnt signaling. Cancer Research. 2009;**69**(8):3278-3282

[41] Ozata DM, Caramuta S, Velazquez-Fernandez D, Akçakaya P, Xie H, Höög A, et al. The role of microRNA deregulation in the pathogenesis of adrenocortical carcinoma. Endocrine-Related Cancer. 2011;**18**(6):643-655

[42] Patel D, Boufraqech M, Jain M, Zhang L, He M, Gesuwan K, et al. MiR-34a and miR-483-5p are candidate serum biomarkers for adrenocortical tumors. Surgery. 2013;**154**(6):1224-8–discussion1229

[43] Patterson EE, Holloway AK, Weng J, Fojo T, Kebebew E. MicroRNA profiling of adrenocortical tumors reveals miR-483 as a marker of malignancy. Cancer. 2011;**117**(8):1630-1639

[44] Perge P, Butz H, Pezzani R, Bancos I, Nagy Z, Pálóczi K, et al. Evaluation and diagnostic potential of circulating extracellular vesicle-associated microRNAs in adrenocortical tumors. Scientific Reports. 2017;**7**(1):5474

[45] Perge P, Decmann Á, Pezzani R, Bancos I, Fassina A, Luconi M, et al. Analysis of circulating extracellular vesicle-associated microRNAs in cortisol-producing adrenocortical tumors. Endocrine. 2018;**59**(2):280-287

[46] Schmitz KJ, Helwig J, Bertram S, Sheu SY, Suttorp AC, Seggewiss J, et al. Differential expression of microRNA-675, microRNA-139-3p and microRNA-335 in benign and malignant adrenocortical tumours. Journal of Clinical Pathology. 2011; **64**(6):529-535

[47] Soon PSH, Tacon LJ, Gill AJ, Bambach CP, Sywak MS, Campbell PR, et al. miR-195 and miR-483-5p identified as predictors of poor prognosis in adrenocortical

cancer. Clinical Cancer Research. 2009;**15**(24):7684-7692

[48] Szabó DR, Luconi M, Szabó PM, Tóth M, Szücs N, Horányi J, et al. Analysis of circulating microRNAs in adrenocortical tumors. Laboratory Investigation. 2014;**94**(3):331-339

[49] Tömböl Z, Szabó PM, Molnár V, Wiener Z, Tölgyesi G, Horányi J, et al. Integrative molecular bioinformatics study of human adrenocortical tumors: MicroRNA, tissue-specific target prediction, and pathway analysis. Endocrine-Related Cancer. 2009;**16**(3):895-906

[50] Velazquez-Fernandez D, Caramuta S, Ozata DM, Lu M, Höög A, Bäckdahl M, et al. MicroRNA expression patterns associated with Hyperfunctioning and non-Hyperfunctioning phenotypes in adrenocortical adenomas. European Journal of Endocrinology. 2014;**170**(4):583-591

[51] Zheng S, Cherniack AD, Dewal N, Moffitt RA, Danilova L, Murray BA, et al. Comprehensive pan-genomic characterization of adrenocortical carcinoma. Cancer Cell. 2016;**29**(5):723-736

[52] Singh P, Soon PSH, Feige J-J, Chabre O, Zhao JT, Cherradi N, et al. Dysregulation of microRNAs in adrenocortical tumors. Molecular and Cellular Endocrinology. 2012;**351**(1):118-128

[53] Sõber S, Laan M, Annilo T. MicroRNAs miR-124 and miR-135a are potential regulators of the mineralocorticoid receptor gene (NR3C2) expression. Biochemical and Biophysical Research Communications. 2010;**391**(1):727-732

[54] Vreugdenhil E, Verissimo CSL, Mariman R, Kamphorst JT, Barbosa JS, Zweers T, et al. MicroRNA 18 and 124a down-regulate the glucocorticoid receptor: Implications for glucocorticoid responsiveness in the brain. Endocrinology. 2009;**150**(5):2220-2228

[55] Sempere LF, Freemantle S, Pitha-Rowe I, Moss E, Dmitrovsky E, Ambros V. Expression profiling of mammalian microRNAs uncovers a subset of brain-expressed microRNAs with possible roles in murine and human neuronal differentiation. Genome Biology. 2004;**5**(3):R13

[56] Mannironi C, Camon J, De Vito F, Biundo A, De Stefano ME, Persiconi I, et al. Acute stress alters amygdala microRNA miR-135a and miR-124 expression: Inferences for corticosteroid dependent stress response. PLoS One. 2013;**8**(9):e73385

[57] Hamzei Taj S, Kho W, Aswendt M, Collmann FM, Green C, Adamczak J, et al. Dynamic modulation of microglia/macrophage polarization by miR-124 after focal cerebral ischemia. Journal of Neuroimmune Pharmacology. 2016;**11**(4):733-748

[58] Hamzei Taj S, Kho W, Riou A, Wiedermann D, Hoehn M. MiRNA-124 induces neuroprotection and functional improvement after focal cerebral ischemia. Biomaterials. 2016;**91**:151-165

[59] Doeppner TR, Doehring M, Bretschneider E, Zechariah A, Kaltwasser B, Müller B, et al. MicroRNA-124 protects against focal cerebral ischemia via mechanisms involving Usp14-dependent REST degradation. Acta Neuropathologica. 2013;**126**(2):251-265

[60] Bretschneider M, Busch B, Mueller D, Nolze A, Schreier B, Gekle M, et al. Activated mineralocorticoid receptor regulates micro-RNA-29b in vascular smooth muscle cells. The FASEB Journal. 2016;**30**(4):1610-1622

[61] Khanna S, Rink C, Ghoorkhanian R, Gnyawali S, Heigel M, Wijesinghe DS,

et al. Loss of miR-29b following acute ischemic stroke contributes to neural cell death and infarct size. Journal of Cerebral Blood Flow and Metabolism. 2013;**33**(8):1197-1206

[62] Cao L, Zhang Y, Zhang S, Jiang T-P, Chen L, Liu J, et al. MicroRNA-29b alleviates oxygen and glucose deprivation/reperfusion-induced injury via inhibition of the p53-dependent apoptosis pathway in N2a neuroblastoma cells. Experimental and Therapeutic Medicine. 2018;**15**(1):67-74

[63] Shi G, Liu Y, Liu T, Yan W, Liu X, Wang Y, et al. Upregulated miR-29b promotes neuronal cell death by inhibiting Bcl2L2 after ischemic brain injury. Experimental Brain Research. 2012;**216**(2):225-230

[64] Rezaei M, Andrieu T, Neuenschwander S, Bruggmann R, Mordasini D, Frey FJ, et al. Regulation of 11β-hydroxysteroid dehydrogenase type 2 by microRNA. Hypertension. 2014;**64**(4):860-866

[65] Simonson B, Das S. MicroRNA therapeutics: The next magic bullet? Mini Reviews in Medicinal Chemistry. 2015;**15**(6):467-474

[66] van Rooij E, Kauppinen S. Development of microRNA therapeutics is coming of age. EMBO Molecular Medicine. 2014;**6**(7):851-864

[67] Srivastava K, Tyagi K. Single nucleotide polymorphisms of microRNA in cardiovascular diseases. Clinica Chimica Acta. 2018;**478**:101-110

Chapter 14

# Post-Translational Modification of MR Activity

*Diego Alvarez de la Rosa and Natalia Serrano-Morillas*

## Abstract

The mineralocorticoid receptor (MR) is a ligand-activated transcription factor that transduces the effects of aldosterone and glucocorticoids in a tissue- and cell type-specific ways. Differential regulation of MR by post-translational modifications (PTMs) has been proposed to play a key role in modulating its function. In addition, modifications of other proteins that physically or functionally interact with MR add an additional layer of regulation to aldosterone or glucocorticoid signaling. In this chapter, we will summarize the main post-translational modifications of MR described so far, discussing their possible implications in the physiological and pathological roles of the receptor. We will also discuss post-translational modulation of other proteins impacting MR function such as heat shock protein 90 or 11ß-hydroxysteroid dehydrogenase type 2.

**Keywords:** mineralocorticoid receptor, aldosterone, glucocorticoids, steroid receptors, protein modification, phosphorylation, Ubiquitylation, SUMOylation, acetylation

## 1. Introduction

The mineralocorticoid receptor (MR) is widely expressed and performs different physiological and pathological roles depending not only on the activating ligand (aldosterone vs. glucocorticoids) but also on context [1–3]. This includes co-expression or not with 11ß-hydroxysteroid dehydrogenase (11ßHSD2) to control local levels of glucocorticoids [4, 5], differential interaction with co-regulators [6] or the physiological mechanism behind the increased circulating levels of aldosterone [7], to name a few.

Multiple levels of regulation controlling MR activity have been described. Transcription of the Nr3c2 gene, coding for the receptor, is modulated by different stimuli and depends on two alternative promoters [1, 8]. Transcriptional control depending on epigenetic mechanisms has also been described [1]. MR transcripts undergo alternative splicing, although the physiological significance of these variants is uncertain [9]. Post-translational control includes regulation of MR mRNA stability by proteins such as Tis11b and HuR [10, 11] or siRNAs such as miR-124 and miR-135a [12–14]. Some MR polymorphisms have been shown to produce different translational efficiencies *in vitro* [15]. Once synthesized, MR activation depends on ligand availability, which in turn can be modulated by co-expression of 11ßHSD2, which creates a low glucocorticoid-microenvironment by metabolizing biologically active glucocorticoids to their 11-keto, biologically inactive derivatives [4, 5]. Activation also depends on the interaction of MR with co-chaperones, including Hsp70 and Hsp90 [16–18]. MR can also be activated in a ligand-independent manner by the

 IntechOpen

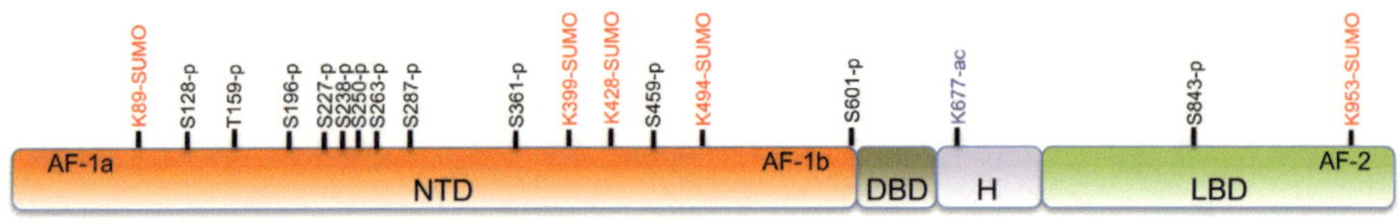


**Figure 1.**
*Schematic representation of MR protein domains and the location of post-translational modifications with demonstrated functional effects. NTD, $NH_2$-terminal domain; DBD, DNA-binding domain; H, hinge domain; LBD, ligand-binding domain; AF, activation function. Phosphorylation sites (p) are shown with black letters; acetylation sites (ac) are shown in blue and SUMOylation sites (SUMO) are shown in red. The length of each domain and the position of each site are drawn to scale.*

GTPase Rac1 [19] or by signaling through the angiotensin II receptor 1 [20]. Once activated, MR forms homodimers or, potentially, heterodimers with related steroid receptors including the glucocorticoid receptor (GR) [21, 22], translocates to the nucleus and interacts with DNA to modulate gene transcription with the help of co-regulators. This provides the biological readout of hormone signaling and involves multiple and complex regulatory steps. In addition, MR activation can initiate rapid signaling events outside the nucleus that modulate cell response and are essential to facilitate transcriptional responses [23, 24].

Every step of MR activation and its impact on cell responses is subject to be modulated by post-translational modifications (PTMs) of the receptor itself or of other proteins physically or functionally interacting with it. PTMs of MR have been previously reviewed in detailed [25] (**Figure 1**). It has long been known that MR is a phosphoprotein [26, 27] and multiple MR residues have been described as potential phosphorylation targets [25]. Most of these amino acids are serine residues, although threonine phosphorylation has been detected using phospho-specific antibodies [28]. One study reported phosphorylation in threonine residues T73[1] and S737 [29], although the functional impact of these modifications has not been studied. Of note, in a more recent study analyzing MR phosphopeptides by liquid chromatography with tandem mass spectrometry, Shibata et al. described 16 different phosphorylated serine residues, but found no evidence of threonine or tyrosine phosphorylation [7]. In addition, other chemical modifications of MR have been described, including ubiquitylation [30–33], SUMOylation [32, 34, 35], acetylation [36] and oxidation [37]. In this chapter, we will update the main known PTMs directly or indirectly affecting MR and focus on their consequences on MR activity.

## 2. Post-translational modifications that alter MR stability

The abundance of naïve MR likely impacts the potency of receptor-mediated cell responses. There are numerous examples in the literature describing alteration of MR steady-state abundance in different physiological or pathological situations [2]. Changes in receptor abundance can arise from changes in its synthesis or in its degradation rates. In addition, an activation-induced MR degradation also seems to participate in controlling hormone responses [33]. Several MR PTMs have been shown to affect receptor half-life in the cell, both in the basal state and after hormonal stimulation.

Basal level of MR expression appears to be controlled by ubiquitylation (**Figure 2**). In the naïve state, MR is monoubiquitylated at an unknown lysine. This modification is stabilized by association to Tsg101 (tumor suppressor gene 101), increasing the half-life of the receptor [31]. This mechanism is shared by related

[1] All amino acid numbers in this chapter refer to the human MR sequence (UniProt P08235).

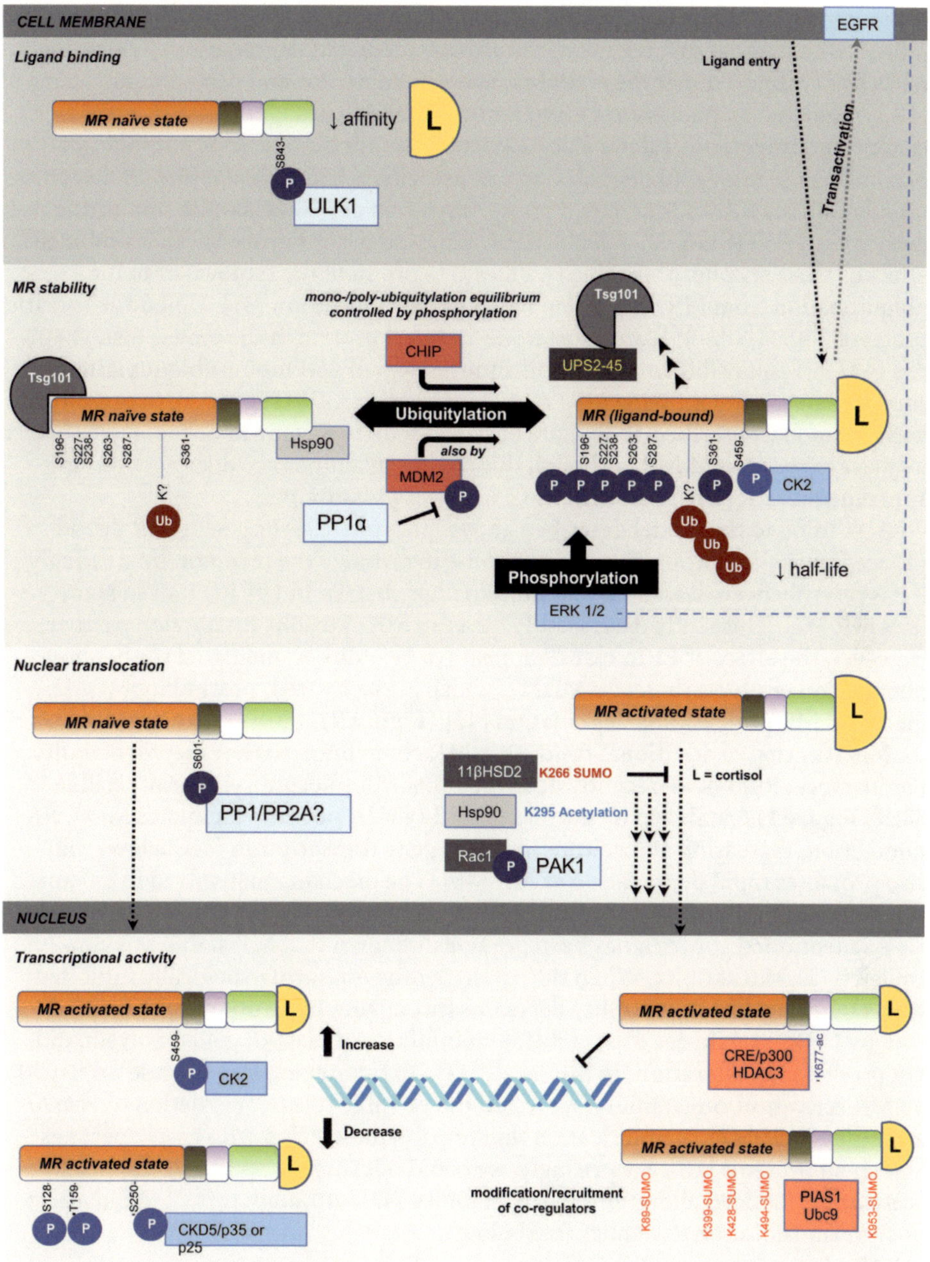


**Figure 2.**
*Schematic representation of well-characterized post-translational modifications affecting mineralocorticoid receptor ligand binding, stability, nuclear translocation or transcriptional activity. MR domain are colored as in* **Figure 1***. L, ligand.*

steroid receptors such as the androgen, glucocorticoid and estrogen receptors [38–40]. In addition, it has been shown that poly-ubiquitylation occurs when Hsp90 activity diminishes and the cytosolic heterocomplex recruits ubiquitin-ligase CHIP decreasing receptor expression level [41]. Taken together, these data suggest that equilibrium between mono- and poly-ubiquitylation contributes to regulating naïve MR abundance.

Ligand activation of MR induces receptor degradation through the proteasome, acting as a brake to attenuate aldosterone responses [33]. Subsequent studies demonstrated that MR is poly-ubiquitylated in response to hormonal stimulation [30–32, 42], a signal that triggers proteasomal-mediated degradation. Interestingly, it has been proposed that the equilibrium between mono- and poly-ubiquitylation of MR is regulated by phosphorylation. Remarkably, MR antagonists such as spironolactone and finerenone totally block aldosterone-induced receptor phosphorylation, preventing the increased degradation rate associated to activation [43]. Aldosterone rapidly induces ERK1/2-mediated phosphorylation of MR at six different serine residues in the NTD (S196, S227, S238, S263, S287 and S361; **Figure 1**). The combined effect of these six phosphoserine residues is to promote the removal of mono-ubiquitylation from MR, triggering receptor destabilization [31]. Ubiquitin-specific protease 2-45 (USP2-45), an aldosterone-induced protein in the mouse distal nephron [44], is responsible for the ligand-induced loss of MR mono-ubiquitylation, simultaneously destabilizing MR/Tsg101 interaction [30] (**Figure 2**). in agreement with the model described above data obtained with *usp2* gene knockout mice showed increase expression of MR, although this change in abundance does not produce apparent alterations in sodium balance or blood pressure [45].

According to the model described above, phosphatases opposing MR ligand-induced phosphorylation should contribute to stabilize the receptor. Interestingly, it has recently been described that protein phosphatase 1α (PP1α) indeed stabilizes MR [42]. This study described PP1α as an MR cytosolic interaction partner. However, the effect of PP1α on MR appears to be indirect, mediated the dephosphorylation of ubiquitin ligase MDM2, which is inactivated, precluding MDM2-mediated MR proteasomal degradation [42] (**Figure 2**).

Modification of additional residues in MR contributes to the receptor stability. For instance, Ruhs et al. recently described that MR phosphorylation at residue S459 (**Figure 1**), catalyzed by casein kinase 2 (CK2), not only facilitates MR-DNA interaction, increasing aldosterone-induced gene transcription (see below), but also promotes rapid degradation of MR [46]. The mechanism involved in enhanced MR degradation by S459 phosphorylation is unknown.

As mentioned above, it has been previously shown that MR stability is controlled by Hps90 activity. When the co-chaperone is pharmacologically inhibited with tanespimycin, MR stability decreases through increase ubiquitylation mediated by CHIP [41]. In contrast, a different inhibitor of Hsp90, geldanamycin, did not produce any alterations in MR levels [17]. To further explore the role on Hsp90 on MR activation and stability, we tested the possible role of acetylation of Hsp90 at residue K295 [47], a modification that impairs interaction with co-chaperones and client proteins [48]. Surprisingly, we could not find any evidence for Hsp90 acetylation-induced alterations in MR stability [47], although this PTM did affect nuclear translocation dynamics (see below).

## 3. Post-translational modifications that directly or indirectly control ligand binding to MR

Ligand binding capacity of MR is not an exclusively intrinsic property of the ligand-binding domain (LBD) of this receptor. It has long been known that MR association to the chaperone Hsp90 is essential for aldosterone binding [49, 50]. In addition, the full-length MR sequence is required to bind aldosterone with high affinity, suggesting that areas outside the LBD contribute to folding of the receptor in a competent state [51]. The idea that PTMs may contribute to regulate MR ligand binding came from the observation that phosphatase treatment of cytosolic extracts greatly diminish aldosterone binding to MR [27]. This suggested that basal phosphorylation in serine/threonine residues is essential for the competency of the receptor to bind ligands. However, these experiments did not allow distinguishing whether the phosphorylation takes place in the receptor itself or in other proteins of the cytosolic heterocomplex containing the naïve receptor. More recently, direct evidence implicating phosphorylation on ligand binding to MR has emerged. Phosphorylation of MR at residue S843 has been shown to diminish the affinity of the receptor for aldosterone and corticosterone [7]. This process is mediated by protein kinase ULK1 [52]. Interestingly, phosphomimetic mutants cannot be activated by aldosterone or cortisol even when the concentration of the hormones is one to two orders of magnitude higher than the calculated *Kd*, indicating that phosphorylation affects not only ligand binding but also ligand-induced receptor activation [53]. Importantly, phosphorylation of MR at residue S843 acts as a dominant-negative modification, inhibiting wild type receptors upon dimerization, which greatly amplifies the impact of this event on total MR activity [53].

Ligand binding to MR is also affected by oxidation. It has long been known that MR is a highly unstable protein and this has been ascribed to sulfhydryl oxidation, which prevents aldosterone binding [37, 54]. In particular, cysteine 849 and 942 appear to be responsible for this effect, since site-directed mutagenesis at these positions eliminate steroid binding to the receptor [55]. This phenomenon appears to be relevant in vivo, since inhibition of glutathione synthetase in mice abrogated aldosterone binding to kidney MR [56]. Since oxidative stress decreases aldosterone binding and activation and aldosterone binding decreases with age, it has been suggested that oxidation of MR could be an important mediator of aging in the kidney [57].

In classic aldosterone tissues like the kidney or the distal colon and in certain neurons, glucocorticoid accessibility to MR is crucially controlled by co-expression of 11ßHSD2, which metabolizes glucocorticoids to produce biologically inactive, 11-keto derivatives [4]. Therefore, transcriptional or post-transcriptional modulations of this enzyme potentially have a large impact on MR activity. We have recently described that 11ßHSD2 is modified by SUMOylation at residue K266 [58] (**Figure 2**). While the effect of SUMOylation on enzymatic activity is mild, its impact on MR activation process is puzzling. In spite of being enzymatically active, non-SUMOylatable mutant 11ßHSD2-K266R was unable to prevent MR nuclear translocation when cells were treated with cortisol, unlike the wild type enzyme [58]. The same was detected when 11ßHSD2 SUMOylation is reversed by co-expression of sentrin-specific protease 1 (SENP1), a protease that catalyzes SUMO deconjugation. However, MR translocated to the nucleus under these conditions does not increase transcriptional response to cortisol and shows diminished recruitment of co-activators [58]. Therefore, 11ßHSD2 SUMOylation drastically alters the ability of this enzyme to regulate MR subcellular localization, although the molecular mechanisms involved in this effect remain to be elucidated.

## 4. Post-translational modifications that alter MR nuclear translocation

Long-term, genomic actions of MR depend on its nuclear localization and interaction with chromatin. While some steroid receptor (ER and PR) are constitutively nuclear, naïve MR is considered to be mainly cytosolic, where it forms part of a heterocomplex with chaperones and other proteins, translocating to the nucleus after ligand binding. In fact, it is most common to find MR evenly distributed between nucleus and cytosol, with a clear nuclear shift when exposed to ligands. This mode of action fits well with data obtained in some models of cultured cell lines, such as COS-7 cells or HEK cells [17, 43, 47, 59] and native tissues [60–62]. In certain tissues and cell types, MR can be found in the nucleus even in the absence of ligand [18, 60, 61]. Therefore, it appears that nuclear translocation plays an important role in MR regulation, although the physiological relevance of this step may strongly vary between different tissues or cell types.

Nuclear translocation has been studied with much more detail in the case of other steroid receptors, including GR, which shares significant sequence homology with MR. In the case of GR, two independent nuclear translocation pathways have been proposed, one that depends on Hsp90 and the attachment of the ligand-bound heterocomplex to microtubules and one where monomers or dimers of GR translocate independently of this machinery [63]. In the case of MR, there is strong evidence indicating that nuclear translocation occurs in an Hsp90-dependent way, with dissociation between the chaperone and the receptor occurring in the nucleus [16, 17]. Inhibition of Hsp90 abrogates hormone binding to MR and nuclear translocation of the receptor, although cells with low levels of Hsp90 expression such as cardiomyocytes present constitutively nuclear MR that can be activated by aldosterone or cortisol [18]. This result suggested that fine-tuning of Hsp90 activity could play a role in controlling MR subcellular localization. Therefore, we decided to explore the role of Hsp90 acetylation at residue K295 in MR nuclear translocation [47]. This modification, regulated by histone deacetylase 6 (HDAC6), inhibits Hsp90 and has been shown to decrease GR and AR activity [48]. In the case of MR, increased acetylation of Hsp90 does not affect ligand binding or transcriptional activity, but alters subcellular dynamics, accelerating MR nuclear import. Given the differential effects of Hsp90 K295 acetylation on MR and GR, it has been proposed that this modification may balance corticosteroid signaling between both receptors when co-expressed in the same cell [47].

Nuclear translocation of MR critically depends on nuclear localization signals (NLS) present in the sequence of the receptor. Three independent NLS has been identified in MR: NL0, 1 and 2 [64]. Among these three, NL0 has been implicated in nuclear localization of the naïve receptor. NL0 was mapped to amino acids 550–602 of human MR. In this area, a cluster of five serine residues and one threonine between amino acids 590 and 602 is important for NL0 activity, since its deletion significantly decreases naïve MR nuclear localization, although it does not abrogate ligand-induced translocation [64]. Interestingly, phosphomimicking mutation S601D (**Figures 1** and **2**) eliminated NL0 activity, resulting in a fully cytosolic MR localization in the absence of ligand. Conversely, non-phosphorylatable mutant S601A resulted in a significant nuclear shift of naïve MR [64]. Therefore, phosphorylation/dephosphorylation balance at S601 may be an important mechanism for controlling MR subcellular distribution in the absence of ligand. The effect of this equilibrium on the physiology of the receptor remains to be studied. Both *in vitro* and *in vivo* experiments indicate that a protein phosphatase from the PP1/PP2A subgroup regulates ligand-induced MR trafficking into the nucleus [65], although it is unclear whether this results from dephosphorylation of MR or other associated proteins such as Hsp90.

Aldosterone-induced nuclear translocation is potentiated by Rac1-mediated phosphorylation of p21-activated kinase 1 (PAK1) (**Figure 2**). This signaling pathway is relevant in the development of chronic kidney disease [19] and in cardiac remodeling and inflammation induced by blood pressure variability in the context of hypertension [66]. It remains to be determined whether PAK1 directly phosphorylates MR and whether it promotes its activity in addition to receptor translocation, as it has been described with estrogen receptors [67].

## 5. Post-translational modifications controlling MR activation and modulating gene transcription

In addition to the mechanisms discussed above modulating MR ligand binding, stability and subcellular localization, additional PTMs regulate the ability of MR to modulate gene transcription, potentially altering the efficacy of the receptor without altering its affinity for agonists. This possibility was suggested after studying a human polymorphism introducing the mutation Y73C, which increases MR transactivation in response to aldosterone by twofold, without changing the $EC_{50}$ [68]. Residue Y73 is placed in AF1a and therefore could modulate interaction with transcriptional co-activators. However, there are no further reports demonstrating that this potential phosphorylation site is actually modified in the protein. Le Moellic et al. proposed a possible role for phosphorylation in controlling MR transcriptional activity [28]. This study found that protein kinase C α (PKCα) mediates rapid MR phosphorylation at serine/threonine residues after stimulation with aldosterone, which presumably acts through a membrane receptor [28]. Blocking PKCα during this early, non-genomic phase precludes the development of the genomic phase. However, whether this effect is directly due to lack of activation of MR or, alternatively modulation of other aspects of the receptor such as aldosterone binding or nuclear translocation was not studied.

More direct evidence of phosphorylation involvement in controlling MR activity came from studying the effect of cyclin-dependent kinase 5 (CKD5) on the receptor. CKD5 has been proposed to phosphorylate two residues in the NTD of MR (S128[2], T159 and S250; **Figure 1**), producing a very powerful decrease in MR transcriptional activity without affecting nuclear translocation [69] (**Figure 2**). The phosphorylation is mediated by direct interaction of the CKD5/p35 or CKD5/p25 complexes with MR LBD in an aldosterone-dependent way [69]. T159 and S250 phosphorylation could be confirmed by mass spectrometry, while phosphorylation at residue S128 was inferred from mutagenesis studies. Mutation of all three residues to alanine was necessary to abolish CKD5-dependent MR inhibition [69].

As indicated above, CK2-dependent MR S459 phosphorylation (**Figure 1**) facilitates MR-DNA interaction, at least in an *in vitro* assay, and increases aldosterone-induced gene transcription [46]. This effect is partially mediated by the NTD of the receptor, where the phosphorylation site is located, possibly by promoting MR-CK2 interaction in a process that needs Hsp90 activity. Interestingly, phosphomimetic mutation S459D not only increased aldosterone-induced responses but also resulted in ligand-independent transcriptional activation (**Figure 2**). Modeling a pro-inflammatory environment by treating cultured cells with a cytokine cocktail increased CK2 expression, resulting in enhanced MR modification, leading to increase receptor activity and activating NFκB signaling and thus enhancing the expression of proinflammatory genes [46]. This could provide a mechanism to help explain the deleterious effects of MR activity in the context of inflammation, as demonstrated in endothelial cells [71]. The mechanism underlying altered MR activity by CK2 phosphorylation remains unclear. The authors speculated that S459 phosphorylation could induce a conformational change that promotes MR-DNA interaction or alternatively enhance MR association with transcriptional co-activators [46]. The latter possibility is plausible, since residue S459 lies in AF-1b within the NTD, a region involved in the interaction between MR and transcriptional co-regulators in a ligand-independent manner [72].

MR acetylation at residue K677 (**Figures 1** and **2**) inhibits its transcriptional activity by preventing MR and RNA polymerase II recruitment to target gene promoters. Surprisingly, K677 acetylation did not affect MR nuclear translocation [36], even though this residue is located in NL1. This study and subsequent work by

---

[2] Human MR has serine residues at positions 127 and 129, but not at position 128. The authors refer to this residue as residing "in the perfect motif of CDK5 phosphorylation site" [69], which is [S/T]PX[K/R/H] [70]. Residue S129 fits this description and therefore it is likely that the authors refer to it instead of residue 128, which is a methionine.

the same group identified CREB-binding protein (CRE)/p300 as the acetylase and HDAC3 as the deacetylase responsible for modifying K677 [36, 73] (**Figure 2**). The molecular basis for the lack of MR binding to target promoters when acetylated at residue K677, which is away from the DBD, is unknown.

Addition of small ubiquitin modifier (SUMO) proteins to five different lysine residues in MR (**Figure 1**), all located within a SUMOylation consensus site, has been proposed to alter its transcriptional activity and co-regulator recruitment [32, 34, 35]. The first description of MR SUMOylation followed the identification of protein inhibitor of activated STAT-1 (PIAS1), a SUMO E3 ligase, as an MR interacting partner using a yeast two-hybrid assay using the NTD of the receptor as bait [34]. The functional consequences of PIAS1-mediated SUMOylation are complex. Co-expression of PIAS1 with MR led to repression of receptor-mediated gene transactivation in two different model promoters, the mouse mammary tumor virus promoter (MMTV) and an artificial glucocorticoid response element (GRE) promoter [34]. However, introducing non-SUMOylatable mutations in the receptor did not produce the expected opposite effects in MMTV, which was unaffected. In contrast, the same mutations increased MR activity on the GRE promoter. Taken together, these results suggest that the effect of PIAS1 on MR is promoter-dependent and may occur through different mechanisms including direct receptor SUMOylation and perhaps SUMOylation of transcriptional co-regulators. In addition, PIAS1 may exert additional modulatory activities independent of its SUMO ligase activity. This possibility is suggested by the observation that a PIAS1 SUMO ligase-dead mutant W363A is still able to inhibit androgen receptor transcriptional activity [74]. The complexity of SUMOylation-dependent regulation of MR activity is illustrated by the fact that the E2 SUMO ligase responsible for its SUMOylation, Ubc9, is able to recruit steroid receptor coactivator-1 (SRC-1) to form a complex with MR and activate its transcriptional activity independently of addition of SUMO residues to the receptor [35]. Therefore, the two enzymes playing a role on MR SUMOylation, PIAS1 and Ubc9 (**Figure 2**), can have opposing effects on the receptor transcriptional activity in a promoter-dependent way, suggesting that many of these actions occur through modification/recruitment of co-regulators.

## 6. Summary and perspectives

Many PTM sites have been identified in MR, but only some of them have been experimentally linked to alterations in MR function (**Figures 1** and **2**). These include modulation of MR ligand-binding ability, stability, nuclear translocation and gene transactivation. In addition, MR-associated proteins such as Hsp90, 11ßHSD2 or ubiquitin ligases such as MDM2 are also modulated by PTMs, adding further regulatory possibilities for fine-tuning MR activity. This complex picture is not unexpected, given the near ubiquitous distribution of MR and the diverse functional roles played by this receptor in response to two different types of ligands, mineralocorticoids and glucocorticoids. Therefore, it will not be surprising to find new PTMs directly or indirectly implicated in the regulation of MR activity. In addition, ligand-dependency of MR PTMs needs to be addressed with more detail. In principle, changes in MR conformation induced by different ligands could affect accessibility to modification sites. Differential PTM in response to different agonists or antagonists could potentially underlie divergent effects of MR-mediated signaling events. Generally, detailed characterization of the functional effects of PTMs is feasible in cultured cells. However, the main challenge remains to elucidate the physiological or pathological importance of these modifications in whole organisms and the clinical relevance that they may have in humans.

Due to the nature of steroid receptors, including MR, they are inherently druggable targets. Excess signaling through MR has now been firmly established as an important factor in hypertension, heart failure and ocular diseases, with compelling evidence indicating further implication in brain, vascular, renal, metabolic and skin diseases [2]. Therefore, there is renewed interest in developing MR modulators with tissue-specific characteristics that may reduce or avoid undesirable side effects. Given the high degree of homology between LBDs of different steroid receptors, a significant effort to develop nonsteroidal inhibitors is underway [75]. In addition, it is possible that allosteric inhibitors or small molecules able to modulate MR protein-protein interactions may provide new strategies to manipulate the system. PTMs may have an important effect on drug binding and future drug development, both for competitive and allosteric modulators. In fact, recent *in silico* approaches have explored this possibility, exploiting the increasing availability of high-throughput PTM screenings and high-resolution protein three-dimensional structures [76]. It can be expected that improved PTM screening, combined with structural and computational methods will provide new testable hypotheses regarding the regulation of steroid receptors and possible new ways of pharmacological modulation of their activities.

## Acknowledgements

This publication is based upon work from the EU COST Action ADMIRE BM1301 in Aldosterone and Mineralocorticoid Receptor Physiology and Pathophysiology www.admirecosteu.com. We would like to thank Dr. N. Faresse for helpful suggestions on the manuscript. The work in the author's laboratory was supported by Ministerio de Economía y Competitividad (MINECO, Spain), grant number BFU2016-78374-R.

## Author details

Diego Alvarez de la Rosa* and Natalia Serrano-Morillas
Department of Basic Medical Sciences (Physiology), Institute of Biomedical Technologies, Universidad de La Laguna, Tenerife, Spain

*Address all correspondence to: dalrosa@ull.edu.es

## References

[1] Gomez-Sanchez E, Gomez-Sanchez CE. The multifaceted mineralocorticoid receptor. Comprehensive Physiology. 2014;**4**(3):965-994

[2] Jaisser F, Farman N. Emerging roles of the mineralocorticoid receptor in pathology: Toward new paradigms in clinical pharmacology. Pharmacological Reviews. 2016;**68**(1):49-75

[3] Shibata S. Context-dependent mechanisms modulating aldosterone signaling in the kidney. Clinical and Experimental Nephrology. 2016;**20**(5):663-670

[4] Chapman K, Holmes M, Seckl J. 11beta-hydroxysteroid dehydrogenases: Intracellular gate-keepers of tissue glucocorticoid action. Physiological Reviews. 2013;**93**(3):1139-1206

[5] Funder JW. Apparent mineralocorticoid excess. The Journal of Steroid Biochemistry and Molecular Biology. 2017;**165**(Pt A):151-153

[6] Fuller PJ, Yang J, Young MJ. 30 years of the mineralocorticoid receptor: Coregulators as mediators of mineralocorticoid receptor signaling diversity. The Journal of Endocrinology. 2017;**234**(1):T23-T34

[7] Shibata S, Rinehart J, Zhang J, Moeckel G, Castaneda-Bueno M, Stiegler AL, et al. Mineralocorticoid receptor phosphorylation regulates ligand binding and renal response to volume depletion and hyperkalemia. Cell Metabolism. 2013;**18**(5):660-671

[8] Viengchareun S, Le Menuet D, Martinerie L, Munier M, Pascual-Le Tallec L, Lombes M. The mineralocorticoid receptor: Insights into its molecular and (patho)physiological biology. Nuclear Receptor Signaling. 2007;**5**:e012

[9] Pascual-Le Tallec L, Lombes M. The mineralocorticoid receptor: A journey exploring its diversity and specificity of action. Molecular Endocrinology. 2005;**19**(9):2211-2221

[10] Lema I, Amazit L, Lamribet K, Fagart J, Blanchard A, Lombes M, et al. RNA-binding protein HuR enhances mineralocorticoid signaling in renal KC3AC1 cells under hypotonicity. Cellular and Molecular Life Sciences. 2017;**74**(24):4587-4597

[11] Viengchareun S, Lema I, Lamribet K, Keo V, Blanchard A, Cherradi N, et al. Hypertonicity compromises renal mineralocorticoid receptor signaling through Tis11b-mediated post-transcriptional control. Journal of the American Society of Nephrology. 2014;**25**(10):2213-2221

[12] Butterworth MB, Alvarez de la Rosa D. Regulation of aldosterone Signaling by MicroRNAs. Vitamins and Hormones. 2019;**109**:69-103. in press

[13] Manníroni C, Camon J, De Vito F, Biundo A, De Stefano ME, Persiconi I, et al. Acute stress alters amygdala microRNA miR-135a and miR-124 expression: Inferences for corticosteroid dependent stress response. PLoS ONE. 2013;**8**(9):e73385

[14] Sober S, Laan M, Annilo T. MicroRNAs miR-124 and miR-135a are potential regulators of the mineralocorticoid receptor gene (NR3C2) expression. Biochemical and Biophysical Research Communications. 2010;**391**(1):727-732

[15] van Leeuwen N, Caprio M, Blaya C, Fumeron F, Sartorato P, Ronconi V, et al. The functional c.-2G>C variant of the mineralocorticoid receptor modulates blood pressure, renin, and aldosterone levels. Hypertension. 2010;**56**(5):995-1002

[16] Galigniana MD, Erlejman AG, Monte M, Gomez-Sanchez C, Piwien-Pilipuk G. The hsp90-FKBP52 complex links the mineralocorticoid receptor to motor proteins and persists bound to the receptor in early nuclear events. Molecular and Cellular Biology. 2010;**30**(5):1285-1298

[17] Grossmann C, Ruhs S, Langenbruch L, Mildenberger S, Stratz N, Schumann K, et al. Nuclear shuttling precedes dimerization in mineralocorticoid receptor signaling. Chemistry & Biology. 2012;**19**(6):742-751

[18] Hernandez-Diaz I, Giraldez T, Arnau MR, Smits VA, Jaisser F, Farman N, et al. The mineralocorticoid receptor is a constitutive nuclear factor in cardiomyocytes due to hyperactive nuclear localization signals. Endocrinology. 2010;**151**(8):3888-3899

[19] Shibata S, Nagase M, Yoshida S, Kawarazaki W, Kurihara H, Tanaka H, et al. Modification of mineralocorticoid receptor function by Rac1 GTPase: Implication in proteinuric kidney disease. Nature Medicine. 2008;**14**(12):1370-1376

[20] Jaffe IZ, Mendelsohn ME. Angiotensin II and aldosterone regulate gene transcription via functional mineralocortocoid receptors in human coronary artery smooth muscle cells. Circulation Research. 2005;**96**(6):643-650

[21] Liu W, Wang J, Sauter NK, Pearce D. Steroid receptor heterodimerization demonstrated in vitro and in vivo. Proceedings of the National Academy of Sciences of the United States of America. 1995;**92**(26):12480-12484

[22] Nishi M, Tanaka M, Matsuda K, Sunaguchi M, Kawata M. Visualization of glucocorticoid receptor and mineralocorticoid receptor interactions in living cells with GFP-based fluorescence resonance energy transfer. The Journal of Neuroscience. 2004;**24**(21):4918-4927

[23] Ruhs S, Nolze A, Hubschmann R, Grossmann C. 30 years of the mineralocorticoid receptor: Nongenomic effects via the mineralocorticoid receptor. The Journal of Endocrinology. 2017;**234**(1):T107-TT24

[24] Thomas W, Harvey BJ. Mechanisms underlying rapid aldosterone effects in the kidney. Annual Review of Physiology. 2011;**73**:335-357

[25] Faresse N. Post-translational modifications of the mineralocorticoid receptor: How to dress the receptor according to the circumstances? The Journal of Steroid Biochemistry and Molecular Biology. 2014;**143**:334-342

[26] Alnemri ES, Maksymowych AB, Robertson NM, Litwack G. Overexpression and characterization of the human mineralocorticoid receptor. The Journal of Biological Chemistry. 1991;**266**(27):18072-18081

[27] Galigniana MD. Native rat kidney mineralocorticoid receptor is a phosphoprotein whose transformation to a DNA-binding form is induced by phosphatases. The Biochemical Journal. 1998;**333**(Pt 3):555-563

[28] Le Moellic C, Ouvrard-Pascaud A, Capurro C, Cluzeaud F, Fay M, Jaisser F, et al. Early nongenomic events in aldosterone action in renal collecting duct cells: PKCalpha activation, mineralocorticoid receptor phosphorylation, and cross-talk with the genomic response. Journal of the American Society of Nephrology. 2004;**15**(5):1145-1160

[29] Hirschberg D, Jagerbrink T, Samskog J, Gustafsson M, Stahlberg M, Alvelius G, et al. Detection of phosphorylated peptides in proteomic analyses using microfluidic compact

disk technology. Analytical Chemistry. 2004;**76**(19):5864-5871

[30] Faresse N, Debonneville A, Staub O. USP2-45 represses aldosterone mediated responses by decreasing mineralocorticoid receptor availability. Cellular Physiology and Biochemistry. 2013;**31**(2-3):462-472

[31] Faresse N, Vitagliano JJ, Staub O. Differential ubiquitylation of the mineralocorticoid receptor is regulated by phosphorylation. The FASEB Journal. 2012;**26**(10):4373-4382

[32] Tirard M, Almeida OF, Hutzler P, Melchior F, Michaelidis TM. Sumoylation and proteasomal activity determine the transactivation properties of the mineralocorticoid receptor. Molecular and Cellular Endocrinology. 2007;**268**(1-2):20-29

[33] Yokota K, Shibata H, Kobayashi S, Suda N, Murai A, Kurihara I, et al. Proteasome-mediated mineralocorticoid receptor degradation attenuates transcriptional response to aldosterone. Endocrine Research. 2004;**30**(4):611-616

[34] Tallec LP, Kirsh O, Lecomte MC, Viengchareun S, Zennaro MC, Dejean A, et al. Protein inhibitor of activated signal transducer and activator of transcription 1 interacts with the N-terminal domain of mineralocorticoid receptor and represses its transcriptional activity: Implication of small ubiquitin-related modifier 1 modification. Molecular Endocrinology. 2003;**17**(12):2529-2542

[35] Yokota K, Shibata H, Kurihara I, Kobayashi S, Suda N, Murai-Takeda A, et al. Coactivation of the N-terminal transactivation of mineralocorticoid receptor by Ubc9. The Journal of Biological Chemistry. 2007;**282**(3):1998-2010

[36] Lee HA, Lee DY, Cho HM, Kim SY, Iwasaki Y, Kim IK. Histone deacetylase inhibition attenuates transcriptional activity of mineralocorticoid receptor through its acetylation and prevents development of hypertension. Circulation Research. 2013;**112**(7):1004-1012

[37] Galigniana MD. Stability study on renal type I mineralocorticoid receptor. Life Sciences. 1996;**59**(7):511-521

[38] Burgdorf S, Leister P, Scheidtmann KH. TSG101 interacts with apoptosis-antagonizing transcription factor and enhances androgen receptor-mediated transcription by promoting its monoubiquitination. The Journal of Biological Chemistry. 2004;**279**(17):17524-17534

[39] Ismaili N, Blind R, Garabedian MJ. Stabilization of the unliganded glucocorticoid receptor by TSG101. The Journal of Biological Chemistry. 2005;**280**(12):11120-11126

[40] La Rosa P, Pesiri V, Marino M, Acconcia F. 17beta-Estradiol-induced cell proliferation requires estrogen receptor (ER) alpha monoubiquitination. Cellular Signalling. 2011;**23**(7):1128-1135

[41] Faresse N, Ruffieux-Daidie D, Salamin M, Gomez-Sanchez CE, Staub O. Mineralocorticoid receptor degradation is promoted by Hsp90 inhibition and the ubiquitin-protein ligase CHIP. American Journal of Physiology. Renal Physiology. 2010;**299**(6):F1462-F1472

[42] Nagarajan S, Vohra T, Loffing J, Faresse N. Protein phosphatase 1alpha enhances renal aldosterone signaling via mineralocorticoid receptor stabilization. Molecular and Cellular Endocrinology. 2017;**450**:74-82

[43] Amazit L, Le Billan F, Kolkhof P, Lamribet K, Viengchareun S, Fay MR, et al. Finerenone impedes aldosterone-dependent nuclear import

of the mineralocorticoid receptor and prevents genomic recruitment of steroid receptor coactivator-1. The Journal of Biological Chemistry. 2015;**290**(36):21876-21889

[44] Fakitsas P, Adam G, Daidie D, van Bemmelen MX, Fouladkou F, Patrignani A, et al. Early aldosterone-induced gene product regulates the epithelial sodium channel by deubiquitylation. Journal of the American Society of Nephrology. 2007;**18**(4):1084-1092

[45] Pouly D, Debonneville A, Ruffieux-Daidie D, Maillard M, Abriel H, Loffing J, et al. Mice carrying ubiquitin-specific protease 2 (Usp2) gene inactivation maintain normal sodium balance and blood pressure. American Journal of Physiology. Renal Physiology. 2013;**305**(1):F21-F30

[46] Ruhs S, Stratz N, Quarch K, Masch A, Schutkowski M, Gekle M, et al. Modulation of transcriptional mineralocorticoid receptor activity by casein kinase 2. Scientific Reports. 2017;**7**(1):15340

[47] Jimenez-Canino R, Lorenzo-Diaz F, Jaisser F, Farman N, Giraldez T, Alvarez de la Rosa D. Histone deacetylase 6-controlled Hsp90 acetylation significantly alters mineralocorticoid receptor subcellular dynamics but not its transcriptional activity. Endocrinology. 2016;**157**(6):2515-2532

[48] Scroggins BT, Robzyk K, Wang D, Marcu MG, Tsutsumi S, Beebe K, et al. An acetylation site in the middle domain of Hsp90 regulates chaperone function. Molecular Cell. 2007;**25**(1):151-159

[49] Caamano CA, Morano MI, Patel PD, Watson SJ, Akil H. A bacterially expressed mineralocorticoid receptor is associated in vitro with the 90-kilodalton heat shock protein and shows typical hormone- and DNA-binding characteristics. Biochemistry. 1993;**32**(33):8589-8595

[50] Nemoto T, Ohara-Nemoto Y, Sato N, Ota M. Dual roles of 90-kDa heat shock protein in the function of the mineralocorticoid receptor. Journal of Biochemistry. 1993;**113**(6):769-775

[51] Hellal-Levy C, Fagart J, Souque A, Rafestin-Oblin ME. Mechanistic aspects of mineralocorticoid receptor activation. Kidney International. 2000;**57**(4):1250-1255

[52] Shibata S, Ishizawa K, Wang Q, Xu N, Fujita T, Uchida S, et al. ULK1 phosphorylates and regulates mineralocorticoid receptor. Cell Reports. 2018;**24**(3):569-576

[53] Jimenez-Canino R, Fernandes MX, Alvarez de la Rosa D. Phosphorylation of mineralocorticoid receptor ligand binding domain impairs receptor activation and has a dominant negative effect over non-phosphorylated receptors. The Journal of Biological Chemistry. 2016;**291**(36):19068-19078

[54] Souque A, Fagart J, Couette B, Rafestin-Oblin ME. Sulfhydryl groups are involved in the binding of agonists and antagonists to the human mineralocorticoid receptor. The Journal of Steroid Biochemistry and Molecular Biology. 1996;**57**(5-6):315-321

[55] Lupo B, Mesnier D, Auzou G. Cysteines 849 and 942 of human mineralocorticoid receptor are crucial for steroid binding. Biochemistry. 1998;**37**(35):12153-12159

[56] Piwien-Pilipuk G, Galigniana MD. Oxidative stress induced by L-buthionine-(S,R)-sulfoximine, a selective inhibitor of glutathione metabolism, abrogates mouse kidney mineralocorticoid receptor function. Biochimica et Biophysica Acta. 2000;**1495**(3):263-280

[57] Piwien-Pilipuk G, Ayala A, Machado A, Galigniana MD. Impairment of mineralocorticoid receptor

(MR)-dependent biological response by oxidative stress and aging: Correlation with post-translational modification of MR and decreased ADP-ribosylatable level of elongating factor 2 in kidney cells. The Journal of Biological Chemistry. 2002;**277**(14):11896-11903

[58] Jimenez-Canino R, Lorenzo-Diaz F, Odermatt A, Bailey MA, Livingstone DEW, Jaisser F, et al. 11beta-HSD2 SUMOylation modulates cortisol-induced mineralocorticoid receptor nuclear translocation independently of effects on transactivation. Endocrinology. 2017;**158**(11):4047-4063

[59] Fejes-Toth G, Pearce D, Naray-Fejes-Toth A. Subcellular localization of mineralocorticoid receptors in living cells: Effects of receptor agonists and antagonists. Proceedings of the National Academy of Sciences of the United States of America. 1998;**95**(6):2973-2978

[60] Ackermann D, Gresko N, Carrel M, Loffing-Cueni D, Habermehl D, Gomez-Sanchez C, et al. In vivo nuclear translocation of mineralocorticoid and glucocorticoid receptors in rat kidney: Differential effect of corticosteroids along the distal tubule. American Journal of Physiology. Renal Physiology. 2010;**299**(6):F1473-F1485

[61] Gomez-Sanchez CE, de Rodriguez AF, Romero DG, Estess J, Warden MP, Gomez-Sanchez MT, et al. Development of a panel of monoclonal antibodies against the mineralocorticoid receptor. Endocrinology. 2006;**147**(3):1343-1348

[62] Han F, Ozawa H, Matsuda K, Nishi M, Kawata M. Colocalization of mineralocorticoid receptor and glucocorticoid receptor in the hippocampus and hypothalamus. Neuroscience Research. 2005;**51**(4): 371-381

[63] Echeverria PC, Picard D. Molecular chaperones, essential partners of steroid hormone receptors for activity and mobility. Biochimica et Biophysica Acta. 2010;**1803**(6):641-649

[64] Walther RF, Atlas E, Carrigan A, Rouleau Y, Edgecombe A, Visentin L, et al. A serine/threonine-rich motif is one of three nuclear localization signals that determine unidirectional transport of the mineralocorticoid receptor to the nucleus. The Journal of Biological Chemistry. 2005;**280**(17):17549-17561

[65] Piwien-Pilipuk G, Galigniana MD. Tautomycin inhibits phosphatase-dependent transformation of the rat kidney mineralocorticoid receptor. Molecular and Cellular Endocrinology. 1998;**144**(1-2):119-130

[66] Yasuoka S, Kai H, Kajimoto H, Kudo H, Takayama N, Anegawa T, et al. Blood pressure variability activates cardiac mineralocorticoid receptor and induces cardiac remodeling in hypertensive rats. Circulation Journal. 2013;**77**(6):1474-1481

[67] Wang RA, Mazumdar A, Vadlamudi RK, Kumar R. P21-activated kinase-1 phosphorylates and transactivates estrogen receptor-alpha and promotes hyperplasia in mammary epithelium. The EMBO Journal. 2002;**21**(20):5437-5447

[68] Marissal-Arvy N, Lombes M, Petterson J, Moisan MP, Mormede P. Gain of function mutation in the mineralocorticoid receptor of the Brown Norway rat. The Journal of Biological Chemistry. 2004;**279**(38):39232-39239

[69] Kino T, Jaffe H, Amin ND, Chakrabarti M, Zheng YL, Chrousos GP, et al. Cyclin-dependent kinase 5 modulates the transcriptional activity of the mineralocorticoid receptor and regulates expression of brain-derived neurotrophic factor. Molecular Endocrinology. 2010;**24**(5):941-952

[70] Borquez DA, Olmos C, Alvarez S, Di Genova A, Maass A, Gonzalez-Billault

C. Bioinformatic survey for new physiological substrates of cyclin-dependent kinase 5. Genomics. 2013;**101**(4):221-228

[71] Davel AP, Anwar IJ, Jaffe IZ. The endothelial mineralocorticoid receptor: Mediator of the switch from vascular health to disease. Current Opinion in Nephrology and Hypertension. 2017;**26**(2):97-104

[72] Yang J, Young MJ. The mineralocorticoid receptor and its coregulators. Journal of Molecular Endocrinology. 2009;**43**(2):53-64

[73] Seo M, Song M, Seok YM, Kang SH, Lee HA, Sohn UD, et al. Lysine acetyltransferases cyclic adenosine monophosphate response element-binding binding protein and acetyltransferase p300 attenuate transcriptional activity of the mineralocorticoid receptor through its acetylation. Clinical and Experimental Pharmacology & Physiology. 2015;**42**(5):559-566

[74] Gross M, Yang R, Top I, Gasper C, Shuai K. PIASy-mediated repression of the androgen receptor is independent of sumoylation. Oncogene. 2004;**23**(17):3059-3066

[75] Martin-Martinez M, Perez-Gordillo FL, Alvarez de la Rosa D, Rodriguez Y, Gerona-Navarro G, Gonzalez-Muniz R, et al. Modulating mineralocorticoid receptor with non-steroidal antagonists. New opportunities for the development of potent and selective ligands without off-target side effects. Journal of Medicinal Chemistry. 2017;**60**(7):2629-2650

[76] Su MG, Weng JT, Hsu JB, Huang KY, Chi YH, Lee TY. Investigation and identification of functional post-translational modification sites associated with drug binding and protein-protein interactions. BMC Systems Biology. 2017;**11**(Suppl 7):132

Chapter 15

# Aldosterone Regulation of Protein Kinase Signaling Pathways and Renal $Na^+$ Transport by Non-genomic Mechanisms

*Warren Thomas and Brian Harvey*


## Abstract

Aldosterone is the key regulating hormone of whole-body fluid and electrolyte homeostasis. Perturbations in aldosterone synthesis and over-activation of the mineralocorticoid receptor (MR) can lead to excess salt reabsorption and hypertension. The cortical collecting duct (CCD) is the main site of action in the kidney for aldosterone regulation of whole-body sodium homeostasis through actions on the epithelial sodium channel (ENaC) and the Na/K-ATPase (Na/K pump). Aldosterone stimulates ENaC trafficking into the apical cell membranes in the CCD and enhances channel stability and open probability, as well as activating the basolateral membrane Na/K pump to produce an overall increase in the transepithelial reabsorption of sodium. Aldosterone/MR regulates the activity of ENaC in the CCD through both rapid non-genomic (secs-mins) and latent genomic (hours-days) signaling pathways. These rapid and slow responses of renal $Na^+$ transport pathways to aldosterone are often treated as distinct and separate events. However, recent evidence points to a close integration between genomic and non-genomic responses to aldosterone to regulate ENaC and Na/K pump activity via protein kinase signaling pathways. Here, we review the integration of aldosterone membrane-initiated non-genomic and nuclear genomic regulations of renal sodium transport via protein kinase signaling pathways and in particular via protein kinase D isoforms.


**Keywords:** aldosterone, non-genomic, protein kinase D, ENaC, Na/K pump, renal $Na^+$ transport

## 1. Introduction

The distal nephron of the kidney is the principal site for salt conservation in the body, and the dysregulation of $Na^+$ homeostasis can contribute significantly to the development of hypertension [1]. Aldosterone is the major salt conservation hormone, and increased circulating levels of the hormone in low $Na^+$ diet, salt-wasting, or hypovolemia such as in hemorrhage produce increased sodium reabsorption in target epithelial tissues of the kidney, distal colon, and sweat gland to restore whole-body salt homeostasis and extracellular fluid volume. The kidney and cardiovascular systems are the principal organs for aldosterone action to regulate blood pressure. Rapid non-genomic and latent genomic actions of aldosterone on both renal and cardiac functions have been described. The main ion transport targets for the natriferic actions of aldosterone in the kidney are the epithelial sodium channel ENaC and the Na/K-ATPase pump. Aldosterone can also affect other epithelial ion transport systems such as potassium and hydrogen ion secretion by activating the ROMK $K^+$ channel and the $H^+$-ATPase pump, respectively [2]. Aldosterone regulates sodium transport in the kidney through its actions on ENaC activity in the distal nephron principal cells of the cortical collecting duct (CCD) as well as activating the basolateral membrane Na/K pump, to produce an overall increase in the transepithelial uptake of sodium. Aldosterone also stimulates $K^+$ recycling at the basolateral membrane through activation of inwardly rectifying $K_{ATP}$ channels which serves to maintain a favorable cell membrane hyperpolarization for sustained $Na^+$ influx via ENaC, in addition to matching $K^+$ recycling rate with Na/K-ATPase pump activity to preserve epithelial cross talk (maintaining equilibrium between apical and basolateral ionic permeabilities) [3].

Aldosterone acts on ENaC via its receptor MR to produce rapid (non-genomic) effects on intermediate cell signaling molecules (protein kinases, MAP kinases, SGK, $Ca^{2+}$, pH, etc.) to enhance ENaC membrane trafficking, channel activity, and stability followed by a latent (genomic) phase to increase the expression of ENaC channel subunits and further stabilization of active channels in the apical membrane [4]. For the past 25 years, it was thought that aldosterone and its receptor MR modulated renal sodium reabsorption principally by preventing the membrane retrieval and degradation of ENaC in the cortical collecting duct via serum glucocorticoid kinase (SGK) [5]. However mouse models deficient in or over-expressing SGK did not show alterations in blood pressure or renal $Na^+$ excretion, pointing to SGK redundancy or other regulatory ENaC pathways more potent than SGK [6]. A novel aldosterone signaling pathway acting through protein kinase D isoforms (PKD) was discovered over a decade ago [7] which is pivotal in transducing aldosterone/MR regulation of ENaC subcellular trafficking and channel activity in CCD, both by rapid non-genomic and latent genomic signaling mechanisms [2, 4]. The role of rapid aldosterone/MR signaling responses in modulating renal sodium reabsorption and whole-body electrolyte balance is still poorly understood; however, recent observations demonstrate that PKD1 activation by aldosterone rapidly regulates ENaC trafficking, one of the earliest physiological responses to the hormone [8]. This review focuses on non-genomic aldosterone regulation of ENaC and renal sodium transport by protein kinase signaling pathways and the impact of rapid kinase signaling, in particular protein kinase D, on the latent genomic responses to influence renal sodium reabsorption in the CCD.

### 1.1 Non-genomic actions of aldosterone on ion transporters

Aldosterone tightly regulates epithelial ion transport in the renal CCD by both genomic and non-genomic processes (**Figure 1**). Aldosterone diffuses across the basolateral membrane of the CCD cell and binds to MR in the cytosol inducing receptor dimerization and the translocation to the nucleus. The hormone-receptor complex can bind to GRE response elements and subsequently recruit other transcription factors. During genomic regulation of ion transport, the aldosterone/MR complex acts as a ligand-dependent transcription factor that can induce the expression of several genes including ENaC, $Na^+/K^+$-ATPase, ROMK, and SGK [9–11]. The binding of aldosterone to MR in the cytosol can also stimulate protein kinase signaling pathways. The rapid activation of certain protein kinases such as MAPK and PKD occurs through the transactivation of EGFR [12, 13].

Rapid activation of signal transduction cascades is amplified via aldosterone-stimulated non-transcriptional responses. Current available evidence indicates that aldosterone non-genomic responses in CCD are dependent on the interaction of aldosterone with cytosolic MR and not via a nonclassical membrane-bound

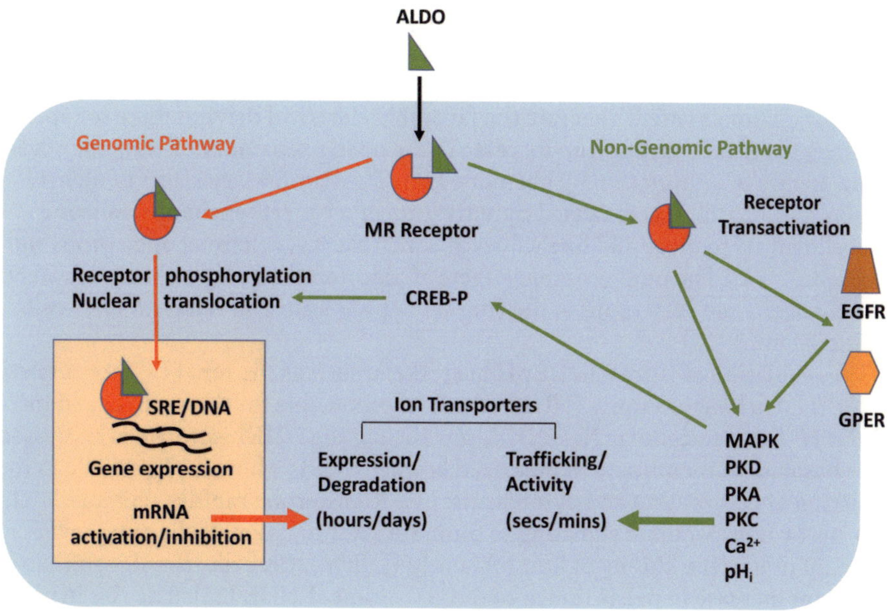


**Figure 1.**
*Genomic and non-genomic actions of aldosterone on epithelial ion transport. In both pathways, aldosterone enters the cytoplasm to bind with MR. A rapid non-genomic signaling pathway is initiated within secs-mins (green arrows) which transactivates the EGFR receptor to produce phosphorylation activation of protein kinases such as MAPK and PKD. Aldosterone may also interact with other receptors such as GPER or directly with specific kinases (PKC and PKA) to modulate intracellular $Ca^{2+}$ or pH. The non-genomic effects of aldosterone result in rapid activation of various ion transporters (ENaC, Na/K pump, Na/H exchanger, $K^+$ channels, and $H^+$-ATPase pumps). Genomic responses occur on a longer time scale of hours-days (red arrows) and are the result of aldosterone/MR translocation to the nucleus, interaction with DNA steroid response elements, mRNA activation/inhibition, and the delayed expression or degradation of ion transporter proteins. Cross talk exists between genomic and non-genomic pathways in both directions. The rapid activation of protein kinases primes the epithelial cells for the latent genomic response by enhancing the trafficking and membrane localization of ion transporters. In addition, non-genomic MAPK and ERK1/2 signaling can activate transcription factors such as CREB which facilitates nuclear translocation of MR and gene transcription to cause expression of protein kinase signaling intermediates [2, 4].*

aldosterone receptor [14]. The signaling cascades which are rapidly activated through the interaction of MR and aldosterone can be inhibited by MR-specific antagonists, for example, spironolactone or eplerenone [15, 16]. There is also strong evidence that, under certain conditions, aldosterone/MR can transactivate other receptors such as the epithelial growth factor receptor EGFR and G-protein estrogen receptor GPER [12, 13, 17].

Non-genomic renal responses to aldosterone have long been described in various experimental animal and cell models. A primary focus of non-genomic aldosterone research has been the rapid actions of aldosterone on the reabsorption of sodium in the distal nephron, in particular rapid regulation of $Na^+$ uptake through ENaC and basolateral extrusion of $Na^+$ via the Na/K pump [2, 4, 29, 30]. The active sodium transport target for aldosterone was first demonstrated in amphibian urinary bladder [31]. One of the earliest reports of rapid actions of aldosterone on sodium transport in the kidney was in 1957 when Cole described the rapid effect of aldosterone administration for 30 min to cause a reduction in urinary loss of $Na^+$ and increased reabsorption by the renal tubules in response to intravenously administered saline in adult male rats [18]. It has also been documented that aldosterone infusion into aldosterone-suppressed rats (by adrenalectomy or infusion with sodium bicarbonate) resulted in the rapid increase in urinary $Na^+$ excretion [19]. The rapid non-genomic actions of aldosterone in vivo were further demonstrated in the intact rat when aldosterone induced a rapid increase in urinary $Na^+$ excretion within 15 min [20].

Aldosterone has been shown to regulate epithelial $K^+$ channels involved in transepithelial $K^+$ secretion and $K^+$ recycling. In the frog skin epithelium which shares similar functional properties to CCD, aldosterone rapidly activated ATP-sensitive $K^+$ ($K_{ATP}$) channels which generate the favorable electrical driving force for apical $Na^+$ entry via ENaC, through an increase in the open probability of $K_{ATP}$ channels within 15 min of stimulation by hormone [21]. The stimulatory effect of aldosterone on $K_{ATP}$ channels was caused by activation of a $Na^+/H^+$ exchanger shifting intracellular pH to more alkaline values at which the $K_{ATP}$ channel open probability was highest [22]. The non-genomic effects of aldosterone on $K_{ATP}$ channels and $Na^+/H^+$ exchanger were very rapid in the frog skin epithelium and renal A6 CCD cells (within 10 min) [23].

The regulation of intracellular pH in epithelia such as the renal CCD occurs via the $Na^+/H^+$ exchanger family (NHE) which is responsible for the exchange of intracellular $H^+$ for extracellular $Na^+$. NHE, specifically the NHE1 isoform, is expressed in the basolateral membrane in polarized epithelial cells where it plays a role in the regulation of cell volume and cytoplasmic pH. Aldosterone rapidly activates NHE isoforms by non-genomic signaling to promote alkalinization of the cytoplasm within 20 min in the kidney of amphibians [24]. In MDCK cells, the aldosterone-dependent increase in $pH_i$ is linked to the activation of NHE [25]. The rise in $pH_i$ is also dependent on the activation of ERK1/2 along with the rapid increase in $[Ca^{2+}i]$ that occurs within 1 min of treatment with aldosterone [26]. Other studies using M1-CCD cells showed that aldosterone induced a NHE-dependent increase in the recovery of $pH_i$ from an acid load within 5 min of hormone treatment. The rapid pH recovery response to aldosterone was reduced by PKCα inhibition or by the activation of MAPK [27]. NHE also has a role in regulating cell volume as well as the induction of proliferation and cell growth. In fact, one of the first pieces of evidence for non-genomic actions of aldosterone on the $Na^+/H^+$ exchanger was reported for cell volume regulation in leukocytes [28].

Another ion transporter target of non-genomic aldosterone signaling in the CCD is the V-type $H^+$ pump ($H^+$-ATPase) which is expressed in intercalated cells of the CCD and is the major mechanism for aldosterone-regulated acid secretion in the kidney. Aldosterone enhances urinary acidification by stimulating $H^+$ efflux via the $H^+$-ATPase pump. This response was first described in turtle bladder [32]. It was later shown in whole-cell patch clamp recordings of mitochondria-rich cells of the frog skin that aldosterone treatment resulted in the rapid exocytotic insertion of $H^+$-ATPase pumps into the luminal membrane within 10 min of hormone stimulation [33]. The rapid insertion of $H^+$ pumps into the membrane was sensitive to PKC inhibition and disruption of the cytoskeleton. In the kidney, the reabsorption of bicarbonate coupled with the release of $H^+$ into the renal ultrafiltrate in the distal nephron accounts for acid-base regulation. Aldosterone has a crucial role in regulating the renal $H^+$-ATPase through non-genomic signaling responses. For example, stimulation with aldosterone for 15 min resulted in the MR-dependent increase in the excretion of $H^+$ from acidic type A intercalated cells of the outer medullary collecting ducts of mice [34]. These responses in the kidney were similar to that observed in the frog skin whereby the increase in $H^+$ pump activity was dependent on the $Ca^{2+}$-induced activity of PKC [33]. Moreover, mice injected with aldosterone displayed an increase in the expression of $H^+$-ATPase in the apical membrane of type A intercalated cells [34] further strengthening the evidence for aldosterone in regulating the trafficking of $H^+$-ATPase pumps in the maintenance of acid-base homeostasis.

In the renal CCD, $K^+$ enters the principal cells through the $Na^+/K^+$-ATPase in the basolateral membrane and is then secreted into the lumen via $K^+$ channels along the apical membrane [35]. The main $K^+$ secreting channel in the kidney is ROMK which is expressed in the apical membrane of cells in the ASDN [36]. The function of ROMK is regulated by aldosterone through SGK1 activity which was found to regulate cell surface expression of the channel [37]. $K^+$ can also enter the cell through $K^+$ channels located in the basolateral membrane of the CCD [38] which may occur due to the stimulation of $Na^+/K^+$-ATPase by mineralocorticoids [39]. ATP-dependent $K^+$ channel ($K_{ATP}$) activity in A6 CCD renal cells was rapidly stimulated by aldosterone (15 min), and this activation modulated the open probability of the channel [21]. Aldosterone has also been shown to produce a non-genomic inhibition of $Ca^{2+}$-dependent intermediate conductance channels ($IK_{Ca}$) located in the basolateral membrane of colonic crypt cells, and this effect was PKC-dependent [40, 41]. Additionally, aldosterone can also activate $Na^+/H^+$ exchange through $Ca^{2+}$- and PKC-dependent signaling pathways that results in an upregulation of $K_{ATP}$ and an inhibition of IKCa channels [42]. Taken together, it is evident that aldosterone can induce rapid signaling responses that impact upon several membrane ion transporter targets by modulating intrinsic biophysical and electrophysiological properties of ion channels, pumps, and exchangers.

### 1.2 Non-genomic actions of aldosterone on protein kinase signaling pathways

Non-genomic effects of aldosterone produce rapid phosphorylation of a wide range of protein kinases such as extracellular stimulus-regulated kinase (ERK) 1/2, protein kinase C (PKC isoforms), cAMP-dependent protein kinase A (PKA), and protein kinase D isoforms (PKD) (**Figure 2**) [2, 4, 29, 42–47]. It is vital to understand how aldosterone stimulation of these signaling cascades augments the activity of sodium ion transporters ENaC and $Na^+/K^+$-ATPase pump in order to establish the physiological relevance of non-genomic signaling for transepithelial $Na^+$ reabsorption processes that are instigated in advance of transcriptional control. For the past 25 years, it was thought that aldosterone and the mineralocorticoid receptor modulated renal sodium reabsorption principally by activating the epithelial $Na^+$ channel ENaC in the cortical collecting duct via serum glucocorticoid kinase (SGK) [5]. However, mouse models deficient in or over-expressing SGK do not show alterations in blood pressure or renal $Na^+$ excretion [6], pointing to redundancy or other regulatory ENaC pathways more potent than SGK.

Aldosterone has been shown to exert rapid non-genomic effects on the activation of several kinase families including PKC, PKD, ERK1/2, and MAPK through the transactivation of EGFR via the non-receptor tyrosine kinase c-Src [2, 4]. The most widely documented mechanism underlying the rapid responses to aldosterone is the activation of protein kinase signaling cascades. Several research groups have investigated the role of ERK1/2 activation in aldosterone-sensitive models such as Madin-Darby canine kidney (MDCK) cells [25], M1-CCD cells [27], vascular smooth muscle cells (VSMC) [48], cardiac myocytes [49], and the mesangial cells of the glomerulus [50]. The activation of ERK1/2 is linked to the variation of cell growth which can occur through hypertrophy [49] or by promoting proliferation [51]. The activation of ERK1/2 is modulated by the simultaneous activation of other signaling cascades. In MDCK cells, the activation of ERK1/2 occurs within 5 min and can be sustained over a period of hours (96). However, in M1-CCD cells, ERK1/2 activation is linked to the transactivation of EGFR and subsequent activation of PKD1 which has been shown to be necessary to maintain the cyclical activation of ERK1/2 beyond 5 min [25]. Additionally, PKD1 involvement in stabilizing ERK1/2 activation occurs in response to growth factors and does not require the direct phosphorylation of ERK1/2 by PKD1 [52]. Aldosterone can also stimulate

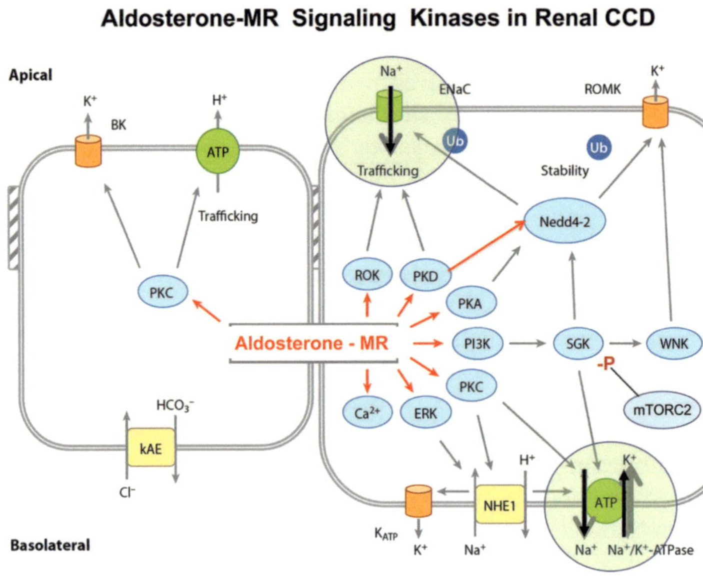


**Figure 2.**
*Aldosterone-induced protein kinase signaling and their modulation of membrane ion transporters in renal CCD. Fundamental signaling intermediates such as protein kinase A (PKA), protein kinase C (PKC), protein kinase D (PKD), phosphoinositide 3-kinase (PI3K), serum- and glucocorticoid-activated kinase (SGK), Rho-activated kinase (ROK), the with no lysine family kinases (WNKs), and the extracellular stimulus-regulated kinase (ERK) are rapidly phosphorylated following treatment with aldosterone. Once activated, these signaling intermediates modulate the activity of ENaC, ROMK, ATP-sensitive $K^+$ channels ($K_{ATP}$), $Na^+/H^+$ exchanger-1 (NHE1), and the Na/K pump ($Na^+/K^+$-ATPase) in the principal cells of the collecting duct. Aldosterone induces rapid stimulation of $H^+$-ATPase pumps in the A-type intercalated cells via PKC-dependent trafficking of the proton pump into the apical membrane. Large-conductance $K^+$ (BK) channel activity is modulated by aldosterone and is involved in the shift of kidney anion exchanger (kAE) activity from the basolateral membrane to the apical membrane (modified from [4]).*

the prolonged activation of ERK1/2 in CCD cells as this process is coupled to Ki-RasA expression where aldosterone can also stimulate Ki-RasA GTPase activity within 15 min of treatment [53]. Another non-genomic kinase signaling target of aldosterone is the p38 MAPK subfamily. The biphasic activation of p38 in vascular smooth muscle cells (VSMC) can occur within 1 min of aldosterone treatment [54], which is followed by a second activation phase measurable after 30 min. The p38 response in VSMC is dependent on the co-activation of MR and c-Src and links p38 to the pro-fibrotic effects of aldosterone on VSMC via the regulation of NADPH. Furthermore, MR-dependent activation of p38 in glomerular podocytes from rats is also promoted by aldosterone, and this p38 activation contributes to the induction of apoptosis [55].

PKC isoforms have diverse roles and regulate critical cellular processes such as proliferation and trafficking. The PKC family of kinases are well-established targets of rapid aldosterone non-genomic responses [2, 4, 43]. For example, aldosterone can promote the activation of PKCα in renal collecting duct cells within 2–5 min after treatment. This activation appears to occur in an MR-independent manner [56, 57] and involves aldosterone binding directly to the kinase [58] along with a simultaneous rise in intracellular $Ca^{2+}$. Additionally, PKCδ and PKCε can also be rapidly activated in response to aldosterone; however, this does not involve the direct binding of the hormone to the kinase but is coupled to MR through EGFR transactivation [12]. The protein kinase D isoform PKD1 activation by aldosterone follows a similar pattern and has been implicated in the induction of proliferation in M1-CCD cells following aldosterone treatment [59] as well as in the stimulation of hypertrophy in cardiac myocytes [60].

Aldosterone can also upregulate serum glucocorticoid kinases; although this activation can be rapid within 20 min, it does not appear to be a non-genomic response but rather dependent on genomic expression of the kinase. ENaC activity is regulated by the aldosterone-targeted kinase serum glucocorticoid kinases which is present in all eukaryotes and exits in multiple isoforms, for example, SGK1, SGK2, and SGK3. All isoforms have been shown to promote ENaC activity with SGK1 and SGK3 being the most potent stimulators of this activity when they have been co-expressed in *Xenopus* oocytes [61, 62]. Aldosterone and other glucocorticoid hormones induce the transcription of SGK1 by acting via nuclear receptors that bind to the response elements in the SGK1 gene. The subsequent rapid increase in SGK1 at both the protein and mRNA level stimulated ENaC-mediated $Na^+$ currents in the epithelium of several tissues such as the kidney, lung, colon, and ocular epithelial cells [5, 63–65]. A rapid increase in ENaC activity by elevation in the channel density at the membrane has been linked to the rapid vesicle trafficking that is coupled to the activation of the RhoA small GTPase [66].

Aldosterone can also promote the activation of second messenger responses such as mobilization of intracellular $Ca^{2+}$, the biosynthesis of cAMP, and the release of nitric oxide. There are many studies documenting the rapid non-genomic rise in intracellular $Ca_i^{2+}$ in response to aldosterone including in CCD cells [67], vascular smooth muscle [68], colonic crypts [42], and the brain [69]. The mechanism by which $Ca^{2+}$ influx occurs in both the colon and the renal nephron has not been fully described; however, $Ca^{2+}$ entry into CCD cells was not sensitive to spironolactone, and $Ca^{2+}$ entry into colonic crypt cells was PKC-dependent via L-type voltage gated channels [70].

The rapid transient activation of cAMP-PKA signaling by aldosterone has been shown in CCD cells, and the phosphorylation of CREB following aldosterone treatment was found to be PKA-dependent [71]. Some research groups have reported aldosterone inducing the activation of PKA; however, they also describe an inhibitory effect between the physiological response stimulated by the cAMP activator forskolin and that stimulated by aldosterone. There is also evidence suggesting that suppressing CREB-dependent transcription occurs via the upregulation of protein phosphatase 2β (PP2β) activation by aldosterone [72]. This could be due in part to the separate activation of isoforms of adenylate cyclase and PKA by forskolin and aldosterone which could result in subcellular compartmentalized signaling. These observations point to a negative feedback loop that is intrinsic to aldosterone signaling thus making cells more refractive to further PKA stimulation after the initial aldosterone-induced response.

### 1.3 Transduction of non-genomic aldosterone responses through the MR

As MR is at present the only widely recognized receptor that is specific to aldosterone, considerable effort has been put in to understand how nuclear receptors such as MR can initiate rapid non-genomic protein kinase signaling cascades, in particular in concert with the transactivation of membrane-associated receptors EGFR and GPER [13, 17, 73]. A number of strands of evidence point to MR as being the receptor responsible for initiating the aldosterone-induced non-genomic rapid signaling cascades in the CCD [74]. The activation of protein kinases such as PKD and ERK1/2 by aldosterone can be inhibited with the use of MR-specific antagonists such as spironolactone and eplerenone [12, 74]. Moreover, rapid actions of aldosterone in MR-null cells can be conferred through exogenous expression of the receptor in Chinese hamster ovarian (CHO) and human embryonic kidney (HEK) cells [74]. MR can be considered to be a multifunctional receptor. If recombinant MR, which lacks its DNA-binding and coactivator-binding domains, is expressed, signaling events can be instigated by a rapid response to aldosterone independent of transcriptional activity [75]. In terms of the intermediate phases that couple the aldosterone-MR interaction with the rapid activation of protein kinases, there are still some questions to be addressed.

Aldosterone/MR can activate non-genomic signaling pathways which regulate renal sodium transport and cell proliferation via transactivation of the membrane-bound epidermal growth factor receptor EGFR [12, 59, 76–79]. Several groups have shown a rapid (<5 min) increase in the phosphorylation of EGFR following the treatment with aldosterone which induces ERK1/2 activation and an increase in intracellular $Ca^{2+}$ [12, 81]. A major signaling pathway that is known to mediate MR transactivation of EGFR is the cytosolic tyrosine kinase c-Src pathway [81, 82]. When c-Src is activated, it phosphorylates EGFR to activate ERK1/2 signaling, and when c-Src is inhibited, the rapid effect of aldosterone is completely abolished indicating that aldosterone transactivation of EGRF and MAPK pathways occurs via c-Src. Phosphorylated ERK1/2 can provoke several cellular responses that range from the activation of $Na^+/H^+$ exchange to cell proliferation [83, 84]. The transactivation of EGFR is not unique to aldosterone and is typically an intermediate step in the transduction of rapid non-genomic membrane-initiated signaling responses stimulated by other steroid hormones such as estrogen [85] and G-protein-coupled receptor agonists [86, 87]. Although it is now well established that the transactivation of EGFR is a fundamental step in linking the initiation of the non-genomic aldosterone/MR signal to aldosterone-responsive downstream kinase signaling intermediates, it has yet to be determined by which molecular mechanism EGFR and its activation are coupled to MR, but it is thought to be ligand-independent EGF. EGFR is phosphorylated by c-Src, within 5 min of treatment with aldosterone, and c-Src phosphorylation could be a significant transducing signal [82]. Cytoplasmic Aldo/MR is recruited into a complex of several proteins including heat shock protein 90 (Hsp90); this complex dissociates on MR activation allowing c-Src phosphorylation of EGFR. The aldosterone-induced phosphorylation of EGFR by c-Src can be blocked by antagonizing Hsp90 interactions with other proteins using the geldanamycin analogue 17-AAG. Inhibiting Hsp90 also suppresses EGFR-dependent downstream signaling events initiated by aldosterone which include the activation of protein kinase D1 [12] and the ERK1/2 mitogen-activated protein (MAP) kinase [25]. The ErbB family of receptor tyrosine kinases (including its member EGFR) can also be activated independently of ligand binding via phosphorylation of specific residues that are distinct from autophosphorylation sites. For example, EGFR can be phosphorylated at Tyr845 by Src tyrosine kinases which result in the activation of EGFR without requiring binding of the receptor to EGF [78, 80, 88].

Other receptors have been implicated in transducing the non-genomic aldosterone actions on protein kinases including stimulation at the membrane that could be initiated via GPCRs, tyrosine kinases, or an as yet "unknown" membrane-associated aldosterone receptor [89]. There is also evidence for direct activation of specific protein kinases by steroid hormones such as vitamin D binding to catalytic domains on the kinase [90], and this appears to be also relevant for aldosterone activation of PKCα [91]. Aldosterone can bind directly to the C2 domain of PKCα, with a binding affinity of between 0.5 and 1 nM, which results in the autophosphorylation of PKCα [58]. There have also been numerous reports proposing GPER (GPR30), a G-protein-coupled estrogen receptor, as a novel non-genomic aldosterone receptor [17, 92, 93]. Some rapid responses to aldosterone in smooth muscle have been linked to GPER-coupled signaling pathway in which the expression of GPER is required for the MR-independent rapid effects of aldosterone [94]. However, the specificity of GPER to bind selectively to steroid hormone ligands remains controversial [95].

## 2. Protein kinase D signaling

Protein kinase D (PKD) is a serine/threonine kinase that includes three isoforms: PKD1/PKCμ, PKD2, and PKD3/PKCν [96]. PKD isoforms contain a tandem repeat of zinc finger-like cysteine-rich motifs at the N-terminus that exhibit a strong affinity for diacylglycerol (DAG) or phorbol ester as well as a pleckstrin homology domain and a C-terminal catalytic domain that has a similar homology with calmodulin-dependent kinases. While the PKD family contain a homologous catalytic domain, each isoform varies with respect to their subcellular localization, expression, and regulation. PKD isoforms are DAG and PKC effectors that facilitate the actions of growth factors, hormones, and other stimuli that can activate phospholipase C (PLC). PKDs have a pair of C1 domains that bind to DAG and phorbol esters. Membrane-associated DAG can bind to and subsequently activate PKD and in turn recruit PKD via its C1 domains. PKC phosphorylates Ser744 and Ser748 in the activation loop of PKD. DAG-stimulated PKCs (δ, ε, θ, and η) have been shown to be PKD dominant activators. However, $Ca^+$- and DAG-activated PKCs α, βi, and βii have also been demonstrated to activate PKD.

PKD isoforms are known to modulate the relative activity of both the ERK and JNK pathways whereby they can attenuate the c-Jun phosphorylation and JNK activation in response to the activation of EGFR while stimulating the ERK and Ras pathways. The PKD family of kinases can regulate budding of secretory vesicles from the trans-Golgi network, and this process is required for locomotion and localization and activity of the Rac1-dependent leading edge in fibroblasts. In addition to a major regulatory role in cell trafficking and motility, PKD also stimulates the recruitment of integrin to newly formed focal adhesions as well as the invasion of cancer cells. Moreover, PKD has been shown to have a role in the regulation of apoptosis, the differentiation of T cells in transgenic models, and reintroduction of DNA synthesis that can be induced by phorbol esters and regulatory peptides that act through Gq-coupled receptors and cardiac hypertrophy [97]. PKD has been implicated as a facilitator of stress and multiple disease states, for example, human hypertrophic cardiomyopathy, the activation of NFκB which is induced by Bcr-Abl in human myeloid leukemia and in oxidative stress responses. PKD isoform involvement in facilitating a wide array of both normal and abnormal biological actions in different subcellular compartments is most likely to be dependent on dynamic alterations in the isoform spatial and temporal localization in combination with their substrate specificity. This is particularly relevant for understanding the physiological role of non-genomic aldosterone activation of PKD in the regulation of renal $Na^+$ transport [2, 4].

Previous studies have shown the PKD isoforms undergo rapid subcellular redistribution in response to cellular stimulation. For example, PKD can be phosphorylated and activated by novel PKC isoforms PKCε and PKCη. We have demonstrated that the aldosterone activation of PKD1 in CCD cells is PKCε dependent [7, 12].

Both PKD1 and PKD2 are known to translocate from the cytosol to DAG-containing microenvironments in the plasma membrane which is followed by PKC-dependent reverse translocation from the membrane to the cytosol where they subsequently accumulate in the nucleus [98]. In contrast to the first two isoforms, PKD3 constantly shuttles between the cytoplasm and the nucleus [99]. The PKD family members can pool and localize at the Golgi complex and the mitochondria. Additionally, PKD1 and PKD2 contain short PDZ-binding motifs in their COOH termini, namely, VSIL in PKD1 and ISVL in PKD2, which can form complexes with regulatory factors in multiple subcellular locations, thereby controlling various cellular activities. The PKD family of kinases are potent regulators of many biological processes such as cell proliferation, polarity, migration, differentiation, reorganization of the actin cytoskeleton, membrane trafficking, vesicle fission, gene expression, inflammation, and hypertrophy [97]. PKD isoforms are also important players in several pathologies associated with both the cardiovascular and renal systems. For example, PKD1 has been implicated in cardiac hypertrophy, while PKD1 and PKD2 activations have been associated with the proliferation of endothelial cells and angiogenesis.

## 2.1 Regulation of cell polarity and trafficking by PKD

The establishment and the maintenance of cell polarity are essential for the functions of several cell types including epithelial cells. In polarized epithelial cells, PKD1 and PKD2 regulate the production of TGN carriers that are intended to locate to the basolateral membrane which suggests that PKD isoforms may have a key role in the generation of epithelial polarity [100].

PKD has been implicated in the many facets of the regulation of subcellular trafficking either by maintenance of the structure in the Golgi or by the regulation of fission at the trans-Golgi network (TGN) [101, 102]. PKD can also regulate Golgi to membrane vesicle trafficking by activating phosphatidylinositol (PtdIns) 4-kinase (PI4KIIIβ) and phosphatidylinositol 4-phosphate 5-kinase (PI4P5K). PKD1 phosphorylates PI4KIIIβ at the Golgi which in turn promotes vesicle fission and subsequently the rate of protein transport to the plasma membrane.

Activated PKD1 phosphorylates and activates phosphatidylinositol 4-kinase IIIb (PI4KIIIb) at the cis- and trans-Golgi promoting the synthesis of phosphatidylinositol-4-phosphate (PI4P) in the Golgi membrane. Ceramide transport protein is released from the endoplasmic reticulum and binds to PI4P, so transporting lipid from the ER to the Golgi. Ceramide is processed at the Golgi to produce sphingomyelin and diacylglycerol. DAG recruits PKD1 and novel PKC isoforms as well as multiple proteins recruited to sites of PI4P biogenesis in the Golgi. These include the arfaptin family proteins. These proteins contain a BAR (Bin/Amphiphysin/Rvs) domain with a concave anionic surface that interacts with negatively charged lipid membranes to facilitate vesicle fission. Other known substrates for PKD1 include actin cytoskeleton regulatory proteins such as cofilin, LIM kinase (LIMK), and rhotekin that contribute to actin-dependent intracellular vesicle trafficking.

## 2.2 Non-genomic aldosterone signaling through protein kinase D pathways

Aldosterone/MR signaling via PKD signaling pathways has been shown to be a key regulator of the transduction of non-genomic responses to the hormone [2, 4]. In renal CCD cells, PKD1 acts as a potent regulator of ENaC and $Na^+/K^+$-ATPase trafficking and activity under basal and aldosterone-stimulated conditions [102]. The activation of PKD1 at the trans-Golgi network (TGN) by aldosterone is an important regulatory mechanism of ENaC trafficking. Aldosterone rapidly (<5 min) induces the interaction between PKD1 and PI4KIIIβ which regulates the signaling of protein kinases and the lipid modification that is essential for vesicle fission. The rapid phosphorylation activation of PKD1 by aldosterone primes the CCD cells for subsequent transcriptional events which increase the expression of ENaC channel subunit proteins. Vital roles of other PKD isoforms including PKD2 and PKD3 in the CCD are emerging with the identification of novel substrates for this kinase family that include other kinases and transcription factors responsible for modulating gene expression and intracellular trafficking. All three PKD isoforms are highly expressed in renal CCD cells and were found to be localized to principal cells in mouse and rat CCD using AQP1 co-localization immunofluorescence assays (**Figure 3**). Rats fed a low $Na^+$ diet for 2 weeks showed increased expression of PKD1 in the CCD principal cells. Confocal immunohistochemistry microscopy revealed the basal expression of PKD1 to be mainly in the trans-Golgi network and cytosolic compartment; PKD2 was localized almost exclusively at the apical membrane, whereas PKD3 was mainly localized in the cytosol and nucleus (**Figure 3**).

The different PKD isoforms exhibit distinct differences in terms of their subcellular localization, which is also influenced by cell type [103]. We have established that PKD1 is expressed throughout the cytosol of principal cells in the renal CCD cells with accumulation in the trans-Golgi network proximal to the nucleus (266). This structure was identified as the TGN with the use of a specific marker, TGN38. PI4KIIIβ is phosphorylated by PKD1 at the TGN with subsequent upregulation in vesicle fission, and we found that PI4KIIIβ was also localized to the TGN in M1-CCD cells [8]. The TGN association of PI4KIIIβ was not affected by the suppression of PKD1 expression. Treatment with aldosterone did not affect the distribution of PKD1 or PI4KIIIβ at the TGN but did promote the formation of an immunoprecipitatable complex between these two kinases within 5 min. This complex remained stable for at least 30 min, consistent with the sustained autophosphorylation of PKD1 detectable following treatment with aldosterone [7]. The interaction between these two kinases was also observed following the long-term aldosterone stimulation ranging between 1 and 24 h.

### 2.3 Integration of aldosterone genomic and non-genomic actions through PKD signaling pathways

Recent work has focused on the physiological role of non-genomic actions of aldosterone, its consequences for genomic responses, and the integration or cross

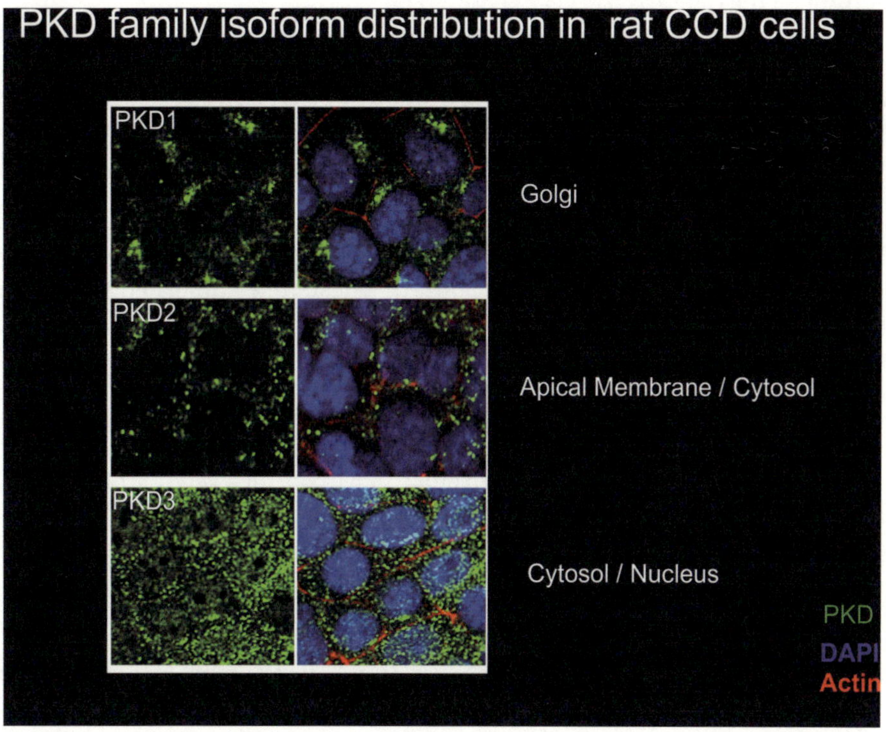


**Figure 3.**
*Subcellular distribution of PKD isoforms in rat renal CCD cells. The PKD isoforms are stained with isoform-specific fluorescence antibodies in green, the nucleus with DAPI stain in blue, and the plasma membrane with actin in red. Following aldosterone treatment, PKD1 rapidly (10 min) localized to apical and basolateral plasma membranes, PKD2 moved out of the apical membrane into the cytosol, and PKD3 became concentrated in the nucleus.*

talk between rapid and latent hormone responses for regulating renal $Na^+$ reabsorption [2, 4, 104, 105].

The activity of crucial rapid signaling intermediates such as PKD, Rho-activated kinase (ROK), protein kinase A (PKA), phosphoinositide 3-kinase (PI3K), PKC, ERK, SGK, and with no lysine family kinases (WNK) can be modulated by aldosterone. Aldosterone activates some or all of these signaling pathways to modulate ENaC channel activity along with other transporters involved in transepithelial sodium reabsorption such as the ATP-sensitive $K^+$ channel and $Na^+/K^+$ pump in principle cells of the CCD. The activation of aldosterone/MR also leads to a suppression of Nedd4-2 ubiquitin ligase activity via SGK which promotes ENaC abundance in the apical membrane [5]. Aldosterone stimulates transcriptional changes in promoting SGK-1 thus inactivating Nedd4-2. This inactivation of Nedd4-2 leads to an increase in ENaC abundance possibly by inhibiting degradation of the channel rather than by membrane insertion or stabilization of the channel complex.

The rapid non-genomic signaling responses induced by aldosterone affect multiple protein kinase signaling pathways, either by directly affecting their activity or indirectly through the modulation of MR-dependent transcription. Both PKCδ and PKCε can be rapidly activated in response to aldosterone; however, this is not reliant on the direct binding of aldosterone to the kinase. The rapid activation is instead coupled to MR via the transactivation of EGFR (109). The rapid activation of PKD1 in response to aldosterone is now known to be a substrate for novel, $Ca^{2+}$-independent PKC isoforms (nPKCs), for example, PKCδ and PKCε. In renal CCD cells, aldosterone stimulates PKD1 activation in the same manner as aldosterone-induced activation of nPKC isoforms. The rapid activation of PKD1 is coupled to MR through the transactivation of EGFR [12].

Aldosterone (rapidly <5 min) activates (phosphorylation) PKD1 in CCD cells through MR transactivation of the EGF receptor involving downstream PKCδ and PKCε and ERK signaling. Aldosterone activation of PKD1 caused translocation of ENaC and Na/K-ATPase pump subunits from the trans-Golgi network to apical and basolateral membrane domains, respectively, within 15 min, via the PKD1-PI4KIIIβ trafficking signaling pathway. Knockdown of PKD1 resulted in a 50% reduction in the basal transepithelial $Na^+$ transport rate concomitant with mislocalization of ENaC to basolateral membranes and Na/K pumps to apical membranes. PKD1 knockdown prevented the genomic response of aldosterone-stimulated transepithelial $Na^+$ reabsorption as measured by the amiloride-sensitive short-circuit current (SCC) in Ussing chambers [8].

Protein kinase D2 is also rapidly activated by aldosterone to modulate ENaC membrane abundance and stability. CCD epithelia in which PKD2 was knocked down showed an increased localization and stabilization of ENaC in apical membranes and an increased basal SCC of fivefold above control levels in wild-type CCD after 24 h. Paradoxically, aldosterone treatment inhibited SCC by 40% after 24 h in PKD2 null M1 cells. However, the SCC levels following aldosterone treatment in PKD2 null CCD epithelia were still 30% higher than the SCC levels observed in aldosterone-treated wild-type CCD. In addition, PKD2 knockdown has revealed a novel inhibitory pathway for aldosterone regulation of ENaC activity which may have a physiological function to "brake" over-stimulation of renal Na reabsorption in the CCD [109].

The protein kinase D3 isoform appears not to mediate non-genomic aldosterone responses. Knockdown of PKD3 in CCD cells did not affect the non-genomic responses to aldosterone on ENaC trafficking but reduced the genomic response to the hormone to increase the expression of ENaC alpha subunits and SGK [109].

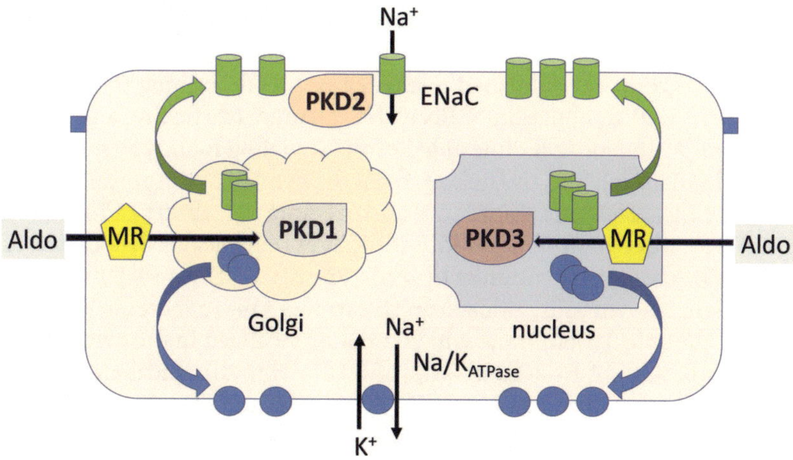


**Figure 4.**
*PKD isoforms regulate ENaC and Na/K pump activity by both non-genomic and genomic aldosterone/MR signaling in the CCD. PKD signaling integrates non-genomic and genomic responses to aldosterone through non-genomic PKD1-stimulated ENaC and Na/K pump trafficking from the trans-Golgi network to apical and basolateral membranes, respectively, and PKD2-dependent ENaC membrane stabilization, and genomic PKD3-stimulated ENaC subunit expression.*

PKD isoforms are a major critical and essential signal transduction pathway for the transduction of both non-genomic and genomic aldosterone/MR regulation of $Na^+$ transport in the CCD. PKD signaling integrates non-genomic and genomic responses to aldosterone through PKD1-stimulated ENaC and Na/K pump trafficking, PKD2-dependent ENaC membrane stabilization, and PKD3-stimulated ENaC subunit expression (**Figure 4**).

## 2.4 Mechanisms of PKD activation by aldosterone

PKD isoforms are downstream targets for active PKCs and can be activated by agonists of G-protein-coupled receptors. Aldosterone induces both rapid phosphorylation and activation of PKD1 [12]. It has been shown that aldosterone activation of PKD1 in CCD cells is PKCε-dependent via aldosterone/MR transactivation of the EGF receptor. The molecular mechanisms of aldosterone activation/phosphorylation of PKD2 and PKD3 isoforms are currently unknown.

## 2.5 The mineralocorticoid receptor is a non-genomic receptor for aldosterone PKD signaling

A number of strands of evidence point to MR as being the receptor responsible for initiating the aldosterone-induced rapid activation of PKD signaling cascades. The activation of protein kinases such as PKD and ERK1/2 by aldosterone, for example, can be inhibited with the use of MR-specific antagonists such as spironolactone and eplerenone. MR can be considered to be a multifunctional receptor. If recombinant MR which lacks its DNA-binding and coactivator-binding domains is expressed, signaling events can be instigated by a rapid response to aldosterone independent of transcriptional activity. The aldosterone/MR-induced phosphorylation of PKD1 via EGFR transactivation by c-Src can be blocked by antagonizing Hsp90 interactions using the geldanamycin analogue 17-AAG. This suppresses EGFR-dependent downstream PKD1 signaling events initiated by aldosterone that include the activation of ENaC trafficking and the ERK1/2 mitogen-activated protein (MAP) kinase [7, 8].

## 3. Aldosterone regulation of ENaC activity via PKD signaling pathways

Our research group has published a series of papers describing the molecular mechanisms of PKD1 modulation of ENaC $Na^+$ channel trafficking and function by aldosterone [2, 4]. Non-genomic aldosterone signaling mainly regulates ENaC activity by stimulating ENaC trafficking from the cytosol to the apical membrane and by enhancing membrane abundance and membrane stability of functional channels. Aldosterone treatment rapidly stimulates the apical translocation of ENaCα, ENaCβ, and ENaCγ subunits in wild-type M1-CCD via PKD1 signaling, but in PKD1 knockdown cells, aldosterone treatment fails to increase ENaC subunit abundance at the apical membrane which remains localized in the cytoplasm. Thus the trafficking process of ENaCα, ENaCβ, and ENaCγ to the apical membrane is defective in CCD cells suppressed in PKD1 expression and indicates a critical role of this protein kinase in regulating subcellular trafficking of ENaC subunits by aldosterone. The rapid effects of aldosterone on ENaC subcellular redistribution precede the genomic increase in the $Na^+$ transport rate through ENaC in CCD cells which is normally detected between 2 and 4 h following treatment with aldosterone and peaks between 16 and 24 h. We have previously reported that the formation of membrane-bound structures that were found to be rich in ENaC subunits was observed following aldosterone stimulation for 5 min. It has been proposed that an ER-Golgi intermediate compartment could be the initial site for the post-ER sorting of proteins. This is consistent with the subcellular redistribution of ENaC channel subunits observed within 2 min of aldosterone stimulation. Previous studies on ENaC-related acid-sensing ion channel (ASIC) suggested that a functional heterodimeric ENaC assembles in the endoplasmic reticulum prior to it undergoing posttranslational modifications as it passes through the Golgi. ENaC is found in vesicles throughout the cytoplasm of cells under high $Na^+$ where its depletion or exposure to aldosterone results in the subsequent translocation of ENaC to the apical membrane without undergoing transcriptional changes [106]. The rapid surface translocation of ENaC and its increased activity has been reported in response to agonists; for example, a twofold increase in the amiloride-sensitive short-circuit current (SCC, transepithelial $Na^+$ current) was observed after 25 min of treatment with forskolin in CCD cells [107]. This increase in SCC coincided with an increase in the apical membrane expression of ENaC. Aldosterone/MR controls the transcription of ENaCα in renal cells, while the remaining subunits, ENaCβ and ENaCγ, are expressed constitutively. We have previously shown that the long-term treatment with aldosterone increases the localization of ENaCα and ENaCβ at the apical membrane in M1-CCD cells which is dependent on PKD1 expression and activation [7]. Further studies showed that aldosterone induces the rapid translocation of ENaCβ and ENaCγ to the plasma membrane within 30 min of treatment and that this translocation, in common with PKD1 activation, was MR-dependent [8].

Aldosterone also induces a rapid phosphorylation (activation) and redistribution of PKD2 from the apical membrane into the cytosol of CCD cells. Genetic suppression of PKD2 in renal CCD cells results in an increase in the abundance of ENaCγ at the apical membrane under both basal and aldosterone-treated conditions. The abundant expression of ENaC at the apical membrane is associated with very high basal $Na^+$ currents through ENaC in PKD2 knockdown CCD epithelia and reveals a tonic inhibition of ENaC function by PKD2 under basal conditions [109]. In its inactive state, PKD2 stimulates the retrieval of the ENaCγ channel subunits out of the apical membrane back into the cytosol thus de-stabilizing ENaC membrane expression and activity. Aldosterone treatment removes this tonic endocytosis of ENaC by phosphorylating PKD2 causing the kinase to be removed from the membrane and inhibiting the retrieval of ENaCγ into the cytosol. In contrast, when PKD2 expression was suppressed by siRNA, the tonic retrieval of ENaC from the apical membrane was removed and ENaC expression was stabilized and enhanced at the membrane resulting in very large basal ENaC-mediated $Na^+$ currents. Moreover, a paradoxical inhibitory effect of aldosterone on ENaC $Na^+$ currents was observed in PKD2 knock-down CCD cells. Given that ENaC activity is a balance between membrane expression and retrieval, the overall regulation of transepithelial sodium transport under basal and aldosterone-stimulated conditions is under the influence of the relative effects of PKD1, PKD2, and SGK1 on ENaC stability in the membrane (**Figure 5**).

### 3.1 Molecular mechanisms of ENaC trafficking regulated by PKD1

Membrane-localized ENaC is subject to constant recycling. The inclusion of ENaC into the apical membrane is a prerequisite for its ubiquitination and retrieval into the subapical pool or its degradation by the proteasome. Nedd4-2 interacts with ENaC through a C-terminal PY internalization motif to facilitate ENaC ubiquitination. The surface expression of ENaC may be equally regulated by deubiquitination by DUBs and ubiquitination by Nedd4-2. However, only PKD1 and PKD2 isoforms provide the composite signaling pathway for the basal control and acute stimulatory effect of aldosterone that influences cellular trafficking dynamics controlling ENaC and Na/K pump membrane targeting, insertion, stabilization, and retrieval (**Figure 6**).

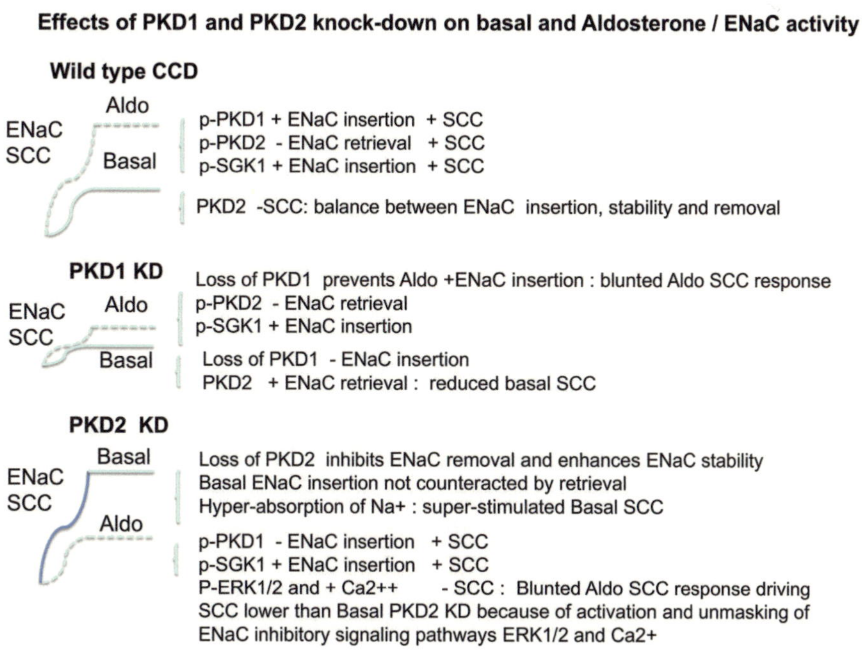


**Figure 5.**
*Effects of PKD1 and PKD2 knockdown on basal and aldosterone-regulated ENaC activity. In wild-type CCD cells, aldosterone induces an increase in the ENaC-dependent transepithelial sodium transport measured by the amiloride-sensitive short-circuit current (Isc) in M1-CCD epithelia mounted in Ussing chambers. Isc is stimulated following aldosterone phosphorylation and activation of PKD1 and SGK1 which together stimulate and stabilize the trafficking of ENaC into the apical membrane. Aldosterone also phosphorylates PKD2 which decreases the retrieval of ENaC back into the cytosol and contributes to the increase in Isc. When PKD1 is suppressed (PKD1 KD), ENaC membrane insertion is decreased, and both basal and aldosterone Isc responses are suppressed. Knocking down PKD2 (PKD2 KD) in CCD cells has an inhibitory effect on the retrieval of ENaC from the apical membrane thus enhancing the stability of the channel resulting in an elevated basal Isc. Paradoxically, hormone stimulation in PKD2 knockdown CCD inhibits Isc and produces a blunted Isc response compared to aldosterone-treated wild-type CCD. Thus PKD2 KD unmasks an inhibitory aldosterone signaling pathway which reduces functional ENaC activity.*

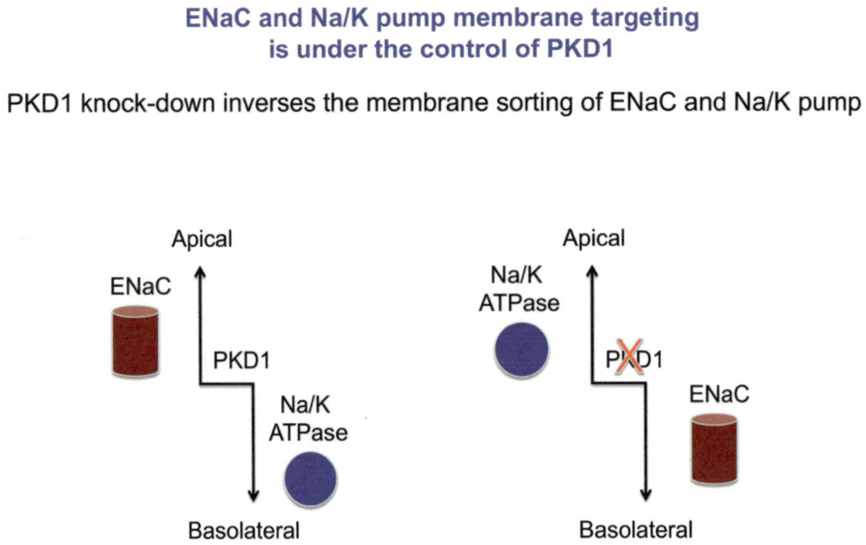


**Figure 6.**
*ENaC and Na/K pump membrane targeting under the control of PKD1. PKD1 regulates the correct targeting of ENaC and $Na^+/K^+$-ATPase to the apical and basolateral membranes, respectively. Knocking down PKD1 expression in CCD cells results in the defective membrane sorting of ENaC and Na/K pump such that their membrane expression polarity is inverted.*

## 3.2 Molecular mechanisms of ENaC trafficking regulated by PKD2

The rapid non-genomic activation of PKD1 by aldosterone has been demonstrated in renal CCD and the implications this has on renal $Na^+$ absorption in terms of trafficking and activity of transporters such as ENaC and $Na^+/K^+$-ATPase pump. To date, less is known about the role of PKD2 in regulating basal ENaC and Na/K pump activity and aldosterone-stimulated renal $Na^+$ reabsorption. There is evidence from transcriptomics studies that the *Pkd2* gene is expressed in the mouse distal convoluted tubule and the collecting duct but not in the connecting tubule [108]. PKD2 protein expression had not been described in the kidney before, and recent studies have shown the expression of PKD2 in mouse and rat distal renal tubules ex vivo and in M1-CCD cells in vitro [109]. The PKD2 isoform was found to be ubiquitously expressed along the length of the distal tubule with the highest expression in the distal convoluted tubule and the connecting tubule and lower levels of expression along the collecting duct. PKD2 was expressed primarily in the principle cells and to a lesser extent in the intercalated cells. The distribution of PKD2 was also determined in rats fed a normal $Na^+$ diet and a diet poor in $Na^+$ in order to elevate plasma levels of aldosterone so as to determine if high aldosterone states can cause shifts in the cellular distribution of PKD2 in the distal nephron. Under basal conditions, the PKD2 cellular distribution appeared mainly localized at the apical membrane (co-localized with AQP2) and showed the lowest expression in the cytosol and was excluded from the nucleus. A similar subcellular distribution of PKD2 was observed in confluent M1-CCD monolayers which also exhibited high PKD2 expression at the plasma membrane and low expression in the cytosol. In high aldosterone states, PKD2 translocates from the apical membrane to a cytosolic compartment. Thus PKD2 shows the opposite pattern of subcellular expression compared to PKD1 under both basal and aldosterone-stimulated conditions. The mechanism by which aldosterone produces a redistribution of PKD2 from the plasma membrane may involve PKC which is also rapidly activated by aldosterone in CCD.

The question arises if PKD2 has a role in regulating the subcellular expression and trafficking of ENaC channel subunits as has been observed for PKD1 in CCD. In other renal tissues, PKD2 has also been shown to function in the basolateral transport of proteins, and knocking down PKD2 affects the membrane trafficking of E-cadherin and β1-integrin [100]. In polarized MDCK cells, the transient expression of a PKD2 kinase-dead mutant resulted in the co-accumulation of E-cadherin, β1-integrin, and the PKD2 mutant at the TGN. It has also been suggested that PKD2 is unlike the other two PKD isoforms because the activation of PKD2 was not shown to induce its redistribution to the nucleus from the cytoplasm. It has also been shown that the activation of NFκB by PKD2 occurs in response to oxidative stress and is not dependent on its catalytic activity. This suggests that PKD2 could have a distinctive regulatory property in comparison to PKD1 and PKD3.

The role of PKD2 in early rapid signaling responses to aldosterone stimulation in $Na^+$ transport has become clearer. Previous work has shown that PKD1 is activated in M1-CCD cells within 5 min in response to aldosterone. A similar activation kinetics has been observed for PKD2 in M1-CCD cells where aldosterone stimulated the autophosphorylation of PKD2 within 10 min coupled with translocation of PKD2 from the cell membrane to the cytosol [109]. Moreover, under low $Na^+$ diet and high aldosterone states, a similar shift in the cellular distribution of PKD2 occurs in the rat distal nephron.

Recent studies have revealed a novel role for PKD2 in the trafficking of ENaC channel subunits [109]. Under basal conditions, ENaCγ is mainly localized in the cytosol. Upon stimulation with aldosterone, ENaCγ is trafficked to the apical membrane, but this response was absent in M1-CCD cells where PKD2 expression was knocked down using siRNA. The genetic silencing of PKD2 in M1-CCD cells produced a higher basal expression of ENaCγ in the apical membrane and a corresponding stimulation of $Na^+$ transport through ENaC. Paradoxically, aldosterone treatment produced a redistribution of ENaCγ out of the apical membrane into the cytosol and a suppressed Isc response in M1-CCD cells deficient in PKD2 (**Figure 5**).

Genetic knockdown of PKD2 in M1-CCD cells results in a stimulation of transepithelial $Na^+$ transport under basal conditions. This increase in ENaC activity corresponds with an increase in basal expression of ENaCγ in PKD2 knockdown CCD when compared to wild-type cells. An inhibition of PKD2-dependent endocytotic retrieval of ENaC channel subunits into the cytosol may result in an increase in both the total ENaC abundance in the membrane and the increase in channel activity. Another possibility for the increase in transepithelial sodium transport in PKD2 knockdown cells could result from an increase in the PKD1-dependent trafficking of ENaC channel subunits. There is also a possibility that PKD1 activity could increase in order to compensate for the absence of PKD2 by upregulating PI4KIIIβ trafficking and therefore affecting ENaC membrane insertion. Unexpectedly, aldosterone treatment stimulated a retrieval of ENaCγ from the apical membrane into the cytoplasm in PKD2-deficient CCD cells. The inhibition of transepithelial $Na^+$ transport by aldosterone in PKD2 knockdown CCD presents a paradox for the classical activation of ENaC by the hormone in wild-type CCD. One would presume that aldosterone could continue to stimulate ENaC activity in the absence of PKD2 in this model due to an upregulation of PKD1- and SGK-dependent ENaC trafficking and membrane stabilization. However, from these findings, we propose that PKD1 and PKD2 exert opposite effects on ENaC membrane abundance and that aldosterone, by activating PKD2 and removing it from the membrane, releases a tonic inhibition of ENaC stability exerted by unphosphorylated PKD2. The translocation and targeting of ENaC and Na/K pump to the apical membrane and basolateral membranes and their membrane stabilization are dependent on cooperative PKD1 and PKD2 non-genomic signaling that may potentiate or synergize with the latent genomic aldosterone effects on ENaC protein expression and membrane abundance. PKD1 is a crucial regulator of the apical membrane-directed trafficking of ENaC. Furthermore, it was shown that PKD1 regulates the membrane localization of the $Na^+/K^+$-ATPase pump, and knocking down PKD1 resulted in the mislocalization of the pump β subunit to the apical membrane and bulk accumulation of the pump protein in the cytosol rather than in the basolateral membranes [8]. Similarly, aldosterone stimulation of PKD1 knockdown M1-CCD cells failed to increase the basolateral membrane abundance of the $Na^+/K^+$ pump normally seen in wild-type cells (**Figure 7**).

### 3.3 PKD1, PKD2, SGK1, and the regulation of ENaC membrane trafficking and stability

The upregulation of SGK1 is the earliest transcriptional and translational response that is elicited by aldosterone, whereas PKD1 and PKD2 are the earliest activated kinases in the non-genomic response to aldosterone in the regulation of ENaC trafficking and stabilization in the apical membrane stabilization. The interactions between aldosterone-stimulated PKD1, PKD2, and SGK have not been investigated; however, certain predictions to guide future research can be proposed and tested (**Figure 8**). Given that PKD1, PKD2, and SGK would be expected to enhance ENaC trafficking, insertion, and stability and to reduce ENaC retrieval and degradation following aldosterone treatment, it would be expected that some cross talk and coordination would exist between these kinases in their kinetics of activation, subcellular localization, and cooperativity. However, from previous

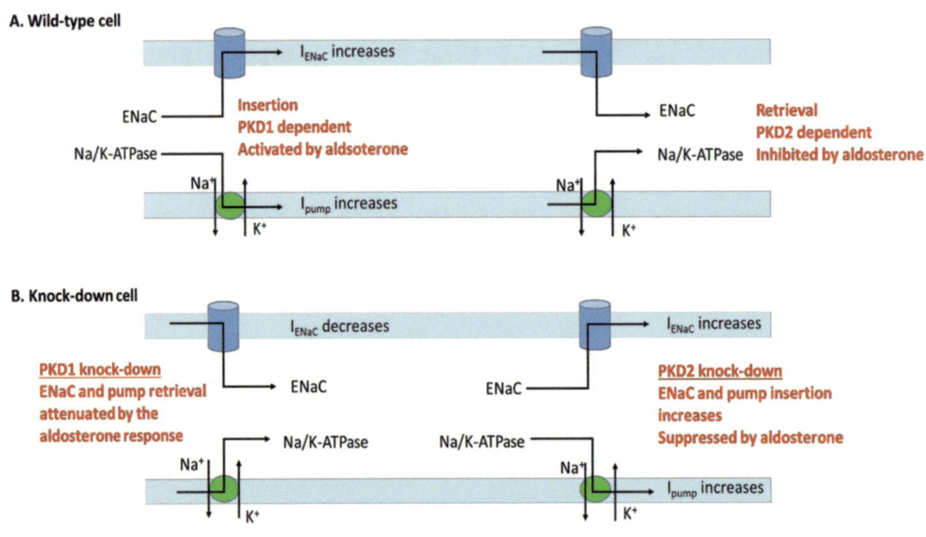


**Figure 7.**
*PKD isoforms exert opposite effects on the membrane abundance and localization of ENaC and Na/K pump with consequences for $Na^+$ transport. The PKD1 isoform regulates the insertion of ENaC channel subunits into the apical membrane of CCD cells. Aldosterone activates the PKD1-dependent trafficking of ENaC subunits to the membrane. In contrast, PKD2 exerts a tonic inhibitory effect on ENaC by stimulating the retrieval of ENaC from the apical membrane into the cytosol under basal conditions. Stimulating PKD2 with aldosterone results in the inhibition of ENaC retrieval back into the cytosol and an increased abundance of ENaC at the apical membrane along with an increase in ENaC activity. Genetic knockdown of PKD1 inhibits ENaC trafficking into the apical membrane under both basal and aldosterone conditions, whereas knockdown of PKD2 releases the tonic inhibition of ENaC activity and suppresses its retrieval by the kinase resulting in a higher abundance and membrane stability of ENaC with consequent elevated $Na^+$ reabsorption ($I_{ENaC}$ and $I_{pump}$). Aldosterone produces a paradoxical inhibition of ENaC membrane abundance and depresses $Na^+$ reabsorption in PKD2 knockdown CCD.*

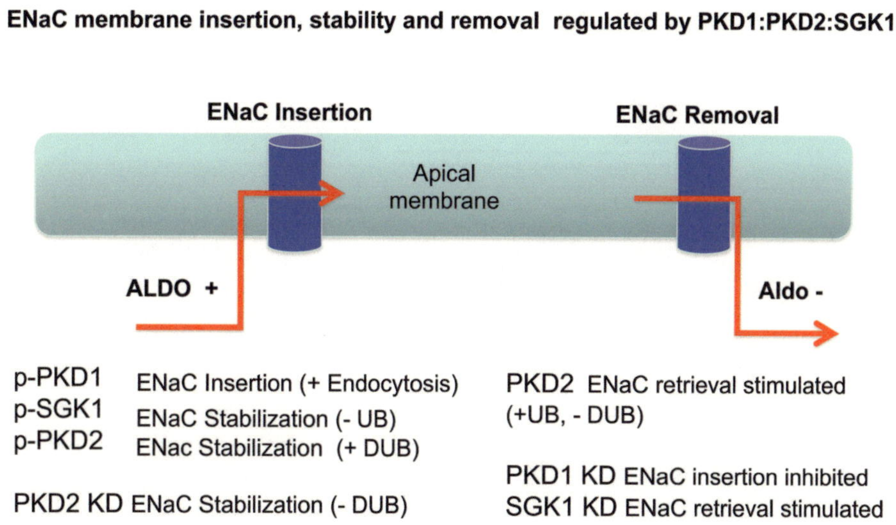


**Figure 8.**
*ENaC membrane insertion, stability, and removal are under the control of interactions between PKD1, PKD2, and SGK1. Aldosterone activates PKD1 to stimulate the insertion of ENaC into the apical membrane. The PKD1-dependent insertion of ENaC increases endocytosis of preformed ENaC subunits into the apical membrane. Additionally, SGK1 is phosphorylated to prevent the ubiquitination of ENaC. In the basal unphosphorylated state, PKD2 tonically stimulates the retrieval of ENaC from the apical membrane. When PKD2 is phosphorylated by aldosterone, the activated PKD2 may increase deubiquitination thus stabilizing ENaC in the membrane. Genetic silencing of PKD2 results in the stabilization of ENaC in the apical membrane which may be due to a decrease in the activity of deubiquitinases. Knocking down SGK1 in CCD cells stimulates the retrieval of ENaC from the membrane while suppressing PKD1 results in the inhibition of ENaC insertion in response to aldosterone.*

work it appears that SGK does not play an essential role in basal or $Na^+$ deprivation-induced renal $Na^+$ transport or ENaC activity, whereas PKD1 and PKD2 expression and activation are absolutely critical for the maintenance of basal and aldosterone-stimulated ENaC function and transepithelial sodium transport.

### 3.4 PKD3 regulation of ENaC and renal $Na^+$ transport

To date, the role of PKD3 in the kidney remains unknown. PKD3 is unlike the other two isoforms whereby it is present in the nucleus as well as the cytoplasm in unstimulated cells. Currently, investigations of PKD3-dependent signaling pathways in the kidney are lacking, while studies in other tissues and cell types have been reliant on the use of non-specific pharmacological inhibitors or the use of small interfering RNA (siRNA). We have used both siRNA and CRISPR/Cas knockdown of PKD3 in M1-CCD cells to obtain some insights into a potential role for PKD3 in the renal transport of sodium. Preliminary data show that PKD3 is primarily localized in the cytoplasm and perinuclear region and translocates to the nucleus under aldosterone treatment or low $Na^+$ diet [109].

PKD3 knockdown resulted in reduced genomic expression of the ENaC$\alpha$ subunit and SGK. Long-term treatment with aldosterone (24–48 h) produced a reduced sodium transport rate in PKD3 suppressed cells compared to wild-type CCD. Knockdown of PKD3 did not interfere with PKD1 nor PKD 2 non-genomic signaling in response to aldosterone nor did it significantly affect basal $Na^+$ transport rates. It thus appears that PKD3 is a genomic signal pathway for aldosterone regulation of ENaC and SGK and may synergize and reinforce with the non-genomic PKD1 and PKD2 modulation of ENaC trafficking and membrane stabilization (**Figure 9**).

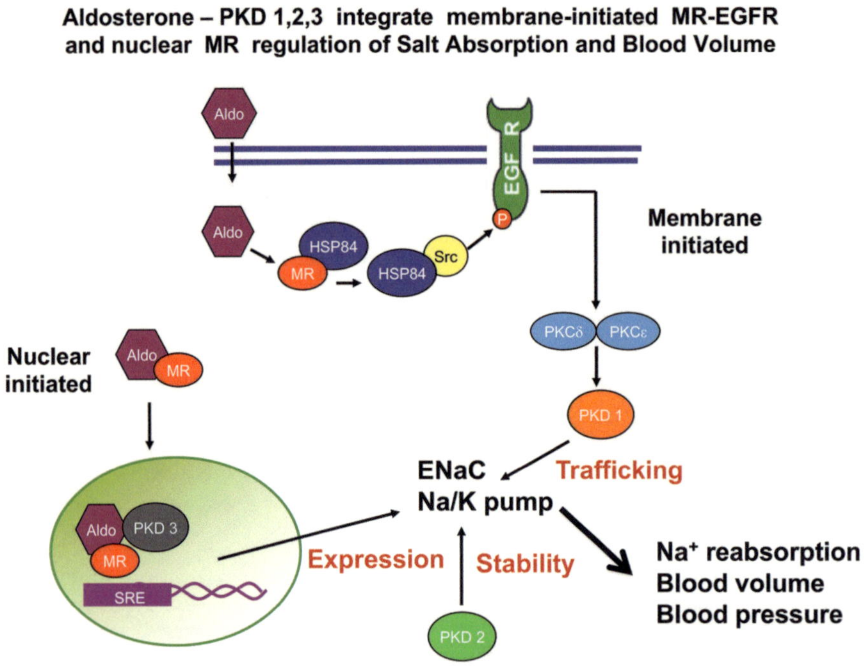


**Figure 9.**
*Regulation of ENaC and Na/K pump by protein kinase D isoforms. PKCδ and PKCε can be rapidly activated in response to aldosterone. The rapid activation of PKC is coupled to MR via the transactivation of EGFR through c-Src. PKD1 is the downstream of PKCδ and PKCε, and once activated, it is responsible for the trafficking of ENaC channel subunits from the cytosol to the apical membrane. PKD2 activation by aldosterone removes a tonic inhibition of ENaC membrane stability and increases the stability of ENaC channels in the membrane. PKD3 activation exerts a stimulatory effect on the expression of ENaC channel subunits and SGK, further amplifying and sustaining the non-genomic response to regulate renal $Na^+$ reabsorption and blood volume/pressure.*

## 4. Conclusions and perspectives

The physiological and pathophysiological roles of PKD isoforms in different biological systems are becoming better understood with the identification of novel substrates for this family of kinases that also interact with other kinases and transcription factors which modulate intracellular trafficking, membrane targeting, and stability of ion transport proteins. These PKD isoform-regulated biological processes fine-tune the aldosterone/MR-dependent transcriptional events and act as important intermediaries between rapid non-genomic signaling and latent transcriptional responses activated by aldosterone to regulate renal electrolyte homeostasis. The development of PKD isoform-specific knockdown or knockout renal CCD cell lines and animal models has the potential to reveal novel rapid non-genomic and genomic roles for PKD isoforms to regulate basal and aldosterone-stimulated ENaC and $Na^+/K^+$-ATPase pump activity in renal CCD cells.

## Acknowledgements

This publication is based upon work from the EU COST Action ADMIRE BM1301 in Aldosterone and Mineralocorticoid Receptor Physiology and Pathophysiology www.admirecosteu.com.

## Author details

Warren Thomas[1,2] and Brian Harvey[1,3]*

1 Department of Molecular Medicine, Royal College of Surgeons in Ireland, Beaumont Hospital, Dublin, Ireland

2 Perdana University, PU-RCSI School of Medicine, Serdang, Selangor, Malaysia

3 Centro de Estudios Cientificos CECs, Valdivia, Chile

*Address all correspondence to: brianharvey@rcsi.com

## References


[1] Pimenta E, Gordon RD, Stowasser M. Salt, aldosterone and hypertension. Journal of Human Hypertension. 2013;**27**(1):1-6. DOI: 10.1038/jhh.2012.27

[2] Harvey BJ, Thomas W. Aldosterone-induced protein kinase signalling and the control of electrolyte balance. Steroids. 2018;**133**:67-74. DOI: 10.1016/j.steroids.2017.10.009. Epub 2017 Oct 24. Review

[3] Urbach V, Van Kerkhove E, Maguire D, Harvey BJ. Cross-talk between ATP-regulated K+ channels and Na+ transport via cellular metabolism in frog skin principal cells. The Journal of Physiology. 1996;**491**(Pt 1):99-109

[4] Thomas W, Harvey BJ. Mechanisms underlying rapid aldosterone effects in the kidney. Annual Review of Physiology. 2011;**73**:335-357. DOI: 10.1146/annurev-physiol-012110-142222

[5] Pearce D. SGK1 regulation of epithelial sodium transport. Cellular Physiology and Biochemistry. 2003;**13**(1):13-20

[6] Fejes-Tóth G, Frindt G, Náray-Fejes-Tóth A, Palmer LG. Epithelial Na+ channel activation and processing in mice lacking SGK1. American Journal of Physiology. Renal Physiology. 2008;**294**(6):F1298-F1305. DOI: 10.1152/ajprenal.00579.2007

[7] McEneaney V, Harvey BJ, Thomas W. Aldosterone regulates rapid trafficking of epithelial sodium channel subunits in renal cortical collecting duct cells via protein kinase D activation. Molecular Endocrinology. 2008;**22**(4):881-892. DOI: 10.1210/me.2007-0225

[8] Dooley R, Angibaud E, Yusef YR, Thomas W, Harvey BJ. Aldosterone-induced ENaC and basal Na+/K+-ATPase trafficking via protein kinase D1-phosphatidylinositol 4-kinaseIIIβ trans Golgi signalling in M1 cortical collecting duct cells. Molecular and Cellular Endocrinology. 2013;**372**(1-2):86-95. DOI: 10.1016/j.mce.2013.03.011

[9] Asher C, Wald H, Rossier BC, Garty H. Aldosterone-induced increase in the abundance of Na+ channel subunits. The American Journal of Physiology. 1996;**271**(2 Pt 1):C605-C611

[10] Beesley AH, Hornby D, White SJ. Regulation of distal nephron K+ channels (ROMK) mRNA expression by aldosterone in rat kidney. The Journal of Physiology. 1998;**509**(Pt 3):629-634

[11] Kolla V, Litwack G. Transcriptional regulation of the human Na/K ATPase via the human mineralocorticoid receptor. Molecular and Cellular Biochemistry. 2000;**204**(1-2):35-40

[12] McEneaney V, Harvey BJ, Thomas W. Aldosterone rapidly activates protein kinase D via a mineralocorticoid receptor/EGFR trans-activation pathway in the M1 kidney CCD cell line. The Journal of Steroid Biochemistry and Molecular Biology. 2007;**107**(3-5):180-190. Epub 2007 Jun 22

[13] Grossmann C, Gekle M. Nongenotropic aldosterone effects and the EGFR: Interaction and biological relevance. Steroids. 2008;**73**(9-10):973-978. DOI: 10.1016/j.steroids.2007.12.008

[14] Dooley R, Harvey BJ, Thomas W. Non-genomic actions of aldosterone: From receptors and signals to membrane targets. Molecular and Cellular Endocrinology. 2012;**350**(2):223-234. DOI: 10.1016/j.mce.2011.07.019

[15] Michea L, Delpiano AM, Hitschfeld C, Lobos L, Lavandero S, Marusic ET.

Eplerenone blocks nongenomic effects of aldosterone on the Na+/H+ exchanger, intracellular Ca2+ levels, and vasoconstriction in mesenteric resistance vessels. Endocrinology. 2005;**146**(3):973-980

[16] Miyata Y, Muto S, Kusano E. Mechanisms for nongenomic and genomic effects of aldosterone on Na+/H+ exchange in vascular smooth muscle cells. Journal of Hypertension. 2005;**23**(12):2237-2250

[17] Feldman RD, Limbird LE. GPER (GPR30): A nongenomic receptor (GPCR) for steroid hormones with implications for cardiovascular disease and cancer. Annual Review of Pharmacology and Toxicology. 2017;**57**:567-584. DOI: 10.1146/annurev-pharmtox-010716-104651

[18] Cole DF. Effect of aldosterone on renal excretion of intravenously administered saline. Endocrinology. 1957;**60**(4):562-565

[19] Musabayane CT, Ndhlovu CE, Forsling ML, Balment RJ. Interaction of aldosterone and oxytocin to influence renal sodium excretion in rats. Experimental Physiology. 1994;**79**(5):763-774

[20] Rad AK, Balment RJ, Ashton N. Rapid natriuretic action of aldosterone in the rat. Journal of Applied Physiology. 2005;**98**(2):423-428

[21] Urbach V, Van Kerkhove E, Maguire D, Harvey BJ. Rapid activation of KATP channels by aldosterone in principal cells of frog skin. The Journal of Physiology. 1996;**491**(Pt 1):111-120

[22] Harvey BJ, Ehrenfeld J. Role of Na+/H+ exchange in the control of intracellular pH and cell membrane conductances in frog skin epithelium. The Journal of General Physiology. 1988;**92**(6):793-810

[23] Harvey BJ, Thomas SR, Ehrenfeld J. Intracellular pH controls cell membrane Na+ and K+ conductances and transport in frog skin epithelium. The Journal of General Physiology. 1988;**92**(6):767-791

[24] Oberleithner H, Weigt M, Westphale HJ, Wang W. Aldosterone activates Na+/H+ exchange and raises cytoplasmic pH in target cells of the amphibian kidney. Proceedings of the National Academy of Sciences of the United States of America. 1987;**84**(5):1464-1468

[25] Gekle M, Freudinger R, Mildenberger S, Schenk K, Marschitz I, Schramek H. Rapid activation of Na+/H+-exchange in MDCK cells by aldosterone involves MAP-kinase ERK1/2. Pflugers Archiv: European Journal of Physiology. 2001;**441**(6):781-786

[26] Gekle M, Golenhofen N, Oberleithner H, Silbernagl S. Rapid activation of Na+/H+ exchange by aldosterone in renal epithelial cells requires $Ca^{2+}$ and stimulation of a plasma membrane proton conductance. Proceedings of the National Academy of Sciences of the United States of America. 1996;**93**(19):10500-10504

[27] Markos F, Healy V, Harvey BJ. Aldosterone rapidly activates Na+/H+ exchange in M-1 cortical collecting duct cells via a PKC-MAPK pathway. Nephron. Physiology. 2005;**99**(1):p1-p9

[28] Wehling M, Käsmayr J, Theisen K. Fast effects of aldosterone on electrolytes in human lymphocytes are mediated by the sodium-proton-exchanger of the cell membrane. Biochemical and Biophysical Research Communications. 1989;**164**(3):961-967

[29] Thomas W, McEneaney V, Harvey BJ. Aldosterone-induced signalling and cation transport in the distal nephron.

Steroids. 2008;**73**(9-10):979-984. DOI: 10.1016/j.steroids.2008.01.013

[30] Ruhs S, Nolze A, Hübschmann R, Grossmann C. 30 years of the mineralocorticoid receptor: Nongenomic effects via the mineralocorticoid receptor. The Journal of Endocrinology. 2017;**234**(1):T107-T124. DOI: 10.1530/JOE-16-0659

[31] Crabbe J. Stimulation of active sodium transport across the isolated toad bladder after injection of aldosterone to the animal. Endocrinology. 1961;**69**:673-682

[32] Al-Awqati Q, Norby LH, Mueller A, Steinmetz PR. Characteristics of stimulation of H+ transport by aldosterone in turtle urinary bladder. The Journal of Clinical Investigation. 1976;**58**(2):351-358

[33] Harvey BJ. Energization of sodium absorption by the H(+)-ATPase pump in mitochondria-rich cells of frog skin. The Journal of Experimental Biology. 1992;**172**:289-309

[34] Winter C, Schulz N, Giebisch G, Geibel JP, Wagner CA. Nongenomic stimulation of vacuolar H+-ATPases in intercalated renal tubule cells by aldosterone. Proceedings of the National Academy of Sciences of the United States of America. 2004;**101**(8):2636-2641

[35] O'Neil RG, Sansom SC. Characterization of apical cell membrane Na+ and K+ conductances of cortical collecting duct using microelectrode techniques. The American Journal of Physiology. 1984;**247**(1 Pt 2):F14-F24

[36] Kohda Y, Ding W, Phan E, Housini I, Wang J, Star RA, et al. Localization of the ROMK potassium channel to the apical membrane of distal nephron in rat kidney. Kidney International. 1998;**54**(4):1214-1223

[37] Yoo D, Kim BY, Campo C, Nance L, King A, Maouyo D, et al. Cell surface expression of the ROMK (Kir 1.1) channel is regulated by the aldosterone-induced kinase, SGK-1, and protein kinase A. The Journal of Biological Chemistry. 2003;**278**(25):23066-23075

[38] Wang WH, Giebisch G. Regulation of potassium (K) handling in the renal collecting duct. Pflugers Archiv: European Journal of Physiology. 2009;**458**(1):157-168

[39] Sansom SC, O'Neil RG. Effects of mineralocorticoids on transport properties of cortical collecting duct basolateral membrane. The American Journal of Physiology. 1986;**251**(4 Pt 2): F743-F757

[40] Bowley KA, Morton MJ, Hunter M, Sandle GI. Non-genomic regulation of intermediate conductance potassium channels by aldosterone in human colonic crypt cells. Gut. 2003;**52**(6):854-860

[41] Bowley KA, Linley JE, Robins GG, Kopanati S, Hunter M, Sandle GI. Role of protein kinase C in aldosterone-induced non-genomic inhibition of basolateral potassium channels in human colonic crypts. The Journal of Steroid Biochemistry and Molecular Biology. 2007;**104**(1-2):45-52

[42] Maguire D, MacNamara B, Cuffe JE, Winter D, Doolan CM, Urbach V, et al. Rapid responses to aldosterone in human distal colon. Steroids. 1999;**64**(1-2):51-63

[43] Baines D. Kinases as targets for ENaC regulation. Current Molecular Pharmacology. 2013;**6**(1):50-64

[44] Thomas W, McEneaney V, Harvey BJ. Rapid responses to steroid hormones

in the kidney. Nephron. Physiology. 2007;**107**(1):p1-p9

[45] Thomas W, McEneaney V, Harvey BJ. Aldosterone-stimulated PKC signaling cascades: From receptor to effector. Biochemical Society Transactions. 2007;**35**(Pt5):1049-1051. Review

[46] Harvey BJ, Alzamora R, Stubbs AK, Irnaten M, McEneaney V, Thomas W. Rapid responses to aldosterone in the kidney and colon. The Journal of Steroid Biochemistry and Molecular Biology. 2008;**108**(3-5):310-317

[47] Harvey BJ, Alzamora R, Healy V, Renard C, Doolan CM. Rapid responses to steroid hormones: From frog skin to human colon. A homage to Hans Ussing. Biochimica et Biophysica Acta. 2002;**1566**(1-2):116-128

[48] Manegold JC, Falkenstein E, Wehling M, Christ M. Rapid aldosterone effects on tyrosine phosphorylation in vascular smooth muscle cells. Cellular and Molecular Biology. 1999;**45**(6):805-813

[49] Okoshi MP, Yan X, Okoshi K, Nakayama M, Schuldt AJ, O'Connell TD, et al. Aldosterone directly stimulates cardiac myocyte hypertrophy. Journal of Cardiac Failure. 2004;**10**(6):511-518

[50] Nishiyama A, Yao L, Fan Y, Kyaw M, Kataoka N, Hashimoto K, et al. Involvement of aldosterone and mineralocorticoid receptors in rat mesangial cell proliferation and deformability. Hypertension. 2005;**45**(4):710-716

[51] Stockand JD, Meszaros JG. Aldosterone stimulates proliferation of cardiac fibroblasts by activating Ki-RasA and MAPK1/2 signaling. American Journal of Physiology Heart and Circulatory Physiology. 2003;**284**(1):H176-H184

[52] Sinnett-Smith J, Zhukova E, Hsieh N, Jiang X, Rozengurt E. Protein kinase D potentiates DNA synthesis induced by Gq-coupled receptors by increasing the duration of ERK signaling in swiss 3T3 cells. The Journal of Biological Chemistry. 2004;**279**(16):16883-16893

[53] Tong Q, Booth RE, Worrell RT, Stockand JD. Regulation of Na+ transport by aldosterone: Signaling convergence and cross talk between the PI3-K and MAPK1/2 cascades. American Journal of Physiology Renal Physiology. 2004;**286**(6):F1232-F1238

[54] Callera GE, Montezano AC, Yogi A, Tostes RC, He Y, Schiffrin EL, et al. c-Src-dependent nongenomic signaling responses to aldosterone are increased in vascular myocytes from spontaneously hypertensive rats. Hypertension. 2005;**46**(4):1032-1038

[55] Chen C, Liang W, Jia J, van Goor H, Singhal PC, Ding G. Aldosterone induces apoptosis in rat podocytes: Role of PI3-K/Akt and p38MAPK signaling pathways. Nephron Experimental Nephrology. 2009;**113**(1):e26-e34

[56] Le Moellic C, Ouvrard-Pascaud A, Capurro C, Cluzeaud F, Fay M, Jaisser F, et al. Early nongenomic events in aldosterone action in renal collecting duct cells: PKCalpha activation, mineralocorticoid receptor phosphorylation, and cross-talk with the genomic response. Journal of the American Society of Nephrology: JASN. 2004;**15**(5):1145-1160

[57] Slater SJ, Kelly MB, Taddeo FJ, Rubin E, Stubbs CD. Evidence for discrete diacylglycerol and phorbol ester activator sites on protein kinase C. Differences in effects of 1-alkanol inhibition, activation by phosphatidylethanolamine and calcium chelation. Journal of Biological Chemistry. 24 Jun 1994;**269**(25):17160-17165

[58] Alzamora R, Brown LR, Harvey BJ. Direct binding and activation of protein kinase C isoforms by aldosterone and 17beta-estradiol. Molecular Endocrinology. 2007;**21**(11):2637-2650

[59] McEneaney V, Dooley R, Harvey BJ, Thomas W. Protein kinase D stabilizes aldosterone- induced ERK1/2 MAP kinase activation in M1 renal cortical collecting duct cells to promote cell proliferation. The Journal of Steroid Biochemistry and Molecular Biology. 2010;**118**(1-2):18-28

[60] Tsybouleva N, Zhang L, Chen S, Patel R, Lutucuta S, Nemoto S, et al. Aldosterone, through novel signaling proteins, is a fundamental molecular bridge between the genetic defect and the cardiac phenotype of hypertrophic cardiomyopathy. Circulation. 2004;**109**(10):1284-1291

[61] Kobayashi T, Deak M, Morrice N, Cohen P. Characterization of the structure and regulation of two novel isoforms of serum- and glucocorticoid-induced protein kinase. The Biochemical Journal. 1999;**344**(Pt 1):189-197

[62] Pao AC, McCormick JA, Li H, Siu J, Govaerts C, Bhalla V, et al. NH2 terminus of serum and glucocorticoid-regulated kinase 1 binds to phosphoinositides and is essential for isoform-specific physiological functions. American Journal of Physiology Renal Physiology. 2007;**292**(6):F1741-F1750

[63] Blazer-Yost BL, Liu X, Helman SI. Hormonal regulation of ENaCs: Insulin and aldosterone. The American Journal of Physiology. 1998;**274**(5 Pt 1): C1373-C1379

[64] Gonzalez-Rodriguez E, Gaeggeler HP, Rossier BC. IGF-1 vs insulin: Respective roles in modulating sodium transport via the PI-3 kinase/ Sgk1 pathway in a cortical collecting duct cell line. Kidney International. 2007;**71**(2):116-125

[65] Watt GB, Ismail NA, Caballero AG, Land SC, Wilson SM. Epithelial Na(+) channel activity in human airway epithelial cells: The role of serum and glucocorticoid-inducible kinase 1. British Journal of Pharmacology. 2012;**166**(4):1272-1289

[66] Pochynyuk O, Medina J, Gamper N, Genth H, Stockand JD, Staruschenko A. Rapid translocation and insertion of the epithelial Na+ channel in response to RhoA signaling. The Journal of Biological Chemistry. 2006;**281**(36):26520-26527

[67] Harvey BJ, Higgins M. Nongenomic effects of aldosterone on Ca2+ in M-1 cortical collecting duct cells. Kidney International. 2000;**57**(4):1395-1403

[68] Wehling M, Ulsenheimer A, Schneider M, Neylon C, Christ M. Rapid effects of aldosterone on free intracellular calcium in vascular smooth muscle and endothelial cells: Subcellular localization of calcium elevations by single cell imaging. Biochemical and Biophysical Research Communications. 1994;**204**(2):475-481

[69] Maggio N, Segal M. Cellular basis of a rapid effect of mineralocorticosteroid receptors activation on LTP in ventral hippocampal slices. Hippocampus. 2012;**22**(2):267-275

[70] Doolan CM, O'Sullivan GC, Harvey BJ. Rapid effects of corticosteroids on cytosolic protein kinase C and intracellular calcium concentration in human distal colon. Molecular and Cellular Endocrinology. 1998;**138**(1-2):71-79

[71] Grossmann C, Wuttke M, Ruhs S, Seiferth A, Mildenberger S, Rabe S, et al. Mineralocorticoid receptor inhibits CREB signaling by calcineurin

activation. FASEB Journal: Official Publication of the Federation of American Societies for Experimental Biology. 2010;**24**(6):2010-2019

[72] Christ M, Meyer C, Sippel K, Wehling M. Rapid aldosterone signaling in vascular smooth muscle cells: Involvement of phospholipase C, diacylglycerol and protein kinase C alpha. Biochemical and Biophysical Research Communications. 1995;**213**(1):123-129

[73] Gros R, Ding Q, Sklar LA, Prossnitz EE, Arterburn JB, Chorazyczewski J, et al. GPR30 expression is required for the mineralocorticoid receptor-independent rapid vascular effects of aldosterone. Hypertension. 2011;**57**(3):442-451

[74] Grossmann C, Benesic A, Krug AW, Freudinger R, Mildenberger S, Gassner B, et al. Human mineralocorticoid receptor expression renders cells responsive for nongenotropic aldosterone actions. Molecular Endocrinology. 2005;**19**(7):1697-1710

[75] Grossmann C, Freudinger R, Mildenberger S, Husse B, Gekle M. EF domains are sufficient for nongenomic mineralocorticoid receptor actions. The Journal of Biological Chemistry. 2008;**283**(11):71gekle09-71gekle16

[76] Grossmann C, Husse B, Mildenberger S, Schreier B, Schuman K, Gekle M. Colocalization of mineralocorticoid and EGF receptor at the plasma membrane. Biochimica et Biophysica Acta. 2010;**1803**(5):584-590. DOI: 10.1016/j.bbamcr.2010.02.008

[77] Grossmann C, Krug AW, Freudinger R, Mildenberger S, Voelker K, Gekle M. Aldosterone-induced EGFR expression: Interaction between the human mineralocorticoid receptor and the human EGFR promoter. American Journal of Physiology. Endocrinology and Metabolism. 2007;**292**(6):E1790-E1800

[78] Grossmann C, Freudinger R, Mildenberger S, Krug AW, Gekle M. Evidence for epidermal growth factor receptor as negative-feedback control in aldosterone-induced Na+ reabsorption. American Journal of Physiology. Renal Physiology. 2004;**286**(6):F1226-F1231

[79] Krug AW, Grossmann C, Schuster C, Freudinger R, Mildenberger S, Govindan MV, et al. Aldosterone stimulates epidermal growth factor receptor expression. The Journal of Biological Chemistry. 2003;**278**(44):43060-43066

[80] Gekle M, Freudinger R, Mildenberger S, Silbernagl S. Aldosterone interaction with epidermal growth factor receptor signaling in MDCK cells. American Journal of Physiology Renal Physiology. 2002;**282**(4):F669-F679

[81] Krug AW, Schuster C, Gassner B, Freudinger R, Mildenberger S, Troppmair J, et al. Human epidermal growth factor receptor-1 expression renders Chinese hamster ovary cells sensitive to alternative aldosterone signaling. The Journal of Biological Chemistry. 2002;**277**(48):45892-45897

[82] Braun S, Losel R, Wehling M, Boldyreff B. Aldosterone rapidly activates Src kinase in M-1 cells involving the mineralocorticoid receptor and HSP84. FEBS Letters. 2004;**570**(1-3):69-72

[83] Gekle M, Freudinger R, Mildenberger S, Silbernagl S. Rapid actions of aldosterone on cells from renal epithelium: The possible role of EGF-receptor signaling. Steroids. 2002;**67**(6):499-504

[84] Quinn S, Harvey BJ, Thomas W. Rapid aldosterone actions on epithelial

sodium channel trafficking and cell proliferation. Steroids. 2014;**81**:43-48. DOI: 10.1016/j.steroids.2013.11.005

[85] Filardo EJ, Quinn JA, Bland KI, Frackelton AR Jr. Estrogen-induced activation of Erk-1 and Erk- 2 requires the G protein-coupled receptor homolog, GPR30, and occurs via trans-activation of the epidermal growth factor receptor through release of HB-EGF. Molecular Endocrinology. 2000;**14**(10):1649-1660

[86] Daub H, Wallasch C, Lankenau A, Herrlich A, Ullrich A. Signal characteristics of G protein-transactivated EGF receptor. The EMBO Journal. 1997;**16**(23):7032-7044

[87] Guerrero J, Santibanez JF, Gonzalez A, Martinez J. EGF receptor transactivation by urokinase receptor stimulus through a mechanism involving Src and matrix metalloproteinases. Experimental Cell Research. 2004;**292**(1):201-208

[88] Stirnweiss J, Valkova C, Ziesche E, Drube S, Liebmann C. Muscarinic M2 receptors mediate transactivation of EGF receptor through Fyn kinase and without matrix metalloproteases. Cellular Signalling. 2006;**18**(8):1338-1349

[89] Wehling M. Rapid actions of aldosterone revisited: Receptors in the limelight. The Journal of Steroid Biochemistry and Molecular Biology. 2018;**176**:94-98. DOI: 10.1016/j.jsbmb.2017.01.016

[90] Slater SJ, Kelly MB, Taddeo FJ, Larkin JD, Yeager MD, McLane JA, et al. Direct activation of protein kinase C by 1 alpha,25-dihydroxyvitamin D3. The Journal of Biological Chemistry. 1995;**270**(12):6639-6643

[91] Alzamora R, Harvey BJ. Direct binding and activation of protein kinase C isoforms by steroid hormones. Steroids. 2008;**73**(9-10):885-888. DOI: 10.1016/j.steroids.2008.01.001

[92] Hermidorff MM, de Assis LV, Isoldi MC. Genomic and rapid effects of aldosterone: What we know and do not know thus far. Heart Failure Reviews. 2017;**22**(1):65-89. DOI: 10.1007/s10741-016-9591-2

[93] Qiao H, Hu B, Zhou H, Yan J, Jia R, Lu B, et al. Aldosterone induces rapid sodium intake by a nongenomic mechanism in the nucleus tractus solitarius. Scientific Reports. 2016;**6**:38631. DOI: 10.1038/srep38631

[94] Bhalla V, Hallows KR. Mechanisms of ENaC regulation and clinical implications. Journal of the American Society of Nephrology: JASN. 2008;**19**(10):1845-1854

[95] Levin ER, Hammes SR. Nuclear receptors outside the nucleus: Extranuclear signalling by steroid receptors. Nature Reviews. Molecular Cell Biology. 2016;**17**(12):783-797. DOI: 10.1038/nrm.2016.122

[96] Rozengurt E, Rey O, Waldron RT. Protein kinase D signaling. The Journal of Biological Chemistry. 2005;**280**(14):13205-13208

[97] Rozengurt E. Protein kinase D signaling: Multiple biological functions in health and disease. Physiology. 2011;**26**(1):23-23

[98] Rey O, Young SH, Cantrell D, Rozengurt E. Rapid protein kinase D translocation in response to G protein-coupled receptor activation. Dependence on protein kinase C. The Journal of Biological Chemistry. 2001;**276**(35):32616-32626

[99] Rey O, Papazyan R, Waldron RT, Young SH, Lippincott-Schwartz J, Jacamo R, et al. The nuclear import of protein kinase D3 requires its catalytic

activity. The Journal of Biological Chemistry. 2006;**281**(8):5149-5157

[100] Yeaman C, Ayala MI, Wright JR, Bard F, Bossard C, Ang A, et al. Protein kinase D regulates basolateral membrane protein exit from trans-Golgi network. Nature Cell Biology. 2004;**6**(2):106-112

[101] Liljedahl M, Maeda Y, Colanzi A, Ayala I, Van Lint J, Malhotra V. Protein kinase D regulates the fission of cell surface destined transport carriers from the trans-Golgi network. Cell. 2001;**104**(3):409-420

[102] McEneaney V, Dooley R, Yusef YR, Keating N, Quinn U, Harvey BJ, et al. Protein kinase D1 modulates aldosterone-induced ENaC activity in a renal cortical collecting duct cell line. Molecular and Cellular Endocrinology. 2010;**325**(1-2):8-17. DOI: 10.1016/j.mce.2010.04.019

[103] Rykx A, De Kimpe L, Mikhalap S, Vantus T, Seufferlein T, Vandenheede JR, et al. Protein kinase D: A family affair. FEBS Letters. 2003;**546**(1):81-86

[104] Le Moëllic C, Ouvrard-Pascaud A, Capurro C, Cluzeaud F, Fay M, Jaisser F, et al. Early nongenomic events in aldosterone action in renal collecting duct cells: PKCalpha activation, mineralocorticoid receptor phosphorylation, and cross-talk with the genomic response. Journal of the American Society of Nephrology. 2004;**15**(5):1145-1160

[105] Yusef YR, Thomas W, Harvey BJ. Physiological techniques in the study of rapid aldosterone effects. Methods in Molecular Biology. 2014;**1204**:219-231. DOI: 10.1007/978-1-4939-1346-6_19

[106] Masilamani S, Kim GH, Mitchell C, Wade JB, Knepper MA. Aldosterone-mediated regulation of ENaC alpha, beta, and gamma subunit proteins in rat kidney. The Journal of Clinical Investigation. 1999;**104**(7):R19-R23

[107] Butterworth MB, Edinger RS, Johnson JP, Frizzell RA. Acute ENaC stimulation by cAMP in a kidney cell line is mediated by exocytic insertion from a recycling channel pool. The Journal of General Physiology. 2005;**125**(1):81-101

[108] Lee JW, Chou CL, Knepper MA. Deep sequencing in microdissected renal tubules identifies nephron segment-specific transcriptomes. Journal of the American Society of Nephrology: JASN. 2015;**26**(11):2669-2677

[109] Quinn S. Aldosterone Regulation of Protein Kinase D and Sodium Reabsorption in the Renal Cortical Collecting Duct [PhD Thesis]. Dublin: Royal College of Surgeons in Ireland; 2018. Available from: https://epubs.rcsi.ie/phdtheses/229/

Chapter 16

# Advances in the Development of Non-steroidal Mineralocorticoid-receptor Antagonists

*Felipe L. Pérez-Gordillo, Maria Jesús Pérez de Vega, Guillermo Gerona-Navarro, Yoel Rodríguez, Diego Alvarez de la Rosa, Rosario González-Muñiz and Mercedes Martín-Martínez*

## Abstract

The mineralocorticoid receptor (MR) belongs to the nuclear receptor superfamily and regulates body fluid and electrolyte balance. In the last years, much effort has been put into the development of non-steroidal MR antagonists that overcome the side effects of the marketed steroid drugs, and can be used for the treatment of hypertension and heart failure, among others. Initially, MR was identified in epithelial cells, however it also plays important roles in non-epithelial tissues. In this sense, it is of interest to discover ligands that might induce different MR conformational changes, leading to specific coregulator interactions, which could confer tissue-specific effects. Different series of non-steroidal ligands with diverse central scaffolds has been described, which shows antihypertensive and cardiorenal protective effects. This review covers a description of different non-steroidal MR antagonist families, with special focus on compounds under clinical development. The analysis of the three-dimensional (3D) structures of non-steroidal MR antagonists in complex with the MR ligand-binding domain (LBD), recently reported, highlights the interactions crucial for binding. The structure-activity relationships of known ligands, together with the insights provided by the 3D structures of ligand - LBD MR complexes, could help in the development of non-steroidal MR antagonists with improved properties.

**Keywords:** mineralocorticoid receptor, MR antagonist, structure-activity relationship, clinical trials

## 1. Introduction

The mineralocorticoid receptor (MR) transduces the effects of the steroid hormone aldosterone on mineral ion homeostasis, extracellular volume, and blood pressure mainly by regulating kidney $Na^+$ reabsorption and $K^+$ and $H^+$ excretion [1]. In addition, MR can also act as a high-affinity receptor for glucocorticoids. In aldosterone target tissues such as the kidney distal nephron, glucocorticoid-mediated activation of MR is limited by co-expression of 11-β-hydroxysteroid dehydrogenase type II (11ßHSD2), which enzymatically limits access of glucocorticoids to the receptor [2]. High corticosteroid circulating levels can overcome this mechanism, producing mineralocorticoid-like effects. Furthermore, MR tissue distribution is much broader than originally expected, and in many cells it is unclear if there are any mechanisms at all providing aldosterone selectivity over glucocorticoids [3]. It is thus reasonable to assume that both aldosterone and glucocorticoids can activate MR in a cell type-specific fashion.

The role of MR in blood pressure regulation and $K^+$ homeostasis has been therapeutically exploited using steroid analogs with competitive inhibitory activity. This strategy is commonly used for treating primary aldosteronism and additional clinical situations where a decrease in extracellular volume is advantageous, such as essential hypertension and edema associated with congestive heart failure or cirrhosis [4]. The interest in MR antagonists has greatly increased in the past two decades. The unexpectedly broad tissue distribution of MR prompted research on possible additional physiological and pathological roles for this receptor [5]. It is now clear that MR has important contributions to the development of fibrosis [6], inflammation [7], and oxidative stress [8], greatly expanding the potential role of MR in human disease. Aldosterone/MR signaling associated with high NaCl intake produces cardiac, vascular, and renal injury independent of changes in blood pressure [9]. The benefits of MR antagonists in patients with heart failure resulted in the approval of their use to treat this condition [10]. Furthermore adipocyte MR activation may be implicated in obesity and metabolic syndrome, opening new possible applications to MR antagonists [11]. New roles of MR in ocular or skin diseases have led to new uses of MR antagonists [5, 12].

Unfortunately, therapeutic interventions aimed at limiting MR actions are hampered by adverse side effects. Ligand-binding domain (LBD) sequence conservation between MR and glucocorticoid, progesterone, and androgen receptors (GR, PR, and AR) implies frequent ligand cross-reactivity. For instance, spironolactone is structurally related to progesterone and acts as a PR agonist and AR antagonist, leading to frequent adverse sexual side effects. This has largely been solved by the use of eplerenone, a second-generation MR antagonist with weaker affinity for AR and PR [13]. The use of MR antagonists is further complicated by their potassium-sparing characteristics. While this activity is desirable in the context of hypertensive patients treated with loop diuretics [14], it is associated with higher mortality in patients with heart failure [15]. Therefore, there is a clear need for developing selective MR modulators that preferably have a nonsteroidal nature and may present selective beneficial actions without undesired side effects [4].

This review aims to delineate the different chemical structural families that have led to MR nonsteroidal antagonists. For a more comprehensive data regarding different compounds in each family, a recent review by Martin-Martinez et al. can be of interest [16]. In this chapter, we also focused on those compounds that entered clinical trials and in the known three-dimensional (3D) structure of nonsteroidal compounds bound to the LBD of MR.

## 2. Nonsteroidal MR ligands

An active search for nonsteroidal MR antagonists has been carried out to overcome the side effects observed with steroidal drugs. In general, starting from a high-throughput screening (HTS), an initial hit compound is identified. Next, a hit to lead optimization process, quite frequently through a structure-based design, leads to compounds with improved binding affinity and pharmacokinetic (PK) properties. Examples of different nonsteroidal MR antagonist families are included in this section. In addition, to facilitate a better understanding through the manuscript, the 2D structures of compounds under clinical trials and/or known 3D structures are described in Sections 3 and 4.

The 1,4-dihydropyridine ring (DHP) has proven to be a rather interesting scaffold and have been explored by Pfizer, Bayer Pharma, and Merck (**Figure 1**). Their studies showed the importance of the stereochemistry at DHP C4 [17, 18], as well as a free DHP amino group [18, 19]. Pfizer described a series of DHP with a phenyl group at C4, with small, nonpolar substituents like F, Cl, or $CF_3$ suitable at this ring [19]. Although a voluminous substituent at C2 led, in general, to lower affinity, the incorporation of tetrazolmethyl group as in **1** resulted in better physicochemical properties while maintaining potency and selectivity over other nuclear hormone receptors (NHRs, $IC_{50}$ > 300 nM for PR, GR, and AR). Compound **1** reduces blood pressure and renal injury in rats. On the other hand, Bayer Pharma, starting from an HTS, and the subsequent optimization, identified DHP **2** (BR-4628) with a chromenone at DHP C4 as a potent MR antagonist with more that 150-fold selectivity over GR, AR and PR and a good PK profile in rats [18]. BR-4628 has been proposed to be a bulky antagonist with a passive mechanism. Docking studies shown that BR-4628 5-acetyl and C6-methyl groups protrude toward the MR helix H12. However, there is also a loss of contacts within this region compared to steroid agonist, which might account for the inability of this complex to recruit co-regulators [20]. Interestingly, for several steroid antagonists, a mechanism based on loss of contacts has been proposed with helix H12 leading to a destabilization of the AF2 region, which is involved in co-regulator interaction [21]. The moderate selectivity of BR-4628 versus L-type $Ca^{2+}$ channels prevented further development. Afterwards, Bayer studies led to a series of heterobicyclic analogs, from which a naphthyridine derivative, named finerenone (**17**, see **Figure 5**), entered clinical trials. DHP has also been the focus of Merck, which patented a series of sub-micromolar binding affinity DHP, as derivative **3** [22].

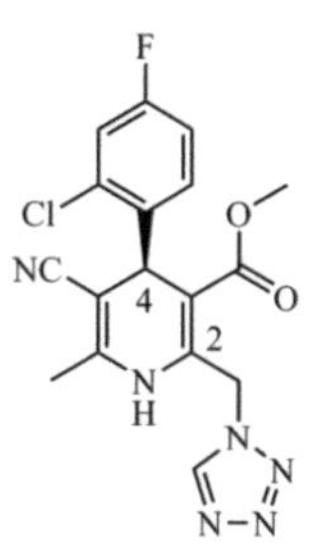

**1**
$IC_{50}$: 52nM[a]
Pfizer

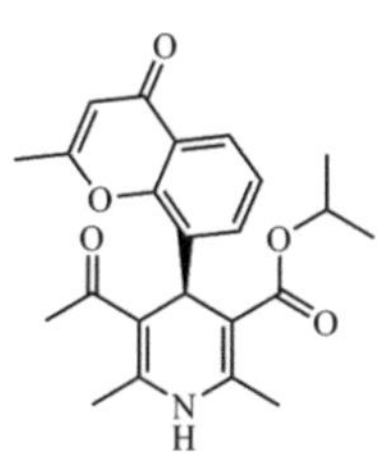

**2, BR-4628**
$IC_{50}$: 28nM[a]
Bayer Pharma

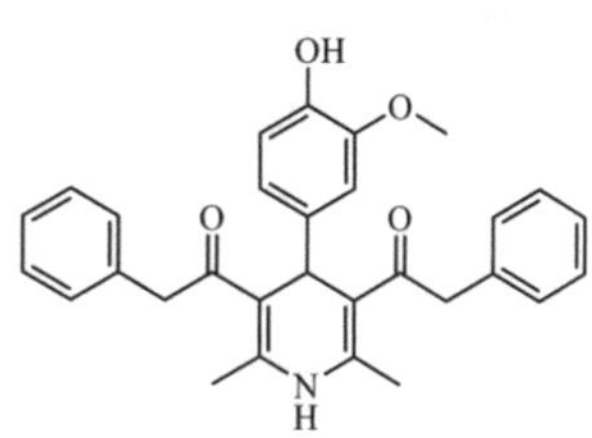

**3**
$IC_{50}$: 21.5 nM[b]
Merck

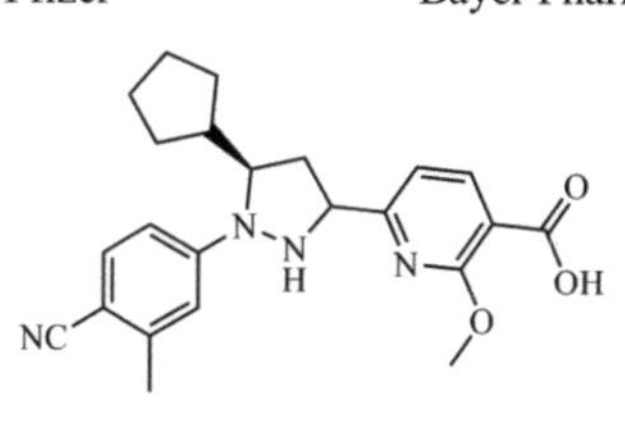

**4**
$IC_{50}$: 4.5 nM[a]
Pfizer

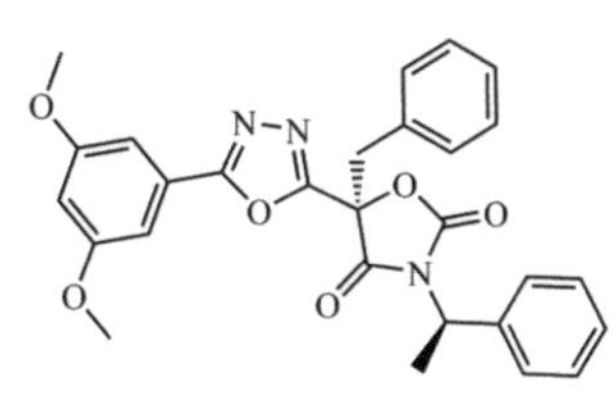

**5**
$IC_{50}$: 39 nM[a]
Merck

**Figure 1.**
*DHP and five-membered heterocyclic rings as scaffolds in MR ligands.* [a]*Cell-based assays.* [b]*Competitive binding assays.*

Five-membered heterocyclic rings have also proven to be quite successful moieties in the search of nonsteroidal MR antagonists. In particular, the pyrrole ring is found in a series of MR ligands developed by Exelixis and Daiichi Sankyo, such as CS-3150 that entered clinical trials (**18**, **Figure 5**) [23]. On the other hand, the pyrazoline ring has been explored by Pfizer, as in compound **4** (**Figure 1**), where the R enantiomer showed higher potency. Compound **4**, with more than 500-fold selectivity over PR, and at least 2000-fold over GR and AR, behaves as an antagonist increasing the urinary $Na^+/K^+$ ratio in rats [24]. The 3-phenyl-pyrazoline cyclization led to a series of conformational restricted pyrazoline derivatives, one of them entered clinical trials, PF-3882845 (**14**, **Figure 5**) [25]. Additionally, starting from an HTS, Merck identified a series of MR antagonists based on the oxazolidine-2,4-dione scaffold. Several derivatives showed potent MR affinity, as compound **5** (**Figure 1**), which has significant selectivity versus other NHRs ($IC_{50}$, PR, AR, GR > 5 µm) [26].

On the other hand, it is worth mentioning the benzoxazinone-derived MR ligands, which have been also broadly explored. An analysis of the X-ray crystal structure of compounds with this bicycle bound to MR LBD provided insights regarding their binding determinants to MR, as explained below (Section 4). In general, in these series there is an additional aromatic ring linked to position 6 of the benzoxazinone moiety, either through linear linkers as in Novartis compound **6** [27] or heteroaromatic rings, like in Takeda derivatives 7, **19–22** (**Figures 2** and **6**) [28, 29]. Compound 7 behaves as antagonist and shows good selectivity over GR, PR, and AR ($IC_{50}$ > 2.5 µM). It is able to decrease urinary $Na^+/K^+$ and has a blood pressure-lowering effect similar to that of spironolactone in a DOCA-salt hypertensive rat model. Interestingly, a carbonyl linker led to AstraZeneca benzoxazinone derivative AZD9977, which is currently in clinical trials (**15**, **Figure 5**). In a recent publication, AstraZeneca describes the thorough structure and property studies that led to the identification of this clinical candidate [30]. Additionally, a benzoxazinone derivative with a rather different pattern of substituents was developed by Mitsubishi Tanabe Pharma leading to apararenone (**16**, **Figure 5**), which is also in clinical trials .

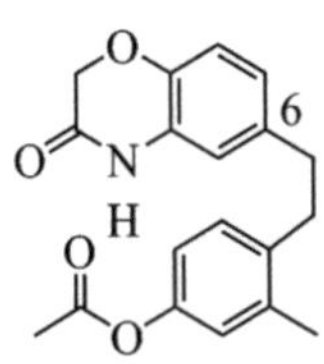

**6**
$IC_{50}$: 1.3 nM[a]
Novartis

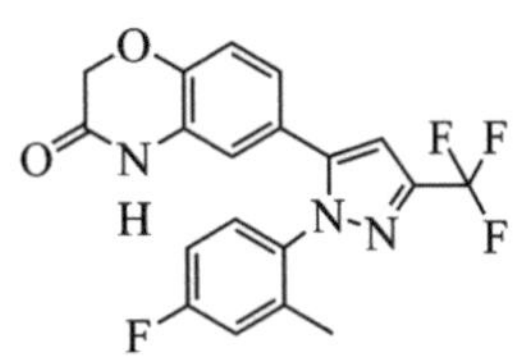

**7**
$IC_{50}$: 41 nM[b]
Takeda pharmaceuticals

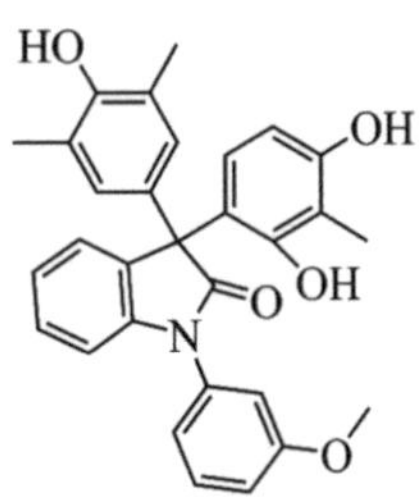

**8**
Ki: 1 nM[b]
Eli Lilly and Company

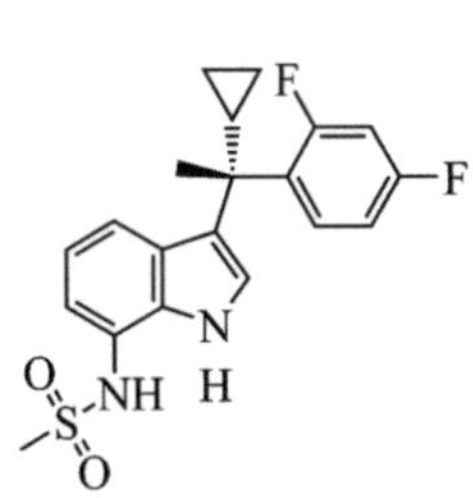

**9**
Ki: 0.49 nM[b]
Eli Lilly and Company

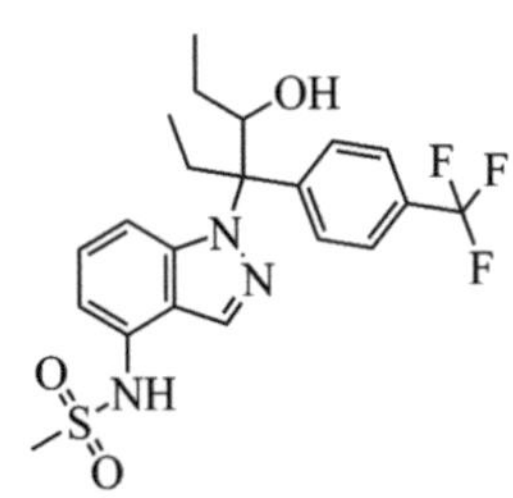

**10**
MR IP: 4 nM[a]
Merck Sharp & Dohme Corp.

**Figure 2.**
*Benzoxazinone-, indole-, and indazole-derived MR ligands. [a]Cell-based assays. [b]Competitive binding assays.*

The indole group was also found as part of two series of potent MR antagonists identified by screening methodologies by Eli Lilly (**Figure 2**). One of them included a 3,3-bisaryloxoindol as central scaffold, where, for example, derivative **8** showed good selectivity over GR, PR, and AR (more than 390-fold) [31]. The other series contained an indole ring, as in compound **9**, which was more potent than eplerenone in lowering blood pressure in a rat hypertension model [32]. A related series containing an indazole ring and an aryl sulfonamide were developed by Merck Sharp & Dohme Corp., for example, compound **10** (stereochemistry not disclosed) that showed a good PK profile in rats [33].

Aryl sulfonamide and urea moieties were also found in compounds **11** and **12**, developed by Sumitomo Dainippon Pharma and Boehiringer Ingelheim, respectively (**Figure 3**) [34, 35]. Recently, a novel byaryl sulfonamide-based MR antagonist was identified in an HTS by AstraZeneca (compound **27**, **Figure 8**). A combination of structure–activity relationship (SAR) exploration and X-ray crystal structure determination subsequently guided the design of related MR antagonist **28** and **29** (**Figure 8**) [36].

Tricyclic scaffolds have also been studied, particularly those containing a central six- or seven-membered ring flanked by differently substituted phenyl moieties. These derivatives are frequently described within patents, and for some of them only scarce pharmacological data is available [16]. Thus, Eli Lilly has developed different families with interesting properties, among them the dibenzooxepine **13** (**Figure 4**), an MR antagonist, with more than 800-fold selectivity over GR, AR, and PR. Compound **13** was studied in combination with tadalafil, a

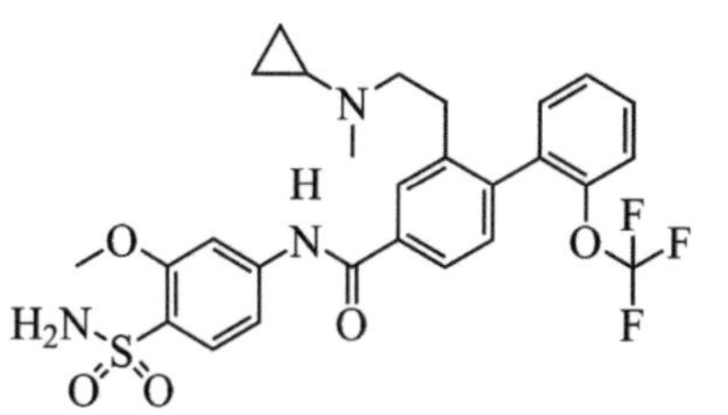

**11**
$IC_{50}$: 22 nM
Dainippon Sumimoto Pharma

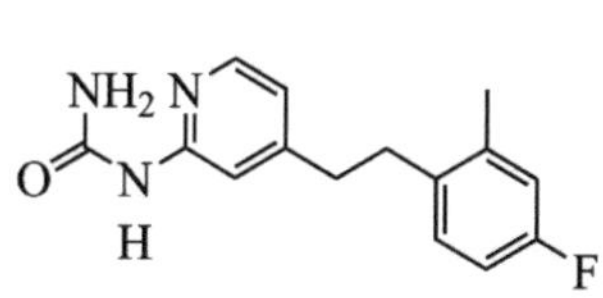

**12**
$IC_{50}$: 4.7 nM
Boehringer Ingelheim International GMBH

**Figure 3.**
*Aryl sulfonamide and urea functionalities in MR ligands. $IC_{50}$ from competitive binding assays.*

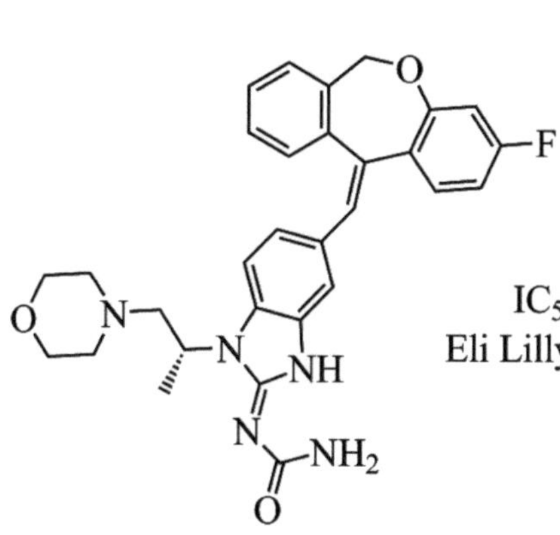

**13**
$IC_{50}$: 0.33 nM
Eli Lilly and Company

**Figure 4.**
*A tricyclic scaffold in MR antagonist. $IC_{50}$ from competitive binding assays.*

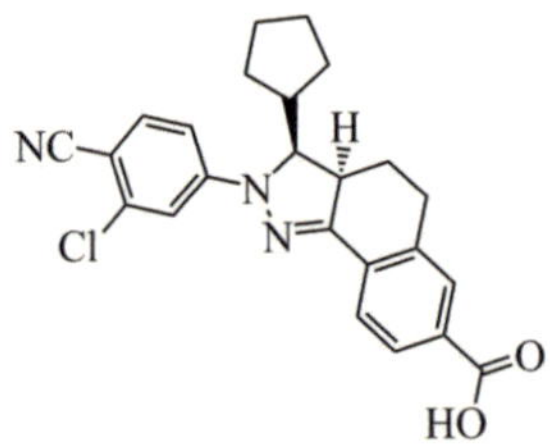

**14, PF-3882845**
$IC_{50}$: 9 nM[a]
Pfizer

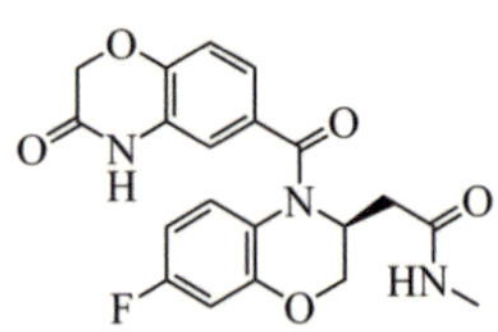

**15, AZD9977**
Ki: 32 nM[b]
AstraZeneca

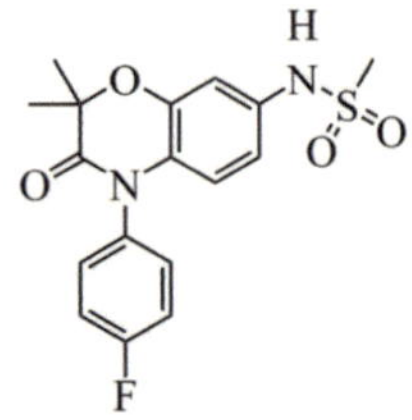

**16, MT-3995, Apararenone**
IC50: <500 nM[b]
Mitsubishi Tanabe Pharma Co

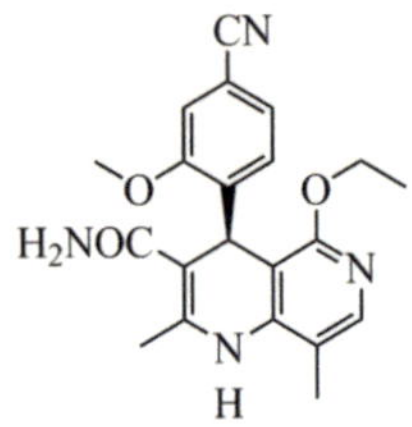

**17, BAY94-8862, Finerenone**
$IC_{50}$: 18 nM[a]
Bayer Pharma

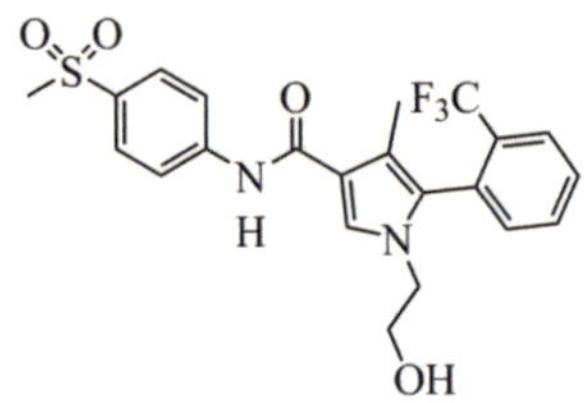

**18, CS-3150, Esaxerenone**
$IC_{50}$: 9.4 nM[a]
Exelisis and Daiichi Sankyo

**Figure 5.**
*MR antagonist that entered clinical trials. [a]Cell-based assays. [b]Binding-based assays.*

A

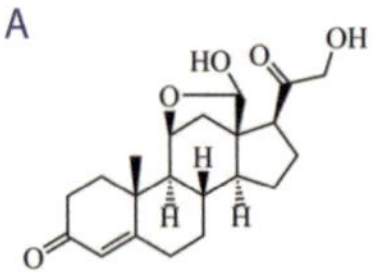

Aldosterona

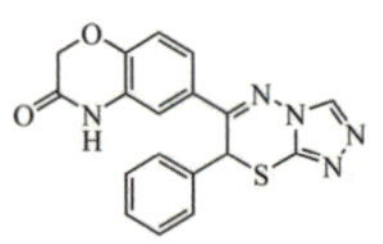

**19**, 3VHV
$IC_{50}$: 510 nM

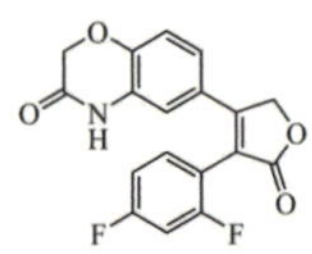

**20**, 3WFF
$IC_{50}$: 660 nM

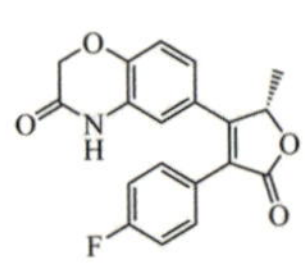

**21**, 3WFG
$IC_{50}$: 120 nM

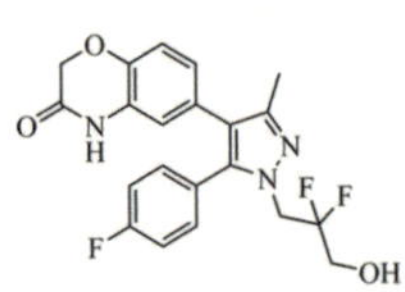

**22**, 4PF3
$IC_{50}$: 43 nM

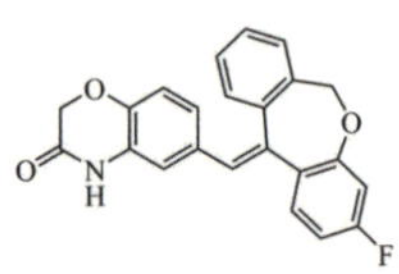

**23**, 5HCV
$IC_{50}$: 2 nM

B

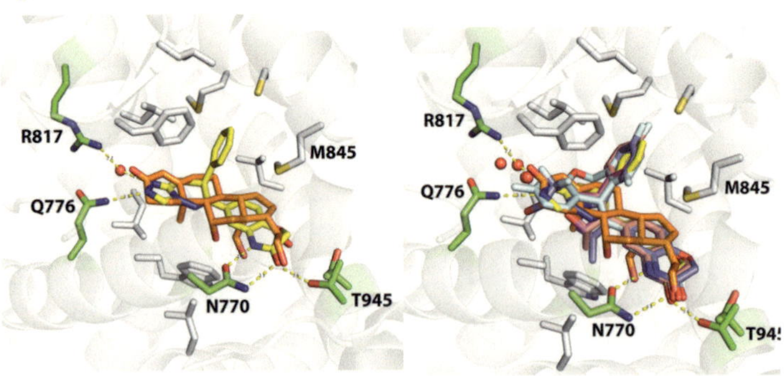


**Figure 6.**
*2D and 3D structures of MR benzoxazine-3-one-based antagonist complexes. (A) 2D molecular structures. (B) Superimposition of the X-ray crystal structures of MR LBD in complex with aldosterone (in orange) and compound **19** (in yellow) (left) and compounds **19** (in yellow), **20** (in red), **21** (in pink), **22** (in blue), and **23** (in cyan) (right) [75]. The hydrogen bonds and water molecules are depicted as yellow dashed lines and red spheres, respectively. $IC_{50}$ from competitive binding assays.*

mild vasodilator, for the treatment of patients with resistant hypertension. These studies showed that their combination led to a greater blood pressure reduction in patients than monotherapies [37]. Some websites associated this compound with LY2623091, which entered clinical trials [38, 39]. Recently, other tricyclic derivatives, with a seven-membered heterocyclic central ring and a benzoxazinone moiety linked to this ring, have been described by Vitae Pharmaceuticals. An example of these latter derivatives is compound **23** whose X-ray crystal structure bound to MR LBD has been solved (**Figure 6**) [40].

## 3. Nonsteroidal MR antagonists that entered clinical trials

The effort devoted to the search of nonsteroidal MR antagonist has led, to the best of our knowledge, to seven compounds entering clinical trials [41–43]. However, two of them, namely, LY2623091 from Eli Lilly and PF03882845 from Pfizer, have been discontinued. Both derivatives are nonsteroidal MR antagonist, selective, and oral bioavailable. LY262309 entered two phase II clinical studies, for patients with chronic kidney disease (CKD) or high blood pressure [44–46], but according to Adis Insight database, this compound was discontinued [47]. PF03882845 (**14**, **Figure 5**) entered phase I clinical studies in patients with type 2 diabetic nephropathy; however the study terminated prematurely due to strategic reasons, according to Pfizer [48, 49].

Recently, AZD9977 from AstraZeneca and KBP-5074 from KBP Biosciences have entered clinical trials. AZD9977 (**15**, **Figure 5**) is a partial MR antagonist in vitro, with cardiorenal protection [50]. It separates organ-protective effects from urinary electrolyte excretion in rodent models, likely reducing hyperkalemia risk. This profile seems to be due to a different pattern of interactions with MR, particularly affecting Met777, which influences the AF2 surface. The AF2 region is key for co-regulator interaction, and a different recruitment compared to eplerenone was observed for this compound. Initial clinical studies showed that AZD9977 was safe and well tolerated; however, compared with rodents, in humans the effects on urinary $Na^+/K^+$ were similar to eplerenone [51]. Yet four phase I clinical trials have been completed with this compound, all in the United Kingdom, the last ones in June 2018 [52]. On the other hand, KBP-5074 is a highly selective and potent MR antagonist. Phase I and IIa studies have been completed in the United States [53]. These studies evaluated safety, tolerability, and PK in healthy volunteers and patients with CKD or renal impairment. A phase IIb trial started in April 2018 for patients with uncontrolled hypertension and advanced CKD.

To date, the most advanced compounds are esaxerenone (CS-3150), finerenone (BAY94-8862), and apararenone (MT-3995). Apararenone (**16**, **Figure 5**, **Table 1**) [42, 54, 55], developed by Mitsubishi Tanabe Pharma Corporation, has completed seven phase II clinical trials for the treatment of diabetic nephropathy; some studies include patients also with albuminuria or with albuminuria and moderately decreased in glomerular filtration rate. There is an active phase II clinical trial in patients with nonalcoholic steatohepatitis (NASH), which will be completed by April 2019.

Finerenone (**17**, **Figure 5**) is a potent, oral bioavailable MR antagonist from Bayer, with more than 500-fold selectivity over AR, PR, or GR [18]. Structural studies indicated that MR Ala773 and Ser810 are the reasons behind its selectivity. These studies also suggested that it is a bulky antagonist that inactivates MR producing a protrusion of LBD helix H12 and avoiding the recruitment of coactivators [56]. Furthermore, it has been found that finerenone modulates MR cofactor binding different from eplerenone. This selective modulation has been suggested as the molecular basis from the different clinical behavior of finerenone compared with eplerenone [57]. Interestingly, it behaves as an antagonist of S810L MR, a mutant that leads to a severe form of familiar hypertension. In preclinical models

| NCT number | Phase | Enrollment | Study start/completion | Location |
|---|---|---|---|---|
| Efficacy and safety of MT-3995 in patients with NASH | | | | |
| NCT02923154 | II | 40 | September 2016/April 2019 | Japan |
| Efficacy and safety of MT-3995 in patients with diabetic nephropathy | | | | |
| NCT02517320 | II | 293 | July 2015/January 2017 | Japan |
| An extended treatment study of MT-3995 in patients with diabetic nephropathy | | | | |
| NCT02676401 | II | 241 | February 2016/August 2017[a] | Japan |

[a]*Primary completion.*

**Table 1.**
*Apararenone (MT-3995) phase II clinical trials completion after 2016 [55].*

| NCT number | Phase | Enrollment | Study start/ completion | Location |
|---|---|---|---|---|
| Efficacy and safety of finerenone in subjects with T2DM and DKD | | | | |
| NCT02540993 FIDELIO-DKD | III | 4800 | September 2015/ October 2019 | Global |
| Efficacy and safety of finerenone in subjects with T2DM and the clinical diagnosis of DKD | | | | |
| NCT02545049 FIGARO-DKD | III | 6400 | September 2015/ February 2020 | Global |
| Efficacy and safety of oral doses of BAY94-8862 in subjects with T2DM and the clinical diagnosis of diabetic nephropathy | | | | |
| NCT01874431 ARTS-DN | II | 823 | June 2013/August 2014 | Global |
| NCT01968668 ARTS-DN Japan | II | 96 | October 2013/ November 2014 | Japan |
| Phase IIb safety and efficacy of different oral doses of BAY94-8862 in subjects with worsening chronic heart failure and left ventricular systolic dysfunction and either T2DM with or without CKD or CKD alone | | | | |
| NCT01807221 ARTS-HF | II | 1058 | June 2013/December 2014 | Global |
| NCT01955694 ARTS-HF-Japan | II | 72 | November 2013/ February 2015 | Japan |
| BAY94–8862 dose finding trial in subjects with chronic heart failure and mild (part A) or moderate (part B) CKD | | | | |
| NCT01345656 ARTS | II | 458 | May 2011/July 2012 | Global |

**Table 2.**
*Finerenone (BAY94-8862) phase III and phase II ARTS clinical trials [68].*

finerenone showed better cardiorenal end-organ protection than spironolactone or eplerenone [58]. Its good properties prompted to further advance it to clinical trials (**Table 2**). In a phase II trial (mineralocorticoid receptor antagonist tolerability study (ARTS)) including subjects with chronic heart failure and mild or moderate CKD, finerenone was at least as effective as spironolactone in decreasing ventricular remodeling but with lower incidence of hyperkalemia and renal adverse effects [59, 60]. The fact that finerenone distributes equally between cardiac and renal tissues in rats, whereas spironolactone and eplerenone show a higher kidney accumulation, might explain the lower incidence of hyperkalemia. The lower accumulation, together with its minimal renal elimination, might open opportunities for the treatment of patients with renal impairment [61, 62]. A subsequent phase II study (ARTS-diabetic nephropathy (ARTS-DN)) analyzed the safety and efficacy of finerenone in subjects with type 2 diabetes mellitus (T2DM) and diabetic nephropathy. In this study the urinary albumin to creatinine ratio (UACR) decreased in patients treated with finerenone compared to placebo, with no significant differences in adverse effects observed between both groups [63, 64]. In the ARTS-heart failure trial (ARTS-HF), different doses of finerenone and eplerenone were compared for patients with worsening heart failure with concomitant T2DM and/or CKD. Finerenone (10–20 mg dose) showed better outcome, including death, cardiovascular hospitalization, or emergency visit [65]. There are two large trials on going (FIDELIO-DKD, FIGARO-DKD) including subjects with T2DM and diabetic kidney disease (DKD) at doses of 10 or 20 mg of finerenone.

Recently, the administration of finerenone to a rat model of metabolic syndrome (Zucker fa/fa) showed that finerenone exerted cardiac protection, as it has been previously described for spironolactone. However, only finerenone afforded renal protection [66, 67].

Esaxerenone (**18, Figure 5**) is a highly potent and selective MR antagonist, with at least 1000-fold higher selectivity over AR, PR, or GR. It has also long-lasting oral activity, longer than steroidal drugs [23]. In addition, it has shown antihypertensive and cardiorenal protective effects in Dahl salt-sensitive hypertensive rats with superior potency than spironolactone or eplerenone and no apparent hyperkalemia [69]. The similar balanced distribution of esaxerenone to the kidney and heart in rats might be the reason of its higher organ-protective effects than marketed drugs. A subsequent study was performed with a model of hypertensive rats, based on a synthetic mineralocorticoid, deoxycorticosterone acetate (DOCA), that induces hypertension and renal injury in combination with salt loading (DOCA rats). In this model, esaxerenone was able to prevent hypertension and the development of renal damage. It has also been suggested that its beneficial actions on renal injury cannot

| NCT number | Phase | Enrollment | Study start/ completion | Location |
|---|---|---|---|---|
| Study of CS-3150 in patients with severe hypertension | | | | |
| NCT02808026 | III | 20 | June 2016/February 2017 | Japan |
| Study of CS-3150 in hypertensive patients with type 2 diabetes and albuminuria | | | | |
| NCT02807974 | III | 51 | June 2016/March 2017 | Japan |
| Study of CS-3150 in combination with ARB or ACE inhibitor in hypertensive patients with moderate renal impairment | | | | |
| NCT02807987 | III | 58 | June 2016/May 2017 | Japan |
| Long-term study of CS-3150 as monotherapy or in combination with other antihypertensive drug in Japanese patients with essential hypertension | | | | |
| NCT02722265 | III | 368 | March 2016/July, 2017 | Japan |
| Study of CS-3150 in patients with essential hypertension | | | | |
| NCT02890173 ESAX-HTN | III | 1001 | September 2016/July, 2017 | Japan |

**Table 3.**
*Esaxerenone (CS-3150) phase III clinical trials [72].*

be only attributed to its antihypertensive effect but also to direct renal protection through antifibrotic, anti-inflammatory, and antioxidant actions. Interestingly, this compound is also able to restore the established renal damage in DOCA rats [70]. Esaxerenone was identified by Exelixis' research collaboration with Daiichi Sankyo. In 2006 they signed an agreement in which Daiichi Sankyo was granted a worldwide license. To date, five phase III studies have been completed related to hypertension, some of them in addition to type 2 diabetes and albuminuria or moderate renal impairment. The combination with other antihypertensive therapies has also been studied (**Table 3**). In February 2018, Exelixis announced that Daiichi Sankyo had submitted a regulatory application to the Japanese Pharmaceutical and Medical Devices Agency for esaxerenone to be approved for the treatment of hypertension [71].

## 4. Structural determinants for nonsteroidal MR antagonists binding to MR LBD

To the best of our knowledge, to date 12 X-ray crystal structures of nonsteroidal ligands bound to MR LBD have been solved. Nine of these reported structures correspond to MR antagonists within the benzoxazinone moiety derivatives class (**Figures 6A** and **7A**) (PDB IDs: compound **15**, 1.82 Å 5MWP [50]; **19**, 1.35 Å 3VHV [28]; **20**, 2.05 Å 2WFF [29]; **21**, 1.40 Å 3WFG [29]; **22**, 1.10 Å 4PF3 [73]; **23**, 2.5 Å 5HCV [40]; **24**, 1.54 Å 6GEV [30]; **25**, 1.8 Å 6GG8 [30]; and **26**, 1.71 Å 6GGG [30]), whereas the remaining three correspond to a sulfonamide aryl moiety (PDB IDs: **27**, 1.86 Å 5L7E; **28**, 2.01 Å 5L7G; and **29**, 2.12 Å 5L7H) (**Figure 8A**) [36].

The X-ray crystal structure of $MR_{C808S/S810L}$-LBD double mutant in complex with compound **19** first revealed the binding mode of benzoxazine-3-one derivatives. The NH group and the carbonyl oxygen of this moiety form hydrogen bonds to Asn770. In addition, the nitrogen atoms of the triazole scaffold establish hydrogen bonds to residue Gln776 and through a water molecule to Arg817 (**Figure 6B**). Similarly, aldosterone, the main MR hormone, is also engaged in hydrogen bonding with both Gln776 and Arg817 through its C3-ketone moiety, as well as with Asn770 through its C21-hydroxyl group (**Figure 6**) [74].

On the other hand, compound **20**, which was reported later [29], also forms hydrogen bonds to Asn770 through the NH group and the carbonyl oxygen of benzoxazine as described for compound **19**. In addition, compound **20** forms a new hydrogen bond to Thr945 through the carbonyl oxygen of the benzoxazine-3-one moiety (**Figure 6B**). The carbonyl oxygen in the dihydrofuran-2-one scaffold establishes hydrogen bonds to residues Arg817 and Gln776 through a water molecule. Overall, compound **20** binds to MR LBD in a similar way as compound **19**. Based on these structural considerations, compound **21**, a dihydrofuran-2-one derivative, was subsequently developed. As expected, the binding mode of compound **21** was similar to that of compounds **19** and **20** (**Figure 6B**).

Later, compound **22**, a benzoxazine-3-one derivative with an azole central ring as core scaffold, was developed [73]. This molecule is a highly potent MR antagonist and also shows remarkable selectivity over other steroid hormone receptors. In addition, it exhibits good PK profile and very low partial agonistic activity [3]. The azole central ring of compound **22** was selected to avoid the formation of water-mediated hydrogen bonding networks, which is known to contribute to partial agonistic activity of some previously reported benzoxazine-3-one derivatives [29, 73]. As expected, the binding mode of compound **22** is similar to that of compounds **19–21**, as observed by the solution of the X-ray crystal structure of its complex with MR LBD (PDB ID: 4PF3) (**Figure 6B**). The NH group and the carbonyl oxygen of the benzoxazine-3-one moiety form hydrogen bonds to Asn770 and Thr945, and the 4-fluorobenzene ring occupies the α-face hydrophobic pocket. The ligand 2,2-difluoropropyl-3-hydroxy moiety points out toward the residues Gln776 and Arg817. Its hydroxyl group directly forms a hydrogen bond to Gln776. The two fluorine atoms do not form any specific hydrogen bonding interactions suggesting that the major contribution of these fluorine atoms to the binding is hydrophobic.

In 2016, Vitae Pharmaceuticals developed compound **23**, a benzoxazine-3-one derivative with a tricyclic scaffold. The X-ray crystal structure of compound **23** in complex with MR LBD showed again a binding mode similar to compounds **19–22**. Similarly, the benzoxazinone moiety is engaged in three hydrogen bonds, two with Asn770, through its NH and CO groups, and another one with Thr945 through its carbonyl oxygen (**Figure 6B**). The tricyclic structure does not engage in any hydrogen bonding with MR LBD [40].

Recently, compound **15** (AZD9977) has been identified as a novel and selective benzoxazine-3-one-based partial MR antagonist [50]. The X-ray crystal structure of compound **15** in complex with $MR_{C808S/C910S}$-LBD double mutant revealed the molecular determinants of its high affinity and selectivity for MR (5MWP). Likewise, compound **15** benzoxamide moiety is also involved in hydrogen bonds with Asn770 and Thr945, whereas compound **15**'s amide extension forms hydrogen bonds with

A

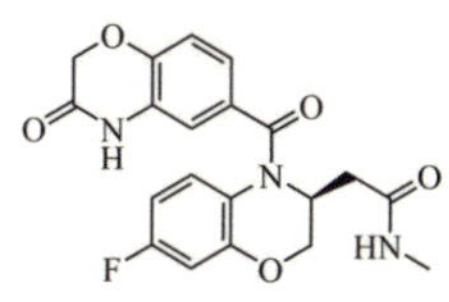

**15**, 5MWP
Ki: 32 nM

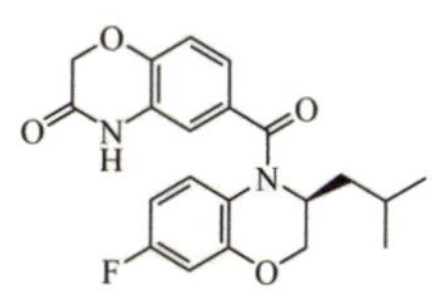

**24**, 6GEV
pKi: 8.7

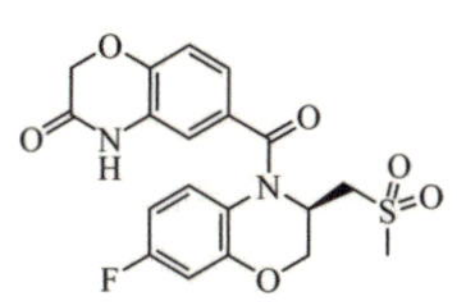

**25**, 6GG8
pKi:9.1

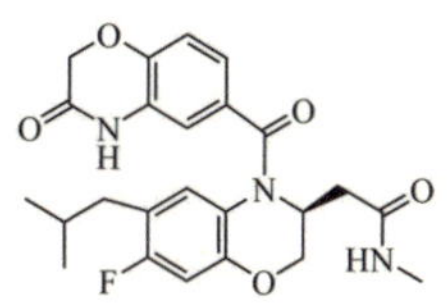

**26**, 6GGG
pKi: 9,2

B

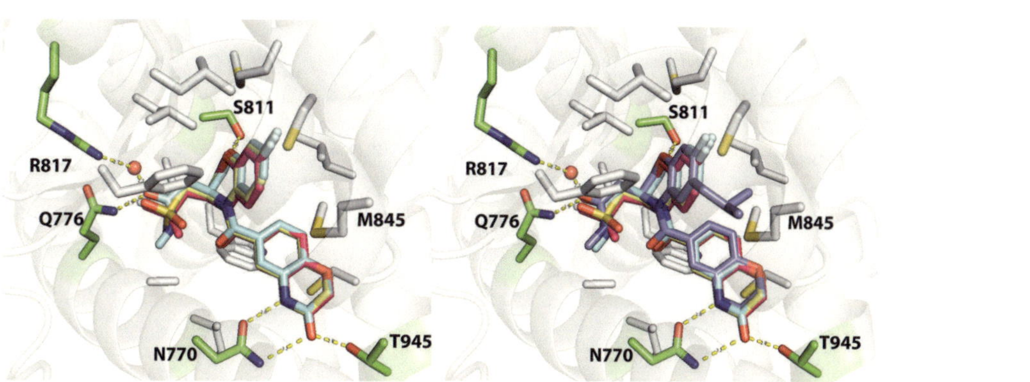


**Figure 7.**
*2D and 3D structures of AstraZeneca benzoxazine-3-one-based antagonist complexes. (A) 2D molecular structures. (B) Superimposition of the X-ray crystal structures of MR LBD bound to compounds **15** (in cyan), **24** (in red), and **25** (in light yellow) on the left and **15** (in cyan), **24** (in red), **25** (in light yellow), and **26** (in purple) on the right [30, 50]. The hydrogen bonds and water molecules are depicted as yellow dashed lines and red spheres, respectively. Ki from competitive binding assays.*

Gln776, Arg817, and Ser810 (**Figure 6B**). An ordered water molecule is also found in the ligand-binding pocket, but it does not seem to mediate hydrogen binding between this compound and MR LBD. The 3,4-dihydro-2H-1,4-benzoxazine oxygen interacts through hydrogen bonding with Ser811. Within the steroid receptor family, Ser811 is unique to MR, which might contribute to the selectivity of compound **15**. The identification of **15** was guided by structure-based design, and in this process three X-ray structures were solved, namely, those of MR LBD bound to derivatives **24**, **25**, and **26**. As it is shown in **Figure 7**, the binding mode of these compounds is rather similar. However, as expected, derivative **24** is not able to interact with Gln776 or Arg817. On the other hand, the isobutyl substituent of **26** causes a rearrangement resulting in an extension of helix H7 and a reposition of helix H6 [30].

Regarding the sulfonamide aryl-based nonsteroidal MR antagonists, in 2017, Nordqvist et al. solved the first X-ray crystal structure of this scaffold-containing derivatives through hit compound **27** in complex with MR LBD (PDB ID: 5L7E) [36]. The 3D structure revealed that the isoxazole is located close to residues Gln776 and Arg817 (**Figure 8**). On the other side of the ligand-binding pocket, compound **27**'s sulfonamide NH also interacts directly with Asn770 through hydrogen bonding. One of the sulfonamide oxygen atoms interacts with both Asn770 and Thr945 through water-mediated hydrogen bond. Interestingly, compound **27** folds back upon itself, pivoting on the sulfonamide motif, to form an intramolecular packing interaction between the two phenyl moieties acquiring a U-shaped binding mode. Following the superimposition of its X-ray crystal structure and that of

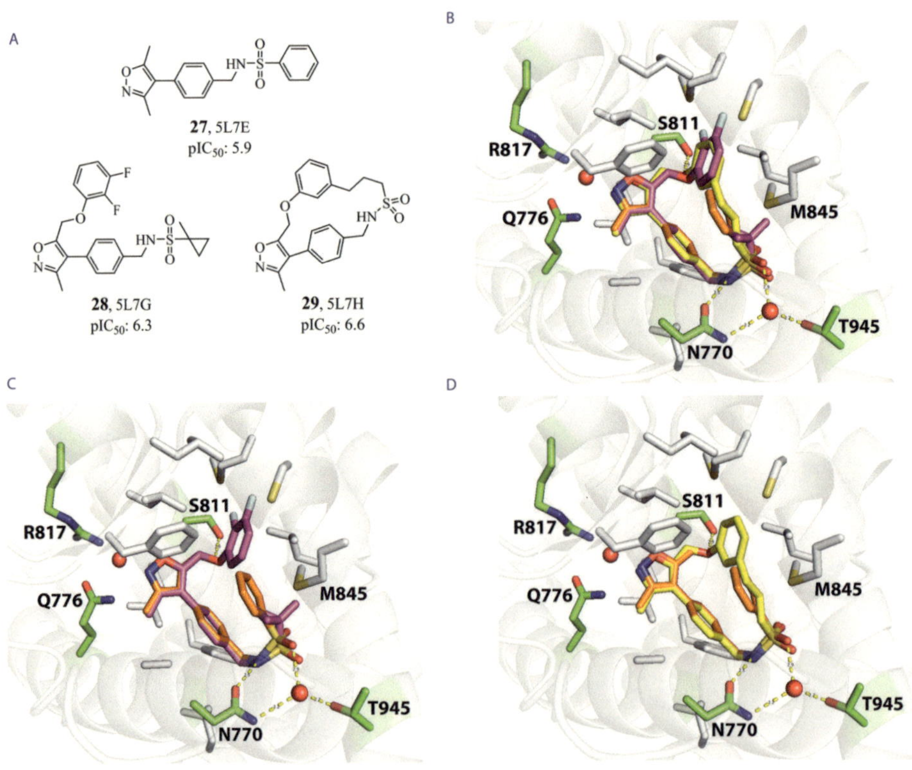


**Figure 8.**
*2D and 3D structures of MR sulfonamide aryl-based antagonist complexes. (A) 2D molecular structures. Superimposition of the X-ray crystal structures of MR LBD in complex with (B) compounds* **27** *(in orange),* **28** *(in magenta), and* **29** *(in yellow), (C) compounds* **27** *and* **28**, *and (D) compounds* **27** *and* **29** *[75]. The hydrogen bonds and water molecules are depicted as yellow dashed lines and red spheres, respectively.* $IC_{50}$ *from human MR reporter gene assays.*

compound **21** (3WFG), it was reasoned to expand the ligand from the isoxazole 5-methyl substituent toward the area around Met852 which is occupied by a phenyl ring of compound **21**. Thus, compound **28** was developed with increased binding affinity toward MR and selectivity over PR and GR. The X-ray crystal structure of MR LBD and compound **28** complex (5L7G) verified that the proposed isoxazole orientation of hit compound **27** was retained and the side chain of Met852 moved to accommodate the 2,3-difluorophenoxymethyl moiety (**Figure 8C**). Afterwards, a deeper analysis of ligand binding modes inspired the design of compound **29**, the first potent macrocyclic oxosteroid receptor antagonist. Despite the conformation constraints imposed by the macrocyclization, the X-ray crystal structure of the complex between MR LBD and compound **29** (5L7H [36]) disclosed that the ligand interactions to the receptor stayed the same as those exhibited by compounds **27** and **28** (**Figure 8D**). It is worth noting that the water molecule mediating hydrogen bond between compounds **27–29** and Ans770 and Thr945 is displaced by the benzoxazine scaffold in compounds 15 and **19–25** (**Figures 6** and 7). For these latter compounds, the benzoxazine scaffold forms a bidentate hydrogen bonding with Asn770 and an additional hydrogen bond with Thr945.

## 5. Conclusions

Since 1959 in which the steroid MR antagonist spironolactone was introduced in the market [42], continuous research has been carried out in attempting to overcome the undesired side effects of this drug. Eplerenone, a second-generation MR antagonist, although more selective for MR, still increases the incidence of hyperkalemia. For this reason, the research was turned toward a third generation of compounds, comprising nonsteroidal antagonists within different chemotypes, which show in general lower side effects. Several examples of this third generation have entered clinical trials as compiled in this review. However, in spite of the last decades of advances, there are still important questions that need further research. Thus, for example, the structural requirements needed for ligands to discriminate the recruitment of different co-regulators and, hence, to fine-tune the transcription of selected genes are still poorly understood. Undoubtedly, a larger body of knowledge in this field will contribute significantly to the future development of novel MR antagonists with improved properties.

## Acknowledgements

This publication is based upon work from the EU COST Action ADMIRE BM1301 in Aldosterone and Mineralocorticoid Receptor (MR) Physiology and Pathophysiology (www.admirecosteu.com). Also supported by grants from Ministerio de Economia y Competitividad (MINECO, Spain; grant SAF2015-66275-C2-2-R and BFU2016-78374-R), CUNY (CCRG-1532), and the Hostos Office of Academic Affairs, US National Institute of Health (NIGMS) SC2GM111231.

**Author details**

Felipe L. Pérez-Gordillo[1], Maria Jesús Pérez de Vega[1], Guillermo Gerona-Navarro[2], Yoel Rodríguez[3,4], Diego Alvarez de la Rosa[5,6], Rosario González-Muñiz[1] and Mercedes Martín-Martínez[1*]

1 Instituto de Química Médica (IQM-CSIC), Madrid, Spain

2 Department of Chemistry, Brooklyn College of The City University of New York, Brooklyn, NY, USA

3 Department of Pharmacological Sciences, Icahn School of Medicine at Mount Sinai, New York, USA

4 Department of Natural Sciences, Hostos Community College of The City University of New York, Bronx, New York, USA

5 Institute of Biomedical Technologies (ITB), Campus de Ciencias de la Salud, Universidad de La Laguna, Tenerife, Spain

6 Department of Basic Medical Sciences, Campus de Ciencias de la Salud, Universidad de La Laguna, Tenerife, Spain

*Address all correspondence to: mmartin@iqm.csic.es

## References

[1] Rossier BC, Baker ME, Studer RA. Epithelial sodium transport and its control by aldosterone: The story of our internal environment revisited. Physiological Reviews. 2015;**95**:297-340

[2] Chapman K, Holmes M, Seckl J. 11beta-hydroxysteroid dehydrogenases: Intracellular gate-keepers of tissue glucocorticoid action. Physiological Reviews. 2013;**93**:1139-1206

[3] Gomez-Sanchez E, Gomez-Sanchez CE. The multifaceted mineralocorticoid receptor. Comprehensive Physiology. 2014;**4**:965-994

[4] Gomez-Sanchez EP. Third-generation mineralocorticoid receptor antagonists: Why do we need a fourth? Journal of Cardiovascular Pharmacology. 2016;**67**:26-38

[5] Jaisser F, Farman N. Emerging roles of the mineralocorticoid receptor in pathology: Toward new paradigms in clinical pharmacology. Pharmacological Reviews. 2016;**68**:49-75

[6] Young MJ, Rickard AJ. Mechanisms of mineralocorticoid salt-induced hypertension and cardiac fibrosis. Molecular and Cellular Endocrinology. 2012;**350**:248-255

[7] Herrada AA et al. Aldosterone as a modulator of immunity: Implications in the organ damage. Journal of Hypertension. 2011;**29**:1684-1692

[8] Queisser N, Schupp N. Aldosterone, oxidative stress, and NF-kappaB activation in hypertension-related cardiovascular and renal diseases. Free Radical Biology & Medicine. 2012;**53**:314-327

[9] Bauersachs J, Jaisser F, Toto R. Mineralocorticoid receptor activation and mineralocorticoid receptor antagonist treatment in cardiac and renal diseases. Hypertension. 2015;**65**:257-263

[10] Kolkhof P et al. Steroidal and novel non-steroidal mineralocorticoid receptor antagonists in heart failure and cardiorenal diseases: Comparison at bench and bedside. Handbook of Experimental Pharmacology. 2017;**243**:271-305

[11] Infante M, Armani A, Mammi C, Fabbri A, Caprio M. Impact of adrenal steroids on regulation of adipose tissue. Comprehensive Physiology. 2017;**7**:1425-1447

[12] Daruich A et al. Central serous chorioretinopathy: Recent findings and new physiopathology hypothesis. Progress in Retinal and Eye Research. 2015;**48**:82-118

[13] Brown R, Quirk J, Kirkpatrick P. Eplerenone. Nature Reviews. Drug Discovery. 2003;**2**:177-178

[14] Alvarez de la Rosa D, Navarro-Gonzalez JF, Giraldez T. ENaC modulators and renal disease. Current Molecular Pharmacology. 2013;**6**:35-43

[15] Roscioni SS, de Zeeuw D, Bakker SJ, Lambers Heerspink HJ. Management of hyperkalaemia consequent to mineralocorticoid-receptor antagonist therapy. Nature Reviews. Nephrology. 2012;**8**:691-699

[16] Martin-Martinez M et al. Modulating mineralocorticoid receptor with non-steroidal antagonists. New opportunities for the development of potent and selective ligands without off-target side effects. Journal of Medicinal Chemistry. 2017;**60**:2629-2650

[17] Arhancet GB et al. Stereochemical requirements for the mineralocorticoid receptor antagonist activity of dihydropyridines. Journal of Medicinal Chemistry. 2010;**53**:4300-4304

[18] Bärfacker L et al. Discovery of BAY 94-8862: A nonsteroidal antagonist of the mineralocorticoid receptor for the treatment of cardiorenal diseases. ChemMedChem. 2012;7:1385-1403

[19] Arhancet GB et al. Discovery of novel cyanodihydropyridines as potent mineralocorticoid receptor antagonists. Journal of Medicinal Chemistry. 2010;**53**:5970-5978

[20] Fagart J et al. A new mode of mineralocorticoid receptor antagonism by a potent and selective nonsteroidal molecule. The Journal of Biological Chemistry. 2010;**285**:29932-29940

[21] Fagart J et al. Antagonism in the human mineralocorticoid receptor. The EMBO Journal. 1998;**17**:3317-3325

[22] Brandish P, Fraley E, Mark E, Hershey JC, Steen JT. Mineralocorticoid receptor modulators. 2009. WO2009/078934A1

[23] Arai K et al. Pharmacological profile of CS-3150, a novel, highly potent and selective non-steroidal mineralocorticoid receptor antagonist. European Journal of Pharmacology. 2015;**761**:226-234

[24] Casimiro-Garcia A et al. Identification of (R)-6-(1-(4-Cyano-3-methylphenyl)-5-cyclopentyl-4,5-dihydro-1H-pyrazol-3-yl)-2-methoxynicotinic acid, a highly potent and selective nonsteroidal mineralocorticoid receptor antagonist. Journal of Medicinal Chemistry. 2014;**57**:4273-4288

[25] Meyers MJ et al. Discovery of (3S,3aR)-2-(3-Chloro-4-cyanophenyl)-3-cyclopentyl-3,3a,4,5-tetrahydro-2H-benzo[g]indazole-7-carboxylic acid (PF-3882845), an orally efficacious mineralocorticoid receptor (MR) antagonist for hypertension and nephropathy. Journal of Medicinal Chemistry. 2010;**53**:5979-6002

[26] Cox JM et al. Mineralocorticoid receptor antagonists: Identification of heterocyclic amide replacements in the oxazolidinedione series. Bioorganic & Medicinal Chemistry Letters. 2014;**24**:1681-1684

[27] Michellys PY, Pei W, Petrassi HM, Richmond W. Compounds and compositions as modulators of steroid hormone nuclear receptors. 2006. WO2006/015259

[28] Hasui T et al. Identification of benzoxazin-3-one derivatives as novel, potent, and selective nonsteroidal mineralocorticoid receptor antagonists. Journal of Medicinal Chemistry. 2011;**54**:8616-8631

[29] Hasui T et al. Design, synthesis, and structure–activity relationships of dihydrofuran-2-one and dihydropyrrol-2-one derivatives as novel benzoxazin-3-one-based mineralocorticoid receptor antagonists. Bioorganic & Medicinal Chemistry. 2013;**21**:5983-5994

[30] Granberg KL et al. Identification of mineralocorticoid receptor modulators with low impact on electrolyte homeostasis but maintained organ protection. Journal of Medicinal Chemistry. 2019;**62**:1385-1406

[31] Neel DA et al. 3,3-Bisaryloxindoles as mineralocorticoid receptor antagonists. Bioorganic & Medicinal Chemistry Letters. 2005;**15**:2553-2557

[32] Bell MG et al. (S)-N-{3-[1-Cyclopropyl-1-(2,4-difluoro-phenyl)-ethyl]-1H-indol-7-yl}-methanesulfonamide: A potent, nonsteroidal, functional antagonist of the mineralocorticoid receptor. Journal of Medicinal Chemistry. 2007;**50**:6443-6445

[33] Cernak TA, Dykstra KD. Mineralocorticoid receptor antagonists. 2014. WO2014/014794A2

[34] Katayama S, Hori S, Hasegawa F, Suzuki K. Biaryl amide derivative or pharmaceutically acceptable salt thereof. 2013. US2013/116227A1

[35] Boyer S, Guo X, Wu D, Wu F. Pyridyl ureas as mineralocorticoid receptor antagonists. 2012. WO2012/064631A1

[36] Nordqvist A et al. Structure-based drug design of mineralocorticoid receptor antagonists to explore oxosteroid receptor selectivity. ChemMedChem. 2017;**12**:50-65

[37] Kowala MC. Combination therapy for resistant hypertension. 2015. WO2015/130568

[38] http://www.chemspider.com/Chemical-Structure.29361352.html [Accessed: July 27, 2018]

[39] https://www.chemicalregister.com/LY2623091/Suppliers/pid705106.htm [Accessed: July 27, 2018]

[40] Lotesta SD et al. Identification of spirooxindole and dibenzoxazepine motifs as potent mineralocorticoid receptor antagonists. Bioorganic and Medicinal Chemistry. 2016;**24**:1384-1391

[41] Kolkhof P, Nowack C, Eitner F. Nonsteroidal antagonists of the mineralocorticoid receptor. Current Opinion in Nephrology and Hypertension. 2015;**24**:417-424

[42] The Practice of Medicinal Chemistry. 3rd ed. Academic Press; 2008

[43] Clinical Trials Information. Available from: https://clinicaltrials.gov/ [Accessed: July 27, 2018]

[44] Wang EB, Chaudhary A, Waterhouse TH, Dickinson GL. Population pharmacokinetics of LY2623091 in patients with hypertension and chronic kidney disease. Journal of Clinical Pharmacology. 2017;**57**:739-746

[45] Dickinson GL, Phillips DL, Posada MM, Chaudhary A, Hall SD. Physiologically based pharmacokinetic modeling to understand the observed drug-drug interaction of LY2623091 with CYP3A inhibitors itraconazole and diltiazem. International Journal of Pharmacokinetics. 2017;**2**:233-245

[46] Clinical Trial Information. Available from: https://clinicaltrials.gov/ct2/results?cond=&term=LY2623091 [Accessed: July 27, 2018]

[47] https://adisinsight.springer.com/drugs/800033156 [Accessed: July 27, 2018]

[48] https://ncats.nih.gov/files/PF-03882845.pdf [Accessed: July 27, 2018]

[49] https://clinicaltrials.gov/ct2/show/NCT01488877 [Accessed: July 27, 2018]

[50] Bamberg K et al. Preclinical pharmacology of AZD9977: A novel mineralocorticoid receptor modulator separating organ protection from effects on electrolyte excretion. PLoS One. 2018;**13**:e0193380

[51] Erlandsson F et al. Clinical safety, tolerability, pharmacokinetics and effects on urinary electrolyte excretion of AZD9977, a novel, selective mineralocorticoid receptor modulator. British Journal of Clinical Pharmacology. 2018;**84**:1486-1493

[52] Clinical Trials Information. Available from: https://www.clinicaltrials.gov/ct2/results?cond=&term=azd9977 [Accessed: July 27, 2018]

[53] Clinical Trials Information. Available from: https://www.clinicaltrials.gov/ct2/results?cond=&term=kbp5074 [Accessed: July 27, 2018]

[54] IIijima TY, Akatsuka H, Kawaguchi T. Benzoxazines and related nitrogen-containing heterobicyclic compounds useful as mineralocorticoid receptor modulating agents. 2007. WO2007/089034

[55] Clinical Trials Information. Available from: https://www.clinicaltrials.gov/ct2/results?term=MT3995 [Accessed: July 27, 2018]

[56] Amazit L et al. Finerenone impedes aldosterone-dependent nuclear import of the mineralocorticoid receptor and prevents genomic recruitment of steroid receptor coactivator-1. The Journal of Biological Chemistry. 2015;**290**:21876-21889

[57] Grune J et al. Selective mineralocorticoid receptor cofactor modulation as molecular basis for finerenone's antifibrotic activity. Hypertension. 2018;**71**:599-608

[58] Kolkhof P et al. Finerenone, a novel selective nonsteroidal mineralocorticoid receptor antagonist protects from rat cardiorenal injury. Journal of Cardiovascular Pharmacology. 2014;**64**:69-78

[59] Pitt B et al. Rationale and design of ARTS: A randomized, double-blind study of BAY 94-8862 in patients with chronic heart failure and mild or moderate chronic kidney disease. European Journal of Heart Failure. 2012;**14**:668-675

[60] Pitt B et al. Safety and tolerability of the novel non-steroidal mineralocorticoid receptor antagonist BAY 94-8862 in patients with chronic heart failure and mild or moderate chronic kidney disease: A randomized, double-blind trial. European Heart Journal. 2013;**34**:2453-2463

[61] Haller H, Bertram A, Stahl K, Menne J. Finerenone: A new mineralocorticoid receptor antagonist without hyperkalemia: An opportunity in patients with CKD? Current Hypertension Reports. 2016;**18**:1-9

[62] Heinig R, Kimmeskamp-Kirschbaum N, Halabi A, Lentini S. Pharmacokinetics of the novel nonsteroidal mineralocorticoid receptor antagonist finerenone (BAY 94-8862) in individuals with renal impairment. Clinical Pharmacology in Drug Development. 2016;**5**:488-501

[63] Bakris GL et al. Effect of finerenone on albuminuria in patients with diabetic nephropathy: A randomized clinical trial. JAMA, the Journal of the American Medical Association. 2015;**314**:884-894

[64] Bramlage P et al. Non-steroidal mineralocorticoid receptor antagonism for the treatment of cardiovascular and renal disease. European Journal of Heart Failure. 2016;**18**:28-37

[65] Filippatos G et al. A randomized controlled study of finerenone vs. eplerenone in patients with worsening chronic heart failure and diabetes mellitus and/or chronic kidney disease. European Heart Journal. 2016;**37**:2105-2114

[66] Lachaux M et al. Short- and long-term administration of the non-steroidal mineralocorticoid receptor antagonist finerenone opposes metabolic syndrome-related cardio-renal dysfunction. Diabetes, Obesity & Metabolism. 2018. p. 1-9

[67] Bender SB et al. Mineralocorticoid receptor antagonism treats obesity-associated cardiac diastolic dysfunction. Hypertension. 2015;**65**:1082-1088

[68] Clinical Trials Information. Available from: https://www.clinicaltrials.gov/ct2/results?term=finerenone [Accessed: July 27, 2018]

[69] Arai K, Tsuruoka H, Homma T. CS-3150, a novel non-steroidal

mineralocorticoid receptor antagonist, prevents hypertension and cardiorenal injury in Dahl salt-sensitive hypertensive rats. European Journal of Pharmacology. 2015;**769**:266-273

[70] Arai K, Morikawa Y, Ubukata N, Tsuruoka H, Homma T. CS-3150, a novel nonsteroidal mineralocorticoid receptor antagonist, shows preventive and therapeutic effects on renal injury in deoxycorticosterone acetate/salt-induced hypertensive rats. The Journal of Pharmacology and Experimental Therapeutics. 2016;**358**:548-557

[71] https://www.businesswire.com/news/home/20180226006626/en/Exelixis-Announces-Collaborator-Daiichi-Sankyo%E2%80%99s-Submission-Regulatory [Accessed: July 27, 2018]

[72] Clinical Trials Information. Available from: https://www.clinicaltrials.gov/ct2/results?term=cs3150 [Accessed: July 27, 2018]

[73] Hasui T et al. Discovery of 6-[5-(4-fluorophenyl)-3-methyl-pyrazol-4-yl]-benzoxazin-3-one derivatives as novel selective nonsteroidal mineralocorticoid receptor antagonists. Bioorganic & Medicinal Chemistry. 2014;**22**:5428-5445

[74] Bledsoe RK et al. A ligand-mediated hydrogen bond network required for the activation of the mineralocorticoid receptor. The Journal of Biological Chemistry. 2005;**280**:31283-31293

[75] Pymol Molecular Graphics System, Version 1.7 Schrödinger, LLC

Chapter 17

# COLT: A New Weapon to Disseminate Knowledge

*Bernard C. Rossier, Michelle Rossier and Jean-Pierre Kraehenbühl*

## Abstract

Too few researchers receive adequate pre- or postgraduate training to conduct a rigorous scientific study. In the digital age, new tools are emerging, and the development of distance education could improve this worrying situation. In this context, Health Science e-Training (HSeT), a nonprofit Swiss foundation, has developed new pedagogical concepts and tools under customized online training (COLT). For the ADMIRE Cost network, we have used an article-based e-learning (ABL) tool that allowed the students to learn how to read in depth and critically a scientific article and to rigorously address the problem of scientific reproducibility. The evaluation of the program by the students and the tutors has been quite positive. In conclusion COLT was well adapted to the needs of the ADMIRE Cost Action, a European network in which students from countries separated by thousands of miles can work at distance under the online supervision of tutors and then meet in a face-to-face session to maximize their learning experience and the interactions between peers and tutors.

**Keywords:** distance learning, article-based e-learning (ABL), customized online training (COLT)

## 1. Introduction

The quality and reproducibility of preclinical and clinical biomedical research have recently been strongly questioned [1, 2]. The causes are multiple: deficient experimental protocols, inappropriate methods and statistical analysis, and incorrect data interpretation. The fundamental problem, however, is deeper: too few researchers receive adequate pre- or postgraduate training to conduct a rigorous scientific study. The quality of education has been debated for centuries and criticized by teachers as well as by the taught. In the digital age, new pedagogical concepts [3, 4] are emerging, and the development of distance education could improve this worrying situation. Benjamin Franklin has found the formula that summarizes the stakes of the problem (**Figure 1**). This review summarizes how the use of new distance learning tools has improved the learning and teaching experience of an educational program proposed to the students (MD, PhD, MD-PhD students, postdoctoral fellows) of the ADMIRE Cost European network.

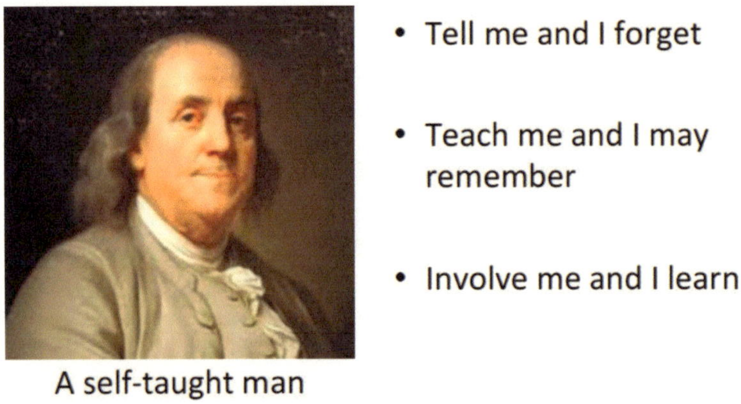
Tell me and I forget
Teach me and I may remember
Involve me and I learn
A self-taught man

**Figure 1.**
*Benjamin Franklin (1706–1790) was an American polymath and one of the founding fathers of the USA. Franklin was a leading author, printer, political theorist, politician, freemason, postmaster, scientist, inventor, humorist, civic activist, statesman, and diplomat. He pioneered and was the first president of the academy and College of Philadelphia which opened in 1751 and later became the University of Pennsylvania. His interest in education is emphasized by this famous quote. (Text and image adapted from Wikipedia https://en.wikipedia.org/wiki/Benjamin_Franklin).*

## 2. COLT: a new pedagogical tool

We have developed customized online training (COLT), a new pedagogical tool. The distance learning module targets a specific audience: pre-graduate (bachelor, master) or postgraduate students (master of advanced studies, diploma of advanced studies, certificate of advanced studies). Each distance learning module is adapted to the target audience according to the requests of the institution. A matrix combines problem-based learning (PBL) and cross-disciplinary approaches. The latter offers online "classical" biomedical disciplines (anatomy, histology, physiology, pharmacology, genetics, etc.) and self-learning/self-assessments. The distance learning is completed with classroom work (courses, seminars, practical work) in the so called "blended" teaching. All these features are housed on a website as described below.

## 3. ADMIRE: cost distance website and learning program

### 3.1 General features of the website

We opened a training website (https://admire.biomedtrain.eu) for the ADMIRE network.

*Intended audience:* the public part of this website is intended as general information to all those interested in the ADMIRE Cost e-learning program. The private part of this website supports many portals, i.e., (i) a portal for the 31 students registered for the entire course, (ii) a portal for the teachers and organizers with access to meeting agendas and related documents regarding the organization of the module, and (iii) a portal for the seven teachers with examples of various e-learning activities developed by HSeT in the module.

*Intended mission of the website:* the intended mission of the portal was to provide (i) organizational and teaching information to the teachers and learners during the 2016 and 2017 sessions, (ii) e-learning and e-teaching content in the module, (iii) several evaluation tools (self-assessment or quizzes) for the students, (iv) several online teaching activities such as "article-based learning" or "case-based learning", and (v) a forum as a communication tool between students or between student and teachers.

*Mandatory activities:* recently published articles in the field of the ADMIRE network selected by the tutors in an annotated article-based learning (ABL) format had to be read critically and in depth by students (individually or in groups).

*Optional activities*: (i) case-based learning (CBL) which uses a web application that drives the learner through intriguing clinical cases to be solved, and (ii) histology practical: a histology practical on the structure of the kidney using a virtual microscope.

### 3.2 Main goal

The main goal was to study basic principles of the mechanisms of action of aldosterone in classical and nonclassical target cells relevant to the treatment of patients suffering from cardiovascular diseases linked to aldosterone-mineralocorticoid receptor (MR) signaling pathways. The principles necessary to understand an article from the scientific literature were reviewed.

### 3.3 Learning objectives

At the end of this e-training module, the trainees were asked to:

- describe the basic concepts underlying the aldosterone-MR signaling pathways in classical (kidney, colon) and nonclassical (vessels, heart, brain) target cells or organs

- describe and apply the basic concepts to solve questions included in ABLs

- critically read, present, and discuss a scientific paper.

### 3.4 Typical pedagogical scenario of a blended ADMIRE cost e-learning module

The general organization and timeline of a typical pedagogical scenario designed for the ADMIRE Cost network are shown in **Table 1**. The individual and team work was organized along a well-defined timeline spanning in this case which is 1 month. Mandatory and optional activities were clearly delineated. Online activities started on Day 1 by the registration of the students, a demonstration how the website works, and an initial quiz to determine the initial level of knowledge of the class.

### 3.5 Article-based learning (ABL)

Five papers [5–9] were selected by the tutors to represent the most interesting and timely questions about the mineralocorticoid receptor signaling pathways.

**Individual work**: each student had to read the *annotated* version of the article and to consider the "thought questions" associated with each section of the article (e.g., abstract, introduction, results, discussion, material, and methods). Annotations enhance the student's understanding of terms and concepts of the paper with links to other helpful resources. If a student was not familiar with the article's topic, he (she) was recommended to read the "related content" section. Most of the links in the annotated version of the article are links to this section.

| Step | Students | Tutors |
|---|---|---|
| 1. **Online**<br>Day 15 | | **Website open to tutors** |
| 2. **Online**<br>Day 1 | **Website open to students**<br>• Registration<br>• How does the website work<br>• Initial quiz | |
| 3. **Online**<br>Day 1 to Day 15 | **Mandatory activities**<br>*Individual assignments*<br>• Read five articles<br>• Read their assigned article-based learning (ABL), and answer the thought questions<br>• Self-learning/self-assessments (online resources)<br>• Interactions with students and tutors through forum | Interactions with students through forum |
| 4. **Online**<br>Day 1 to Day 30 | **Optional activities**<br>• Case-based learning (CBL)<br>• Renal histology (annotated) (virtual microscope) | Interactions with students through forum |
| 5. **Online**<br>Day 15 to Day 30 | **Mandatory activities**<br>*Team assignments*<br>Each group of students (5–6) work on specific team assignments<br>• Preparation of their presentation for the face-to-face session | Interactions with students through forum |
| 6. **Face-to-face**<br>Day 30 | **Plenary session**<br>Students and tutors<br>• Each group presents its ABL<br>• General discussion led by tutors | |
| 7. **Online**<br>Day 30 | • Final quiz<br>• Module evaluation questionnaire | Module evaluation questionnaire |
| 8. **Online**<br>Day 31 to Day 40 | Reporting from HSeT/tutors to the students about<br>• Their individual and team assignments<br>• Their results to the quizzes<br>• Their feedbacks (course evaluation) | |

**Table 1.**
*Typical pedagogical scenario of a distance "blended" learning module.*

**Team work**: each group of students had:

1. to identify the strength and weaknesses of their paper

2. to identify the main unanswered question(s) raised by the article

3. to propose experimental strategies to address these questions left open

4. to address the issue of scientific reproducibility

5. to rate the quality of the article on a scale from 1 to 5 (1 = poor; 2 = fair, interesting but many flaws in the experimental design and data presentation; 3 = good, worthwhile reading despite many mistakes and flaws; 4 = excellent,

DOI: http://dx.doi.org/10.5772/intechopen.87235

must be read by scientists in this field; 5 = outstanding, goes beyond its specialized field, establishes new paradigms)

6. to prepare an oral presentation for the face-to-face session.

### 3.6 Related content and self-assessments

Content directly related to the ABL topics was available. For instance, related to the paper by Choi et al. [5], the students had access to a number of pages dealing with hypertension together with self-assessment quizzes. Having completed the quiz, the student received a feedback explaining why she or he did not check the right answer and a link to the corresponding page from which the question was issued.

### 3.7 Online resources

The online resources covered important aspects of renal and cardiovascular anatomy, histology, cell and molecular biology, genetics, physiology, and pathophysiology.

### 3.8 Optional activities

Optional activities included CBL entitled "Ms Long QT" and "The Walker's Cramp" allowing the students to study the problems of arrhythmias and atherosclerosis, respectively. The students could also familiarize themselves with the microscopic structure of the kidney thanks to a virtual microscope and relate the structure of the organ to its function.

### 3.9 Distance tutoring (forum) and monitoring

**A general forum** allowed general interactions between students and tutors from Day 1.

**Group forums** were open to students for their team work and the preparation of their presentation. They could interact with their group tutor from Day 15 to Day 30.

### 3.10 Students and tutors

Forty-two students from 11 countries (Denmark, France, Germany, Hungary, Ireland, Italy, Poland, Scotland, Slovenia, Spain, and Turkey) attended the 2016–2017 courses supervised by seven tutors.

### 3.11 Face-to-face sessions

There were two face-to-face sessions one in Dublin on March 1, 2017, and one in Paris on November 17, 2017, attended by 26 and 16 students, respectively.

### 3.12 Evaluation of the work of the students

Online quizzes were carried out in the first day of the course and compared to the results obtained at the end of the face-to-face return session, allowing to objectively quantify the progress made by each trainee. The initial quiz on Day 1 (fall 2016) (maximum possible score, 120 points) was carried out by 14 students with a mean score of 61% (range, 35–85%). According to our experience, this score indicated already a rather good level of knowledge in this specific field, not surprisingly taking in account that all student came from laboratories highly specialized in the field of mineralocorticoid receptor signaling pathways. The final quiz on Day 30 (spring 2017) showed a mean score of 68% (range, 52–90%) indicating an improvement of 7 points and a narrowing of the range. According to our previous experience, we expected 10–15 points of improvement, but the explanation may reside in the student's motivation probably not optimal for reasons described below. The tutors could evaluate the class performance for each question and determine the specific weaknesses (questions with correct answers <25%) and the strengths (questions with correct answers >75%) of the class.

### 3.13 Evaluation of the e-learning module by students and tutors

The students and the tutors evaluated the online course. Both gave a positive evaluation. The benefits were obvious for both students and teachers.

The evaluation of the answers by the students (17 respondents) was scored on a qualitative scale (no, rather no, rather yes, yes, no opinion) and was overall quite positive for the website navigation (**Figure 2**), the online resources and self-learning tools, and the ABL individual and team assignments.

Some of the most interesting individual comments and suggestions are:

*"I would incrementally allow access to the online resources- allowing for a gradual accumulation of the material. I think this would make studying this material seem less of a mountain to climb and if each resource came with an email to state that it was available it would remind the users that the material is there. I think this would promote a wider utilization of these superb learning materials..."*

*"I think the self-assessments were too difficult and not linked to the resources provided. Sometimes after reading the resources provided and selecting the answers based on the resources you would get the wrong answer. I think the multiple choice should only have one answer not multiple correct answers as this made it very confusing to answer..."*

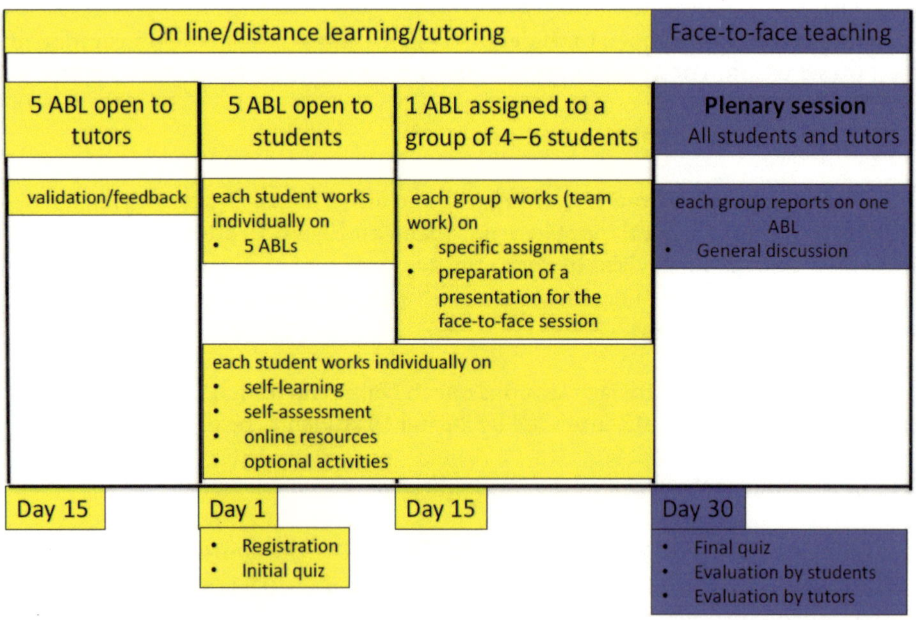


**Figure 2.**
*Evaluation of the e-learning module navigation by the students.*

*"I would add video lessons to make easier the comprehension of the most complex issues with a global correction of every question we had to answer, it would have help us for oral presentation..."*

*"In my opinion, should be perform in more time. It is really well organized, but at least from my point of view we need more time to do all the quizzes/assesments and read the articles..."*

*"I will be happy to see more interaction with tutors..."*

*"Overall, I have found the e-learning website very useful, user-friendly and well-organized. The approach taken to teach the course was very fruitful as it was helping people from various background of the field. The course has given me the very best introduction to the field in the beginning of each topic then it was progressing and enabling to gain in-depth knowledge of the field. For improving the website, I would not put the quizzes not to the very end and I would rather put each quiz at the end of each topic and/slide show not let the student proceed to next chapter/topic until each session is completely finished. This will further "pressurize" the e-learning and keep the students more actively on the website..."*

Most of the remarks, criticisms, and suggestions made by the students and the tutors have been considered for further improvements of the module.

On the positive side, "*We have to work more but we learn more...*" is a common remark from students of various backgrounds taking different modules (COLT format).

"*I would like to maintain my access to the website after the end of the e-learning module...*" is also a frequent request that we take a sign of success. Our policy has always been to grant this access as long as the student wishes.

## 4. Discussion

A number of new forms of distance learning/teaching have emerged during the last 10 years [10, 11]. Many universities and institutions around the world are examining the potential of online technology to develop new and more efficient teaching methods and, ideally, to decrease costs.

### 4.1 MOOCs

The most prominent and visible e-learning courses are "massive open online courses" (MOOCs). There has been a lot of talk about MOOCs, an "educational buzzword" according to John Daniel [12]. Are the MOOCs going to transform higher education and science as suggested by Mitchell Waldrop [13]? The first MOOC was created in Canada in 2008 (G. Siemens and S. Downes) based on the theory of *connectivism*, which favors collaboration and interaction between participants, hence the acronym cMOOC [14]. The activities of a cMOOC typically comprise four elements: (1) to gather/compile the interesting contents, (2) to archive them in a personal document by sharing it by a blog, (3) to appropriate the contents by explaining its own understanding, and (4) to spread the personal work. To succeed in a cMOOC, it is obviously necessary for a participant to do more than read and watch videos and requires his or her active participation (involvement). A cMOOC is considered to work when it feeds on itself through the contributions and contents of the participants, even beyond the course [15]. In 2011, S. Thrun (Stanford) launched a first distance course on the Coursera platform on the theme of artificial intelligence, open to all and accessible worldwide. The success was considerable: more than 160,000 students enrolled.

This course was offered in parallel with the classic one given locally to Stanford students. This is the beginning of xMOOCs (x referring to the MITx platform launched in December 2011 by MIT). The xMOOCs are more traditional in their pedagogical approach (the so-called behaviorist). The market is dominated by three course providers (Udacity, Coursera, and edX). The teaching materials include short video courses, online exercises and tests, student interactions (forum), and online peer reviews (Coursera). Some platforms (Coursera) even allow the analysis of free text responses. Following the success of xMOOCs from major American universities, several initiatives have emerged in Europe and Asia. Some projects come from French-speaking universities (i.e., EPFL in Switzerland and University of Geneva, using the Coursera platform, or the University of Lyon 1 in collaboration with the Catholic University of Louvain who has developed their own open-source LMS platform). In February 2014, the Class Central site [16] which lists the available MOOCs included 476 courses, 70% of which use the Coursera platform. Forty-four percent of the courses came from computer science and mathematics and only 24% from science, health, and medicine. As of 2018, the Class Central site listed over 2700 courses, a very rapid increase since 2014. The current limits of xMOOCs are (1) the small percentage of students who finish the course and obtain certification (5–15% in general), which however in absolute value often represents several thousand students; (2) low penetration on the African continent and in countries that do not have optimal access to the web; and (3) the difficulty of checking exams allowing accreditation. There is also a risk of cultural "imperialism" imposing the concepts of some elite institutions, a threat to cultural diversity.

### 4.2 Inverted classroom or flipping the lecture

Teachers have also used online lectures open to their students to "flip" their class. In other words the students must follow the online lectures and carry out the associated assignments and quiz before a face-to-face session with the teacher focusing on discussing the points that have been the least understood during the online session. This model may be cost-effective and efficient and does not require that the recorded lecture be made publicly available avoiding the problem of copyrights that is encountered with MOOCs.

### 4.3 COLT and SPOCs

There are other approaches to developing distance education, tailored to the needs and culture of each training institution, and that could (it is fashionable) be grouped under the acronym COLT described above. How to read a scientific article? How to write a scientific article? How to write a research grant application? How to design and perform a clinical trial? These are topics that can be treated very effectively with the COLT approach. This model of teaching obviously only affects a small number of students, but at present many institutions in Switzerland, Europe, the USA, and Africa have used such a type of teaching in collaboration with HSeT. Interestingly a recent report from the University of Princeton strongly favors a similar approach they termed "small private online courses" (SPOCs). In summary, MOOCS and COLT represent two different but complementary approaches. The first should arouse the interest of a very wide audience for a theme, while the second allows the deepening and accreditation of knowledge acquired by a target audience, admittedly small but most often highly motivated.

### 4.4 Economic challenges of digital distance education

The economic challenges of digital distance education could be significant and, of course, influence access to education and training around the world. In fact, the economic model of the MOOCs is still very vague, and J.R. Young [17] has summarized the situation prevailing in the USA: "it is following a common approach of Silicon Valley start-ups: build fast and worry about money later." No one will deny that Google, Facebook, and others have been particularly successful in adopting this strategy. As far as COLT is concerned, it falls within the usual framework of academic teaching and does not require any additional resources, provided that this approach replaces conventional teaching and does not add to it.

### 4.5 Perspectives and future improvements

As mentioned, the motivation of the students could has been higher provided they could obtain not only a certificate attesting their attendance to the course but a certain number of European Credit Transfer and Accumulation System (ECTS) credits if the final examination is passed. ECTS is a standard means for comparing the "volume of learning based on the defined learning outcomes and their associated workload" for higher education across the European Union and other collaborating European countries. Ideally a European university (some have shown some interest) might be asked to take the lead (leading house) and propose to the European students a certificate of advanced study (CAS) in the field of aldosterone and its receptor. The CAS will be officially accredited by the university and the number of ECTS attributed precisely defined. One unsolved difficulty encountered by all universities is to determine the equivalence between an ex cathedra hour of teaching and the time spent by tutors to teach the students online.

## 5. Conclusion

In conclusion COLT is well adapted to a European network in which students from different countries can work online under the supervision of their tutor and then meet in a face-to-face session to maximize the learning experience and interactions between students and tutors.

## Acknowledgements

This publication is based upon the work from the EU COST Action ADMIRE BM1301 in aldosterone and mineralocorticoid receptor (MR) physiology and pathophysiology (www.admirecosteu.com).

Our thanks to Catherine El Bez for useful comments and thoughtful suggestions.

## Author details

Bernard C. Rossier[1,2*], Michelle Rossier[1] and Jean-Pierre Kraehenbühl[1,2]

1 Health Science e-Training Foundation, Epalinges, Switzerland

2 University of Lausanne, Lausanne, Switzerland

*Address all correspondence to: bernard.rossier@unil.ch

## References

[1] Abbott A. Doubts over heart stem-cell therapy. Nature. 2014;**509**:15-16

[2] Prinz F, Schlange T, Asadullah K. Believe it or not: How much can we rely on published data on potential drug targets? Nature Reviews. Drug Discovery. 2011;**10**:712

[3] Bourhy H, Troupin C, Faye O, Meslin FX, Abela-Ridder B, Sall AA, et al. Customized online and onsite training for rabies-control officers. Bulletin of the World Health Organization. 2015;**93**:503-506

[4] Rossier BC, Kraehenbuhl JP, Rossier M. Role of distance learning in the education and the training of the investigator. Medical Science (Paris). 2014;**30**:603-604

[5] Choi M, Scholl UI, Yue P, Bjorklund P, Zhao B, Nelson-Williams C, et al. K+ channel mutations in adrenal aldosterone-producing adenomas and hereditary hypertension. Science. 2011;**331**:768-772

[6] Fraccarollo D, Berger S, Galuppo P, Kneitz S, Hein L, Schutz G, et al. Deletion of cardiomyocyte mineralocorticoid receptor ameliorates adverse remodeling after myocardial infarction. Circulation. 2011;**123**:400-408

[7] McCurley A, Pires PW, Bender SB, Aronovitz M, Zhao MJ, Metzger D, et al. Direct regulation of blood pressure by smooth muscle cell mineralocorticoid receptors. Nature Medicine. 2012;**18**:1429-1433

[8] Shibata S, Rinehart J, Zhang J, Moeckel G, Castaneda-Bueno M, Stiegler AL, et al. Mineralocorticoid receptor phosphorylation regulates ligand binding and renal response to volume depletion and hyperkalemia. Cell Metabolism. 2013;**18**:660-671

[9] Zhang J, Rudemiller NP, Patel MB, Karlovich NS, Wu M, McDonough AA, et al. Interleukin-1 receptor activation potentiates salt reabsorption in angiotensin II-induced hypertension via the NKCC2 co-transporter in the nephron. Cell Metabolism. 2016;**23**:360-368

[10] Allen IE and Seaman J. Grade Change. Tracking Online Education in the United States; 2014. Available from: https://www.onlinelearningsurvey.com/reports/gradechange.pdf

[11] Siemens G, Gasevic D, Dawson S. Preparing for the Digital University: A Review of the History and Current State of Distance, Blended, and Online Learning. Athabasca University: Bill and Melinda Gates Foundation; 2015. Available from: https://www.classcentral.com/report/george-siemens-preparing-for-digital-university/

[12] Daniel J. Making sense of MOOCs: Musings in a maze of myth, paradox and possibility. Journal of Interactive Media. 2012;(3):18. DOI: 10.5334/2012-18

[13] Waldrop MM. Online learning: Campus 2.0. Nature. 2013;**495**:160-163

[14] Siemens G. What is the Theory that Underpins Our Moocs? (online). 2012. Available from: http://www.elearnspace.org/blog/2012/06/03/what-is-the-theory-that-underpins-our-moocs/

[15] El-Bez C. Les MOOCs: Entre opportunités et défis: Premiers Retour d'expérience. University of Lausanne; 2013. pp. 1-65

[16] Class-Central. Class Central Free Online Education. Available from: https://www.class-central.com/

[17] Young JR. Inside the Coursera Contract: How an Upstart Company Might Profit From Free Courses. 2012. Available from: http://chronicle.com/article/How-an-Upstart-Company-Might/133065/